TRENDS IN INFECTIOUS DISEASES

Edited by **Shailendra K. Saxena**

Trends in Infectious Diseases
http://dx.doi.org/10.5772/57062
Edited by Shailendra K. Saxena

Contributors

Ramesh Rai, Georgios Meletis, Hiromi Takahashi-Omoe, Katsuhiko Omoe, Silpi Basak, Monali Narayanrao Rajurkar, Nora Hilda Rosas-Murrieta, Irma Herrera-Camacho, Lourdes Millán-Pérez-Peña, Francisca Sosa-Jurado, Gerardo Santos-López, Veronica Vallejo-Ruiz, Julio Reyes-Leyva, Helena Lucia Barroso Dos Reis, Thais Camporez Pimentel, Dennis de Carvalho Ferreira, Phillippe Godefroy, Mauro Romero Leal Passos, Ana Beatriz Azevedo Queiroz, Antonio Chambo Filho, Juliana Bittencourt Pessoa, Danielle Camisasca, Silvia Paula De Oliveira, Sutapa Biswas Majee, GOPA ROY BISWAS, Shailendra K. Saxena

Published by InTech
Janeza Trdine 9, 51000 Rijeka, Croatia

Publishing Process Manager Iva Lipovic
Technical Editor InTech DTP team
Cover InTech Design team

First published May, 2014
Printed in Croatia

Additional hard copies can be obtained from orders@intechopen.com

Trends in Infectious Diseases, Edited by Shailendra K. Saxena
p. cm.
ISBN 978-953-51-1312-6

For EU product safety concerns:
IN TECH d.o.o., Prolaz Marije Krucifikse Kozulić 3, 51000 Rijeka, Croatia,
info@intechopen.com or visit our website at intechopen.com.

Meet the editor

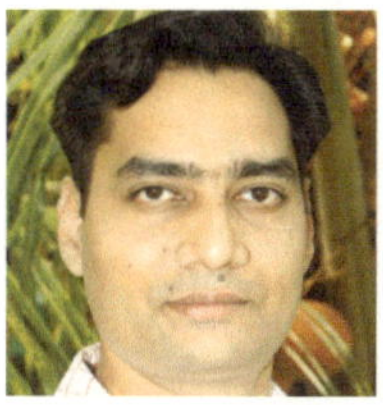

Dr Shailendra K. Saxena is a Medical Microbiologist at CSIR-Centre for Cellular and Molecular Biology (CCMB) in India. The main research interests of his group are to understand the epidemiology and molecular mechanisms of host-defense during human viral infections and to develop new predictive, preventive and therapeutic strategies for them using JEV and HIV as a model. His research work has been published in various high impact factor journals with high citation. He has received many awards and honors in India and abroad including various Young Scientist Awards, BBSRC India Partnering Award and named as "Global Leader in Science" by The Scientist magazine (USA).

Contents

Preface

In spite of development in public health, medicine, and expertise, infectious diseases remain a foremost source of illness and death globally. Characteristic of infection is the incursion of host mechanism by infectious pathogens. The connection of pathogens with disease is a complex process which may require long time to be understood and answered. One of the most destructive epidemics in the last century occurred in 1918 when influenza pandemic broke, resulting in deaths of millions in less than a year. Similarly, HIV infection is causing continuous disaster affecting ~34 million people and causing ~13.9 million deaths. These examples display the fright of infectious disease unpredictability and their reemergence.

Pathogens hijack the synchronized metabolic activities and use host factors as substrate for the process of their multiplication and flourishment. Not only pathogens, but their products like proteins and secreted toxins, damage host tissues. Infectious diseases are the outcome of the described process; they are transmissible diseases and can jump from one host to another with the help of vectors; biological vectors (low vertebrates, insects, avians, etc.) or physical vectors (air, water soil, fomites, etc). Infectious agents are microorganisms such as viruses, bacteria, nematodes, fungi and macro parasites. Discovery of disease-causing pathogens is medically and clinically important. Infectious diseases on onset display various symptoms of illness resulting into severe from the infection, morbidity and sometimes fatality also gets reported. Infectious diseases continue to be foundation for more risky and fatal health threats globally, giving serious challenges to the scientific community to control, cure and prevent them from causing diabolical effects on human race.

Majority of infectious diseases attack immune compromised hosts like infants, old aged and sick people. They cause fatal epidemics with huge extent and severity, emergence and reemergence, reassortment and destroy economies globally. Research activities report that infectious diseases like influenza, Japanese encephalitis, measles, hepatitis, cholera, dysentery, TB, typhoid fever, yellow fever, and malaria have been spine breaking for economy. Novel technologies and for molecular characterization of pathogens and studying their morphology, genome, epidemiology, serology and advancement in vaccines development, are necessary to eradicate the pathogens effectively. These problems can be controlled only by timely diagnosis and control measures.

The need of the hour is to efficiently combat infectious disease which requires onerous and combinatorial efforts between individuals, researchers, analysts, drug developers and funding agencies. Lack of specific vaccines and therapeutics increases the risk potential of infectious disease, hence the development of effective therapeutics and strategies is extremely urgent. Disease control may be enhanced by improvements in prevention, sanitation and hygiene. Introduction of vaccination, antibiotics, other antimicrobial medicines, technological advances in detecting and monitoring infectious diseases like serological testing, pathogen isolation and tissue culture techniques are promising and support infectious disease surveillance and control. We need to tackle diverse challenges of the emergence of new infectious diseases, re-emergence of old diseases and outbreaks. Answering the questions about role of infectious agents in causing acute or chronic diseases, cancers and various other conditions is crucial.

This book covers a collection of chapters by brilliant researchers who have devoted their time to combat against infectious diseases. This book gives a comprehensive overview of recent trends in infectious diseases, as well as general concepts of infections, immunopathology, diagnosis, treatment, epidemiology and etiology of current clinical recommendations in management of infectious diseases, highlighting the ongoing issues, recent advances, with future directions in diagnostic approaches and therapeutic strategies. The book focuses on various aspects and properties of infectious diseases, whose deep understanding is very important for safeguarding human race from more loss of resources and economies due to pathogens.

The authors and editors of the book hope that this work might increase the interest in this field of research and that the readers will find it useful for their investigations, management and clinical usage. Also, I would like to thank Council of Scientific and Industrial Research (CSIR-CCMB), Director CCMB Dr CM Rao, colleagues, family, and parents who gave me a lot of encouragement and support during the work on this book.

Shailendra K. Saxena, PhD, DCAP, FAEB,
CSIR-Centre for Cellular and Molecular Biology,
Hyderabad, India

Section 1

Viral Infectious Diseases

Chapter 1

Japanese Encephalitis: A Neglected Viral Disease and Its Impact on Global Health

Shailendra K. Saxena, Parth T. Agrawal and
Madhavan P.N. Nair

Additional information is available at the end of the chapter

http://dx.doi.org/10.5772/58529

1. Introduction

Japanese encephalitis (JE) is among the most significant viral encephalitis in Asia, particularly in rural and suburban areas where rice culture and pig farming coexist. It has also occurred rarely and occasionally in northern Australia and some parts of the western pacific. JE is caused due to infection with the JE virus (JEV), a mosquito borne flavivrus. The main JEV transmission cycle involves *Culex tritaeniorhynchus* mosquitoes and similar species that lay eggs in rice paddies and other open water resources, with pigs and aquatic birds as principal vertebrate amplifying hosts [Han *et al.*, 2012]. Humans are generally considered as dead-end JEV hosts i.e. they rarely develop enough viremia to infect feeding mosquitoes. Nearly 20-30% of JE cases are fatal and 30-50% of survivors have major neurological disorders [Bhattacharyya *et al.*, 2013]. JE is mostly a disease of children but other age groups may be affected [Kundu *et al.*, 2013; Griffiths *et al.*, 2013; Larena *et al.*, 2013]. In most temperate areas of Asia, JEV is transmitted mainly during summer season, when large epidemics can occur. In the tropics and subtropics region, transmission can occur throughout the year but often increases during the rainy season [Campbell *et al.*, 2011]. The first epidemic of JE was recorded in Japan in 1871. Major outbursts have been seen in nearly every 10 years. In 1924 more than 6,000 cases were reported in a major outbreak in Japan [Solomon *et al.*, 2000]. The disorders caused by JEV began from Southeast Asia and now it's affecting people worldwide [Liu *et al.*, 2013; Li *et al.*, 2013]. Nearly 30 million people are at danger of JEV infection [Saxena *et al.*, 2003]. Though intensive care and support are able to lower the death rate but patients continue to suffer from this disease for a long period of time. Some effects such as learning difficulties and behavioral problems can remain masked for several years.

2. Epidemiological features

JE is believed to be originated in Indonesia and Malaysia long back in mid 1500s [Weaver *et al.*, 1999; Sinniah *et al.*, 1989]. JEV leads to major outbreaks in both temperate regions of Asia like China, Japan, Korea, Philippines, Taiwan and tropical regions like Bangladesh, India, Sri Lanka and Nepal [Bista *et al.*, 2005]. The cases of JE are also reported in newer geographical regions in the Torres Strait islands of Australia and in Papua New Guinea [Fig. 1]. The reason for this wide spread of JE is unknown but it may be due to population shift or variations in agricultural practices, animal husbandry, climate, ecology or migratory birds patterns. In India the first case of JE was seen in 1955. JE is reported to be endemic in many parts such as Assam, Bihar, Madhya Pradesh, Tamil Nadu, Uttar Pradesh and West Bengal.

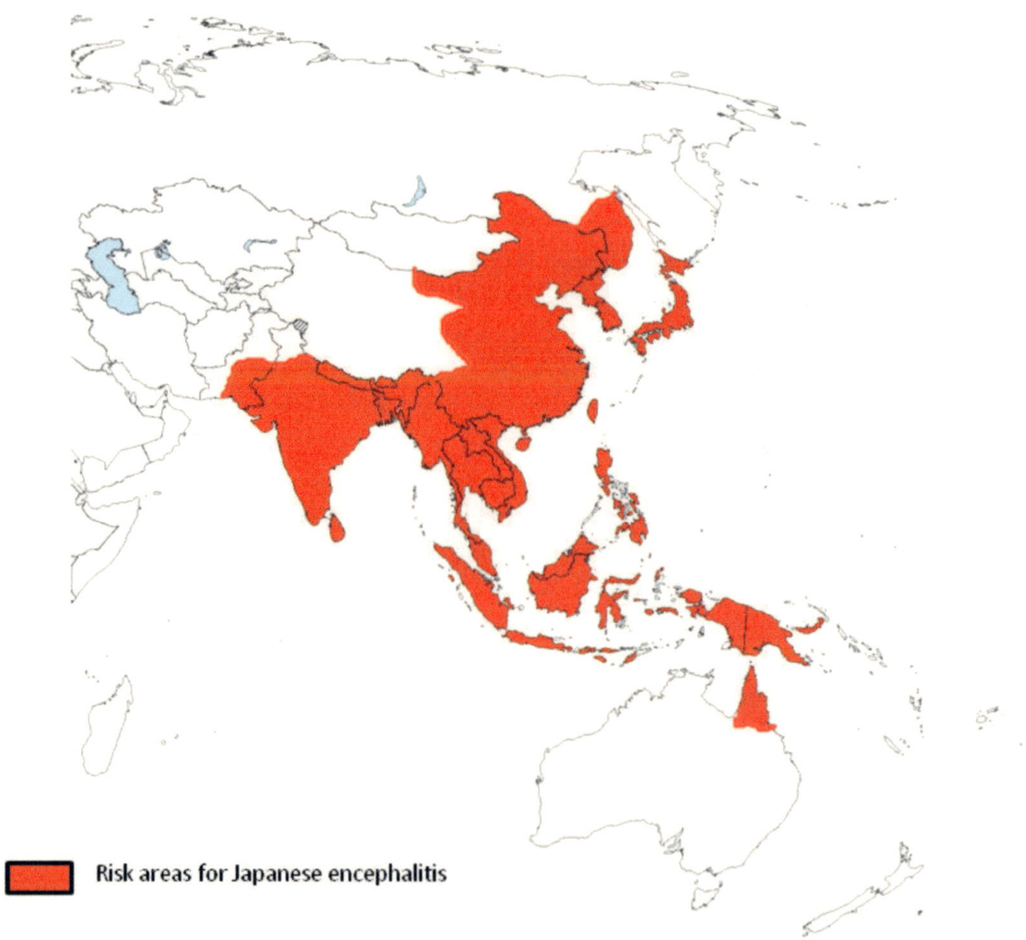

Figure 1. Epidemiology of JE globally. The areas highlighted in red display the endemic regions affected by JE.

3. Viral replication and morphogenesis

JEV virion comprises of a single strand of positive-sense RNA of around 11kb, enclosed in a nucleocapsid and surrounded by envelope made up of glycoproteins [Agrawal *et al.*, 2013; Ye *et al.*, 2012]. The RNA consists of a short 5′ untranslated region (UTR), a longer 3′ UTR and a single open reading frame between them. It encodes 3432 aminoacid polyprotein, which is translationally and post translationally cleaved by viral and host proteases into three structural proteins (core-C, pre-membrane-PrM and envelope-E) and seven nonstructural (NS) proteins (NS1,NS2A,NS2B,NS3,NS4A,NS4B and NS5) [Fig 2][Yang *et al.*, 2013].

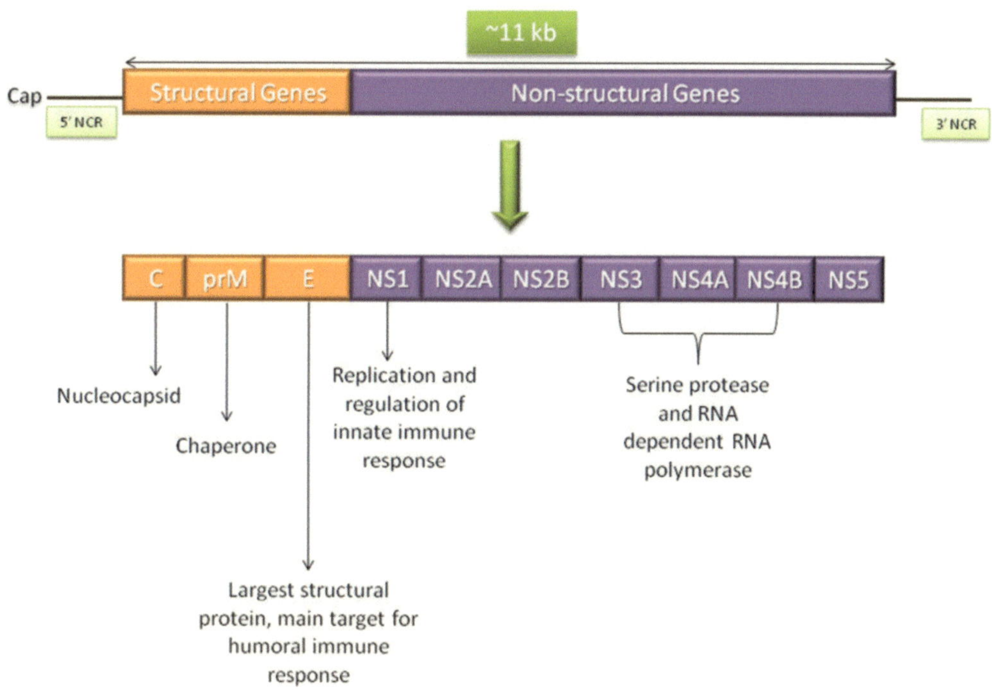

Figure 2. Organization of the JEV genome

The C protein of 12-14 kDa in size is highly basic and fuses with the RNA to form the nucleocapsid. The PrM is in close proximity with the E protein, forming a heterodimer and is believed to act as a 'chaperone' to it, hindering its function until after virion release. Just before the virion release, the PrM protein is cleaved by a protease to its mature M protein form. This alteration contributes for the formation and activation of E protein homodimers. Researchers suggested that the extremely conserved N glycosylation motif N^{15}-X^{16}-T^{17} in JEV PrM and its N-glycan substituents are essential for several stages of JEV biology: PrM biogenesis, virus release and pathogenesis. The E protein is the largest structural protein, comprising of approximately 500 aminoacids, with up to two potential glycosylation sites. It is the main target for the humoral immune response and is believed to play a vital role in viral entry into host cells [Solomon *et al.*, 2003]. The xlink protein is involved in virus replication and regulation of the innate immune response [Li *et al.*, 2012; Zhang *et al.*, 2012]. The functions of NS3 and NS4 are prominent, they code for serine protease and RNA dependent RNA polymerase (RdRp) [Lu *et al.*, 2013]. There is a high rate of mutation in JEV because RdRp is expected to have some error which leads to vast alterations in genomic sequences of JEV worldwide [Saxena *et al.*, 2008]. Since all flaviviral NS proteins are essential for viral replication, any one of them can be selected as target for selective inhibitors of viral replication for therapeutic intervention [Anantpadma *et al.*, 2011; Mastrangelo *et al.*, 2012].

4. Pathogenesis

The development of JEV infection, beginning from its entry till reaching its site of action, the central nervous system (CNS) is not well understood. Studies with other flaviviruses have brought us to the belief that upon entry through mosquito bite, the virus infects dendritic cells in the skin and is carried to the nearest draining lymph nodes, thereby initiating a round of early immune response. But this response is not enough to counter the virus. Meanwhile the virus spreads to secondary lymphoid organs before entering the blood circulation through the efferent lymphatic system. During the subsequent transient viremia, peripheral organs such as kidney, liver and spleen are known to be infected first, after which the neurotropic virus spreads to the CNS. It is still not clear how JEV is able to escape the host's peripheral immune response. After the virus escapes the immune system, it crosses the Blood Brain Barrier to enter the CNS. JEV may cross the BBB by passive transport across the endothelium, by active replication in endothelial cells or by a 'Trojan Horse' mechanism in which the virus is carried into the brain by infected inflammatory cells. Monocytes and macrophages are considered to be the feasible carriers of the virus in the CNS as the virus can survive for a prolonged time and effectively replicate within these cells. During the entry of infected monocytes and macrophages through the BBB, change in the structural and functional integrity of the BBB, leads to production of matrix metalloproteases released by endothelial cells of BBB. This further result in deterioration of BBB stability. BBB stability. Due to the compromised functioning of the BBB, peripheral inflammatory cells are recruited to the infected brain that extends the neuronal impairment.

JEV causes neuronal damage in the brain. However in several cases, JEV is possibly not directly involved in the destruction of brain tissue but it may activate microglia and trigger cell-mediated immune response. Microglial cells are the resident immune cells of the CNS and have a crucial role in host defense against invading microorganisms. Microglial activation is considered as an adaptive response whereby microglia release neuroprotective factors to ease the recovery of injured neurons. They also perform phagocytosis for dying or damaged neurons, before they lyse and release toxic agents into surrounding areas. JEV infection activates microglia both morphologically and functionally, *in vivo,* which causes rise in the level of pro-inflammatory mediators, such as IL-6, TNF-α, RANTES and MCP-1 [Thongtan *et al.*, 2012]. These proinflammatory mediators and cytotoxins released from activated microglia are involved in inducing neuronal death that complements JE. Neuronal death by secreted TNF is mediated by the TNF receptor-associated death domain protein (TRADD), which there upon regulates a downstream apoptotic cascade, in neurons [Swarup *et al.*, 2007]. During JEV infection, nitric oxide (NO) is released by macrophages and plays a significant role in inflammation, even though NO itself is a strong antimicrobial agent, researchers have suggested that it strongly inhibits synthesis of viral RNA, protein accumulation and virus release from infected cells. NO production is higher in the JEV infected brain, and plays a crucial role in the innate immunity of the host and its ability to restrict the initial stages of JEV infection in the CNS [Saxena *et al.*, 2000].

In addition to neuronal and microglial cells, astrocytes are also infected by JEV. Astrocytes are known to maintain homeostasis in the CNS and support the survival and information processing function of neurons. They respond fast to CNS infection and help regulate neuroinflammation. JEV infection results in astrocyte activation, but the infection overpowers the capacity of activated astrocytes to maintain metabolic homeostasis, resulting in an over accumulation of toxic byproducts of metabolism that are injurious to neuronal viability. However JEV infection triggers metabolic reprogramming by upregulating the expression of many proteins such as IP-10, ceruloplasmin and glutamine synthase by astrocytes, involved in the metabolic pathways vital for maintaining neuronal health. This increase is deficient to meet the increased demand that accompanies JEV infection. Astrocytes help in the transmission of JEV from peripheral tissues to the cerebrospinal fluid.

Disease course	Incubation period	Signs and symptoms
Prodromal stage	1-6 days	Fever, muscle pain, headache along with vomiting. In children gastrointestinal symptoms like nausea, vomiting, diarrhea and abdominal pain may be prominent.
Acute encephalitic stage	7-13 days	Photophobia, hyperexcitability, focal and neurological signs, muscular rigidity, dull, mask like face with wide unblinking eyes, tremor, widespread hyertonia, cogwheel rigidity, other irregularities in movement, upper motor neuron signs, cerebellar signs and cranial nerve paralysis sometimes leading to coma
Late convalescent stage	14-15 day onwards	Fever subsides, neurological signs may improve, and eventually either death may occur, or a long term psychoneurological condition may persist, if patient survives.

Table 1. Duration, signs and symptoms of Japanese encephalitis

JE usually develops in patients after an incubation period of 5-15 days [Table 1]. In humans, most JEV infections are asymptomatic, with about 1 in 300 JEV infections resulting in symptoms ranging from non-specific mild fever to severe meningoencephalitis categorized by fever, lessened consciousness, seizures and focal neurological signs. At later stages, poliomyelitis-like flaccid paralysis and parkinsonian syndrome develop, which exhibit the standard description of JE like dull, flat and mask-like face with wide, unblinking eyes, tremor, widespread hypertonia, cogwheel rigidity and other irregularities in movement [Dutta *et al.*, 2010]. Paralysis of the upper body is more common than that of legs. Nearly 30% of survivors have genuine persistent motor deficits and approximately 20% have severe cognitive and language impairment [Mackenzie *et al.*, 2004].

5. Transmission

The JE virus exists in a zoonotic transmission cycle between mosquitoes and pigs and/or water birds; humans get infected only accidentally when bitten by an infected mosquito [Fig 3] and are a dead-end host [Gould *et al.*, 2008]. JEV has been isolated from many mosquito species in field studies, and even though the major mosquito vectors differ in diverse geographical regions, the most important is *Culex tritaeniorhynchus*. For Eastern Asia, Southern Asia and Southeastern Asia, the chief vector is *C. tritaeniorhynchus* [Rao *et al.*, 2001]. For Northern Australia, the chief vector is *C. annulirostris.* From India's outlook, there are several other secondary vectors such as *Anopheles peditaeniatus, A. subpictus, C. epidesmus, C. gelidus, C. pseudovishnui, C. whitemorei, Mansonia uniform* and *M. Indiana* [Borah *et al.*, 2013]. Pigs are the key component in the transmission cycle with respect to human infection, while egrets, herons and other ardeid birds are significant maintenance hosts [Hecker *et al.*, 2013; Sarkar *et al.*, 2013]. Of other vertebrates, horses can develop CNS infection but are a dead-end host; Other domestic animals may also get infected, but do not show any evidence of viremia. Rodents are refractory to infection; and amphibians, bats and reptiles can be infected experimentally and virus can persist, but the role of these species in hibernating and maintaining the virus in the environment is undisclosed.

There are two epidemiological forms of transmission: an endemic form in tropical areas with virus circulation almost throughout the year, but with a wide seasonal peak probably due to irrigation practices; and an epidemic form in more temperate areas with clear summer seasonality [Schuh *et al.*, 2013; Gao *et al.*, 2013]. Subsequently, JE is mainly a rural disease, where *Cx. tritaeniorhynchus* mosquitoes breed in rice paddies and pigs provide the main source of blood meals, with the consequence of transmission cycles in close proximity to human habitation.

6. Diagnosis

Patients with JE present many signs of acute encephalitic syndrome. There are various possible causes of acute encephalitic syndrome; therefore laboratory confirmation is crucial for the accurate diagnosis of JE [Table 2], which is a tough task because of very low viremia. Reverse passive hemagglutination, immunofluorescence and staphylococcal coagglutination tests using polyclonal or monoclonal antibodies have proved the value of antigen detection in Cerebrospinal fluid (CSF) for rapid diagnosis of JE. Advanced methods like Immunogold silver staining (IGSS), have been effectually used in the detection of antigen in mononuclear cells of peripheral blood and CSF of patients. Immunohistochemistry has been used to detect viral

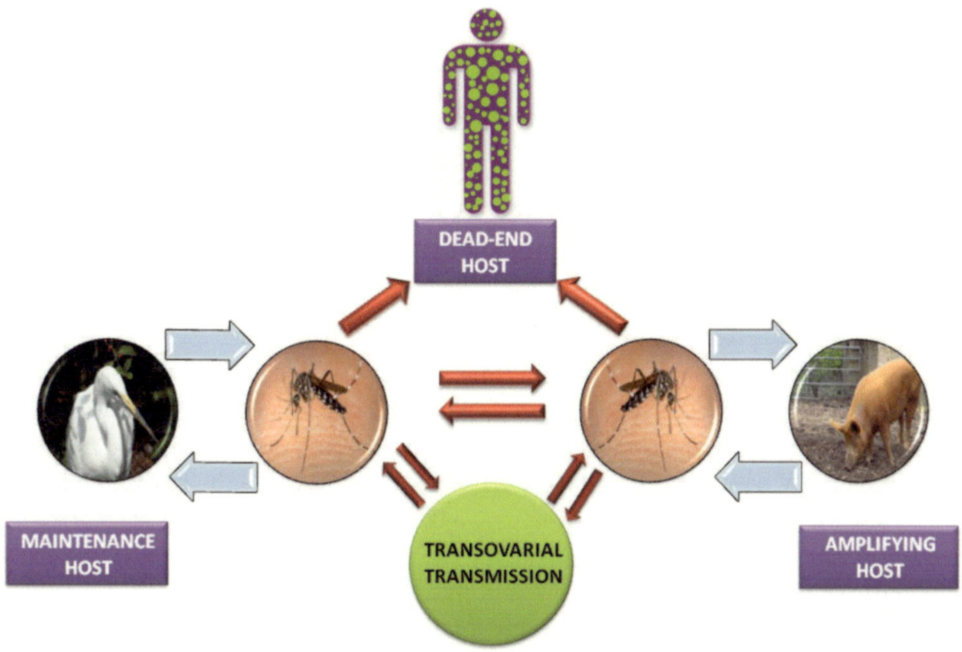

Figure 3. Transmission cycle of Japanese encephalitis virus. Infected Culex mosquitoes (vectors) play the role in the spread of JEV. Pigs are the amplifying hosts and birds (egrets) are the maintenance hosts while humans are the dead-end hosts.

antigens in the CNS. Histopathology inspection is also very obliging for clinical association and diagnosis of JEV. Diagnosis is accordingly targeted towards the detection of antibodies in serum and cerebrospinal fluid. Cases like cross-reactivity of antibodies to other flaviviruses cause confusion in the diagnosis of JEV. IgM capture ELISA has been the most extensively used diagnostic method for JE detection [Hobson-Peters *et al.*, 2012; Palani *et al.*, 2013; Borthakur *et al.*, 2013]. Currently, dipstick method, JEV-CheX and reverse transcriptase PCR are some of the methods which are used for the early detection of JEV [Yang *et al.*, 2013; Seo *et al.*, 2013; Zheng *et al.*, 2013].

Diagnostic tool	Detects
Immunogold Silver Staining (IGSS)	Antigens in mononuclear cells peripheral blood and CSF
Hemagglutination test	Antigens in CSF
MAC-ELISA	IgM antibodies
Dipstick method, JEVCheX	Antibodies
RT-PCR, RT-LAMP	Universal oligonucleotide primers

Table 2. Laboratory diagnostic tools for Japanese encephalitis

7. Treatment

Currently there is no therapy for JE [Saxena *et al.*, 2009]. Presently, chemotherapy during JE is mainly supportive and not targeted towards JEV specifically. Interferon therapy has not proved to be a great success [Tiwari *et al.*, 2012]. Naturally occurring compounds such as arctigenin, a phenylpropanoid and rosmarinic acid, which is a phenolic compound found in many *Labiatae* provide protection to mice against JEV GP78 by noticeably decreasing JEV induced neuronal apoptosis, activation of microglial cells, active caspase activity and induction of proinflammatory mediators in the brains of the infected animals.

An *in vivo* study has shown that minocycline reduces neuronal apoptosis, activation of microglial cells, active caspase activity, proinflammatory mediators and viral titer on later stages after infection. Another compound, N-methylisatin-β-thiosemicarbazone derivative is known to inhibit JEV replication completely *in vitro*. Glucosidase inhibitors of the endoplasmic reticulum such as N-nonyl-deoxynojirimycin, which block the trimming step of N-linked glycosylation, have been shown to eliminate the production of many endoplasmic reticulum-budding viruses, including dengue type-II and JEV. Another recent study carried out in mice using RNA interference showed that a single intracranial organization of lentiviruses delivering short hairpin RNA or lipid-complexed small interfering RNA (siRNA) either before or after the viral challenge was sufficient to provide protection against lethal encephalitis. From the study it was clear that by precise drug design of the conserved site, a single siRNA treatment could suppress viral infection across species, thus enhancing the treatment of acute viral infections with overlapping clinical symptoms [Ghosh *et al.*, 2009].

8. Protection

The control of JE is based mainly on three measures: mosquito control, avoiding human exposure and immunization. Mosquito control has failed to be an effective measure and suffers from the lack of research into new pesticides. Avoiding complete exposure from infected mosquitoes is not practically possible. Accordingly, immunization is the only effective method for long-term protection. To prevent JE, it is crucial to apply a large scale vaccination for the human population in JE prone areas [Tiwari *et al.*, 2012]. There are many groups of vaccines [Table 3] which are presently in use such as purified, formalin-inactivated mouse brain derived and cell culture derived live attenuated vaccine [Lin *et al.*, 2013]. Several vaccines are still in different stages of development such as DNA vaccines, recombinant virus based/chimeric vaccines [Li *et al.*, 2013]. In most countries, the currently available vaccine for use is an inactivated vaccine derived from mouse brain, which is manufactured in many regional countries, but it is costly, involves three doses, needs boosting at quite frequent intervals, may be less effective due to antigenic variation and gives rise to a number of vaccine related adverse reactions [Yun *et al.*, 2013].

Vaccine	Source	Characteristics
(i) Formalin-inactivated mouse brain derived	Nakayama strain	Costly, less effective and side effects are seen
(ii) Inactivated hamster kidney cell vaccine	Beijing strain	Very less side effects are seen
(iii) Live attenuated hamster kidney cell line vaccine	SA14-14-2 strain, China	Costly but effective and very less side effects are seen

Table 3. Comparison of vaccine for Japanese encephalitis

There are several side effects of JE vaccination. Side effects which are mainly seen after vaccination are redness, swelling and tenderness. Rarely systematic adverse reactions are also seen after vaccination like headache, myalgia, abdominal pain and skin rash. Some recipients of the vaccine had very rare major neurological side effects [Sohn *et al.*, 2000]. To avoid some of the adverse reactions, vero cell grown inactivated vaccines are being examined and some of them are currently in clinical trials. Live attenuated vaccines seem to offer good hope; some of the advantages are that these provide long lasting immunity and are very sensitive. Currently, the only potential vaccine is the Chinese SA 14-14-2 strain [Verma *et al.*, 2012]. Protein-protein interaction is essential for various cellular functions and impeding such interactions using synthetic composites is a very noteworthy idea for formulation of new pharmaceuticals [Haridas *et al.*, 2013].

9. Conclusion

JE is a neurological disease caused by a mosquito-borne JEV. Unlike smallpox and polio, JEV cannot be completely eradicated because of its enzootic nature of transmission. Ever since its discovery, JEV has continued to expand its activity into new regions, while many JE vaccines have been made commercially available in different parts of the world. Concern about its spread has been emphasized by the recent emergence and spread of JEV in northern Australia, making it a major concern for global public health. Currently, prevention of infection with most arboviruses relies primarily on efforts to control vector populations by spraying repellents, wearing protective clothing and reducing breeding places.

One of the most important research areas is the development of an ideal JE vaccine: one that is nontoxic, less expensive and more effective and that provides life-long protection with a single dose. The development of such a vaccine will be greatly aided by a expanding our knowledge of JEV replication and pathogenesis at the molecular level, which has now become technically possible with the use of infectious JEV SA14-14-2 cDNA technology. This technology also has huge potential for developing JEV SA14-14-2 as a vaccine vector to deliver foreign gene(s), as has already been accomplished with infectious YFV 17D cDNA technology.

Acknowledgements

Authors are grateful to Dr Ch. Mohan Rao, Director, CSIR-Centre for Cellular and Molecular Biology (Council of Scientific and Industrial Research, India), for the encouragement and support for this work. NIH Awards (R37DA025576; R01MH085259) support S.K.S. and M.P.N.

Author details

Shailendra K. Saxena[1*], Parth T. Agrawal[1] and Madhavan P.N. Nair[2]

1 CSIR-Centre for Cellular and Molecular Biology (CCMB), Hyderabad, AP, India

2 College of Medicine, Florida International University, Miami, FL, USA

References

[1] Agrawal T., Sharvani V., Nair D. & Medigeshi G.R. (2013) Japanese encephalitis virus disrupts cell-cell junctions and affects the epithelial permeability barrier functions. *PLoS One*, 8(7), e69465, doi: 10.1371/journal.pone.0069465.

[2] Anantpadma M. & Vrati S. (2011) siRNA-mediated suppression of Japanese encephalitis virus replication in cultured cells and mice. *J. Antimicrob. Chemother*, 67(2), 444-451.

[3] Bhattacharyya S., Sen U. & Vrati S. (2013) Regulated IRE1-dependent decay pathway is activated during Japanese encephalitis virus-induced unfolded protein response and benefits viral replication. *J Gen Virol*, doi: 10.1099/vir.0.057265-0.

[4] Bista MB & Shrestha JM. (2005)Epidemiological situation of Japanese encephalitis in Nepal. *JNMA J Nepal Med Assoc*, 44(158), 51-56.

[5] Borah J., Dutta P., Khan S.A. & Mahanta J. (2013) Epidemiological concordance of Japanese encephalitis virus infection among mosquito vectors, amplifying hosts and humans in India. *Epidemiol Infect*, 141(1), 74-80.

[6] Borthakur A., Das N. & Bora B. (2013) Data from the World Health Organization (WHO) National Network Laboratory for Japanese encephalitis. *J Glob Infect Dis*, 5(2), 76-79.

[7] Campbell G.L., Hills S.L., Fischer M., Jacobson J.A., Hoke C.H., Hombach J.M., Marfin A.A., Solomon T., Tsai T.F., Tsu V.D., Ginsburg A.S. (2011) Estimated global incidence of Japanese encephalitis: a systematic review, *Bull World Health Organ*, 89(10), 766-774.

[8] Dutta K., Rangarajan P.N., Vrati S. & Basu A. (2010) Japanese encephalitis: pathogenesis, prophylactics and therapeutics. *Current Science*, 98 (3), 326-334.

[9] Gao X., Liu H., Wang H., Fu S., Guo Z. & Liang G. (2013) Southernmost Asia is the source of Japanese encephalitis virus (genotype 1) diversity from which the viruses disperse and evolve throughout Asia. *PLoS Negl Trop Dis*, 7(9):e2459, doi: 10.1371/journal.pntd.0002459.

[10] Ghosh D, Basu A (2009) Japanese Encephalitis—A Pathological and Clinical Perspective. *PLoS Negl Trop Dis*, 3(9): e437. doi:10.1371/journal.pntd.0000437.

[11] Gould E.A. & Solomon T. (2008) Pathogenic flaviviruses. *Lancet*, 371(9611), 500-509.

[12] Griffiths M.J., Lemon J.V., Rayamajhi A., Poudel P., Shrestha P., Srivastav V., Kneen R., Medina-Lara A., Singh R.R. & Solomon T. (2013) The functional, social and economic impact of acute encephalitis syndrome in Nepal – a longitudinal follow-up study. *PLoS Negl Trop Dis*, 7(9), e2383, doi:10.1371/journal.pntd.0002383.

[13] Han Y.W., Singh S.K. & Eo S.K. (2012) TThe roles and perspectives of Toll-like receptors and CD4 (+) helper T cell subsets in acute viral encephalitis.*Immune Netw*, 12(2), 48-57.

[14] Haridas V., Rajgokul K.S., Sadanandan S., Agrawal T. & Sharvani V. (2013) Bispidine-amino acid conjugates act as a novel scaffold for the design of antivirals that block Japanese encephalitis virus replication. *PLoS Negl Trop Dis*, 7(1): e2005. doi: 10.1371/journal.pntd.0002005.

[15] Hecker K., El Kurdi S., Joshi D. & Stephen C. (2013) Using network analysis to explore if professional opinions on Japanese encephalitis risk factors in Nepal reflect a socio-ecological system perspective. *Ecohealth*, 10(4), 415-422.

[16] Hobson-Peters J. (2012) Approaches for the development of rapid serological assays for surveillance and diagnosis of infections caused by zoonotic flaviviruses of the Japanese encephalitis virus serocomplex. *J Biomed Biotechnol*, 2012:379738, doi: 10.1155/2012/379738.

[17] Kundu K., Dutta K., Nazmi A. & Basu A. (2013) Japanese encephalitis virus infection modulates the expression of suppressors of cytokine signaling (SOCS) in macrophages: implications for the hosts' innate immune response. *Cell Immunol*, 285(1-2), 100-110.

[18] Larena M., Prow N.A., Hall R.A., Petrovsky N. & Lobigs M. (2013) JE-ADVAX vaccine protection against Japanese encephalitis virus mediated by memory B cells in the absence of CD8(+) T cells and pre-exposure neutralizing antibody. *J Virol*, 87 (8), 4395-4402.

[19] Li J., Chen H., Wu N., Fan D., Liang G., Gao N. & An J. (2013) Characterization of immune responses induced by inactivated, live attenuated and DNA vaccines against Japanese encephalitis virus in mice. *Vaccine*, 31(38), 4136-4142.

[20] Li S.H., Li X.F., Zhao H., Deng Y.Q., Yu X.D., Zhu S.Y., Jiang T., Ye Q., Qin E.D. & Qin C.F. (2013) Development and characterization of the replicon system of Japanese encephalitis live vaccine virus SA14-14-2. *Virol J*, 10, 64, doi: 10.1186/1743-422X-10-64.

[21] Li Y., Counor D., Lu P., Duong V., Yu Y. & Deubel V. (2012) Protective immunity to Japanese encephalitis virus associated with anti-xlink antibodies in a mouse model. *Virol J*, 9:135. doi: 10.1186/1743-422X-9-135.

[22] Lin C.W., Chang C.Y., Chen W.L., Lin S.C., Liao C.C., Chang J.Y., Liu C.C., Hu A.Y., Lu T.C., Chou A.H., Wu S.C., Chong P. & Huang M.H. (2013) Formulation and immunological evaluation of a trivalent vaccine comprising emulsified submicron particles and inactivated virions of H5N1/EV71/JEV. *Hum Vaccin Immunother*, 9(11), 2378-2385.

[23] Liu W.J., Zhu M., Pei J.J., Dong X.Y., Liu W., Zhao M.Q., Wang J.Y., Gou H.C., Luo Y.W. & Chen J.D. (2013) Molecular phylogenetic and positive selection analysis of Japanese encephalitis virus strains isolated from pigs in China. *Virus Res*, doi:pii: S0168-1702(13)00294-3. 10.1016/j.virusres.2013.09.002.

[24] Lu G. & Gong P. (2013) Crystal Structure of the full-length Japanese encephalitis virus NS5 reveals a conserved methyltransferase-polymerase interface. *PLoS Pathog*, 9(8):e1003549. doi: 10.1371/journal.ppat.1003549.

[25] Mackenzie J.S., Gubler D.J. & Petersen L.R. (2004) Emerging flaviviruses : the spread and resurgence of Japanese encephalitis, West Nile and dengue viruses. *Nat Med*, 10 (12 Suppl), S98-109.

[26] Mastrangelo E., Pezzullo M., De Burghgraeve T., Kaptein S., Pastorino B., Dallmeier K., de Lamballerie X., Neyts J., Hanson A.M., Frick D.N., Bolognesi M. & Milani M. (2012) Ivermectin is a potent inhibitor of flavivirus replication specifically targeting NS3 helicase activity: new prospects for an old drug. *J Antimicrob Chemother*, 67(8), 1884-1894.

[27] Palani G., Padmanabhan P.P., Ramesh K., Asadullah K.S., Sambasivam M., Arunagiri K. & Krishnasamy K. (2013) Development and evaluation of flavi-immunoglobulinM capture enzyme-linked immunosorbent assay. *Indian J Pathol Microbiol*, 56(3), 269-271.

[28] Rao P.N. (2001) Japanese encephalitis. *Indian Pediatr*, 38(11), 1252-1264.

[29] Sarkar A., Banik A., Pathak B.K., Mukhopadhyay S.K. & Chatterjee S. (2013) Envelope protein gene based molecular characterization of Japanese encephalitis virus clinical isolates from West Bengal, India: a comparative approach with respect to SA14-14-2 live attenuated vaccine strain. *BMC Infect Dis*, 13(1), 368, doi: 10.1186/1471-2334-13-368.

[30] Saxena S.K. (2008) Japanese encephalitis: perspectives and new developments. *Future Neurol*, 3(5), 515-521.

[31] Saxena S.K., Mathur A. & Srivastava R.C. (2003) Inhibition of Japanese encephalitis virus infection by diethyldithiocarbamate is independent of its antioxidant potential. *Antivir Chem Chemother.*, 14(2), 91-98.

[32] Saxena S.K., Singh A. & Mathur A. (2000) Antiviral effect of nitric oxide during Japanese encephalitis virus infection. *Int. J. Exp. Path*, 81(2), 165–172.

[33] Saxena S.K., Mishra N., Saxena R., Singh M. & Mathur A. (2009) Trend of Japanese encephalitis in North India: evidence from thirty-eight acute encephalitis cases and appraisal of niceties. *J Infect Dev Ctries*, 3(7), 517-530.

[34] Schuh A.J., Ward M.J., Brown A.J. & Barrett A.D. (2013) Phylogeography of Japanese encephalitis virus: genotype is associated with climate. *PLoS Negl Trop Dis*, 7(8):e2411. doi: 10.1371/journal.pntd.0002411.

[35] Seo H.J., Kim H.C., Klein T.A., Ramey A.M., Lee J.H., Kyung S.G., Park J.Y., Cho Y.S., Cho I.S. & Yeh J.Y. (2013) Molecular detection and genotyping of Japanese encephalitis virus in mosquitoes during a 2010 outbreak in the Republic of Korea. *PLoS One*, 8(2):e55165. doi: 10.1371/journal.pone.0055165.

[36] Sinniah M. (1989) A review of Japanese-B virus encephalitis in Malaysia. *Southeast Asian J Trop Med Public Health*, 20(4), 581-585.

[37] Sohn Y.M. (2000) Japanese encephalitis immunization in South Korea: past, present, and future. *Emerg Infect Dis*, 6(1), 17-24.

[38] Solomon T. (2003) Recent advances in Japanese encephalitis. *J Neurovirol*, 9(2), 274-283.

[39] Solomon T., Dung N.M., Kneen R., Gainsborough M., Vaughn D.W. & Khanh V.T. (2000) Japanese encephalitis. *J Neurol Neurosurg Psychiatry*, 68(4), 405-415.

[40] Swarup V., Das S., Ghosh S. & Basu A. (2007) Tumor necrosis factor receptor-1-induced neuronal death by TRADD contributes to the pathogenesis of Japanese encephalitis. *J Neurochem*, 103(2), 771-783.

[41] Thongtan T., Thepparit C. & Smith D.R. (2012) The involvement of microglial cells in Japanese encephalitis infections. *Clin Dev Immunol.*, 2012:890586. doi: 10.1155/2012/890586.

[42] Tiwari S., Chitti S.V.P., Mathur A. & Saxena S.K. (2012) Japanese encephalitis virus: an emerging pathogen. *Am J virol*, 1, 1-8.

[43] Tiwari S., Singh R.K., Tiwari R. & Dhole T.N. (2012) Japanese encephalitis: a review of the Indian perspective. *Braz J Infect Dis*, 16(6), 564-573.

[44] Verma R. (2012) Japanese encephalitis vaccine: need of the hour in endemic states of India. *Hum Vaccin Immunother*, 8(4), 491-493.

[45] Weaver S.C., Powers A.M., Brault A.C. & Barrett A.D. (1999) Molecular epidemiological studies of veterinary arboviral encephalitides. *Vet J,* 157(2), 123-138.

[46] Yang K., Li Y., Duan Z., Guo R., Liu Z., Zhou D., Yuan F. & Tian Y.(2013) A one-step RT-PCR assay to detect and discriminate porcine reproductive and respiratory syndrome viruses in clinical specimens. *Gene,* 531(2), 199-204.

[47] Yang S., He M., Liu X., Li X., Fan B. & Zhao S. (2013) Japanese encephalitis virus infects porcine kidney epithelial PK15 cells via clathrin- and cholesterol-dependent endocytosis. *Virol J,* 10:258. doi: 10.1186/1743-422X-10-258.

[48] Ye Q., Li X.F., Zhao H., Li S.H., Deng Y.Q., Cao R.Y., Song K.Y., Wang H.J., Hua R.H., Yu Y.X., Zhou X., Qin E.D. & Qin C.F. (2012) A single nucleotide mutation in NS2A of Japanese encephalitis-live vaccine virus (SA14-14-2) ablates xlink' formation and contributes to attenuation. *J Gen Virol,* 93(Pt 9), 1959-1964.

[49] Yun S.I. & Lee Y.M. (2013) Japanese encephalitis: The virus and vaccines. *Hum Vaccin Immunother,* 10(2), 263-279.

[50] Zhang T., Wu Z., Du J., Hu Y., Liu L., Yang F. & Jin Q. (2012) Anti-Japanese-encephalitis-viral effects of kaempferol and daidzin and their RNA-binding characteristics. *PLoS One,* 7(1):e30259. doi:10.1371/journal.pone.0030259.

[51] Zheng H., Shan T., Deng Y., Sun C., Yuan S., Yin Y. & Tong G. (2013) Molecular characterization of Japanese encephalitis virus strains prevalent in Chinese swine herds. *J Vet Sci,* 14(1), 27-36.

Chapter 2

Oral HPV Related Diseases: A Review and an Update

Helena Lucia Barroso dos Reis,
Silvia Paula de Oliveira, Danielle Resende Camisasca,
Juliana Bittencourt Pessoa,
Ana Beatriz Azevedo Queiroz,
Mauro Romero Leal Passos, Philippe Godefroy,
Dennis de Carvalho Ferreira,
Thais Camporez Pimentel and
Antonio Chambo Filho

Additional information is available at the end of the chapter

1. Introduction

Human papilloma virus (HPV) is responsible for the most common sexually transmitted infections. It is estimated that two thirds of people who have unprotected sexual intercourse with a HPV carrier are infected [1].

Since HPV has tropism for epithelial tissue [2-4], it can affect both skin and mucosa [3, 4]. It causes several types of injuries, ranging from asymptomatic infection and benign warts to invasive injuries [5]. HPV infection has been found in a wide range of anatomical sites: genital and anal tract, urethra, upper airway, tracheobronchial mucosa, nasal paranasal cavities, and oral cavity. HPV on oral mucosa presently afflicts 1% to 43% of the general population, depending on the diagnosis method used [5], and may be even associated with oral malignancies [6].

The aim of this review article is to offer the academic community an updated review of HPV, emphasizing its importance as a public health matter. This review encloses HPV epidemiology, virology description of different oral lesions, clinical picture, oncogenesis and, diagnostic tools. We have also reviewed current treatment choices and prophylaxis, as well as vaccines against HPV.

2. The biology of human papillomavirus — Virion structure

HPV is a small DNA virus belonging to *Papillomaviridae* family [1, 2, 7, 8]. Its virion consists of a non enveloped, singular double stranded DNA molecule [5, 8, 9], of about 7.9kb [8], involved by a capsid, of about 55 nm in diameter [8, 9], containing only two structural proteins [8].

HPV genome presents a notable organization. It weighs $5.2x10^6$D and contains 7.200 – 8.000 pairs of nitrogenous bases (pnb) [9]. All putative open reading frames (ORFs) are limited to only one strand of DNA [8]. Non-coding strand probably forms a second, which bears pieces of preserved ORFs, irrespective of localization and composition [8], Chlaudhary et al (2009) have suggested that the basis of the HPV molecule DNA can be divided in three parts. The first part, with 4.000 pnb, accounts for viral replication and cell transformation while the second part, with 3.000 pnb, represents an important codification zone, since it encodes the viral particle structural proteins. The last one, with only 1.000 pnb, contains a non-coding zone; it is, however, fundamental, since the viral origin of replication belongs to this part [9].

2.1. Genome structure

The difference of HPV types is due to the variation of E6 and E7 sequence of nitrogenous bases. This variation can produce either an easier to inhibit gene or a harder to inhibit one, thus stratifying the virus oncogenic phenotype into high, intermediate and low risk types [7].Besides its oncogenic potential, the HPV types vary according to tissue tropism and their association with these tissues [10]. Over a 100 HPV types [7] have been identified, but only 25 (HPV - 1, 2, 3, 4, 6, 7, 10, 11, 13, 16, 18, 31, 32, 33, 35, 40, 45, 52, 55, 57, 58, 59, 69, 72, 73) were associated with benign or malignant lesions [3, 10]. Low-risk HPV (6, 11, 38, 40, 42, 54, 55, 61, 62, 64, 67, 69, 70, 71, 72, 81, 83, 84, 89) [11] causes injuries which produce abnormal cell growth [8]; however, they are unlikely to undergo malignant neoplastic transformation. High-risk HPV (16, 18, 26, 31, 33, 35, 39, 45, 51, 52, 53, 56, 58, 59, 66, 68, 73, 82) [11] are likely to induce malignant neoplastic transformation [3, 11]. Recently HPV- 26, 53, 66 have been found to be among the potentially high-risk types [12].

HPV - 6, 11 are related to condyloma *acuminatum* and, in children, laryngeal papilloma, conjuntival papilloma and genital warts [13]. HPV – 16, 18, mainly, but also 31, 32 and 35 are associated with squamous cell carcinoma [11]. Although benign forms rarely developed into malignant, they can concurrently present with the high-risk malignant injury [9].

3. Prevalence and incidence

The American Cancer Society has estimated that more than 6 million people are infected by HPV each year, with 3 million affecting the 15- 25 age group [14].

Asymptomatic oral and oropharynx HPV prevalence at oral cavity has not yet been established [15], probably because different methods were used in different studies [3]. Methods have varied in terms of size of samples, collecting procedures, test sensibility and use of PCR or PCR inhibitors. This may explain the huge variation in HPV detection rate: 22 to 60% or 0 to 81.1%, depending on the methods and on the studied population [15].

Recent meta-analysis has demonstrated that HPV is an isolated risk factor for the development of oral carcinoma [2]. Oral squamous cell carcinoma is known to be linked with both heavy drinking and smoking and it has been related to HPV [6, 7].

3.1. Oral human papillomavirus infection

When oral mucosa is considered normal, the epithelium may serve as a container of HPV which would be activated at some point in time and induce injury [16]. A huge number of different oral diseases may be associated with oral HPV, but they rarely cause lesions [17]. Lesions may range from benign warts, which are far more common, to malignant injuries [6].

3.2. Sexual and nonsexual transmission

Many studies have discussed HPV transmission, but the mechanisms involved remain unknown. Unprotected sexual intercourse is its leading cause, particularly oral-genital sex, when the genital mucosa is infected by the virus, which will be present both clinically and subclinically [1, 16] in adolescent and adults. Early sexual relationships, high number of sexual partners, parity, smoking and another sexually transmitted infection may elevate the rate of virus infection [6, 18, 19].

Oral HPV can be transmitted by direct skin-skin contact [3] and self-inoculation [1, 4]. Upper airway transmission has not yet been established [8].

Infant HPV is mainly transmitted at birth by infection of the maternal cervix. Thus, the recurrent laryngeal papillomatosis seems to be acquired by such manner [19, 20]. However, another transmission route is mother-fetus, before, during or after the child-birth [1, 4, 8] that may be made possible by infected amniotic fluid and umbilical cord blood [21].

The transmission of HPV through fomites may also occur [22].

4. Risk and protective factors

In the social sphere, people who have yet to initiate sex life have a low probability of HPV infection. On the other hand, people who started their sex life earlier or have a promiscuous sexual life are more likely to have sexually transmitted infections, including HPV. In the economical sphere, it has been found that low levels of HPV infection were strongly related with higher income levels [4].

Early age initial sexual activity, oral sex, more than one sexual partner, not wearing condoms, infrequent use of condoms all pose important risks to any sexually transmitted infection, such as HPV. Homosexuals tend to have greater number of sexual partners than heterosexuals, and as such, they should be more commonly infected than heterosexuals, but studies have yet to confirm this trend [4, 8].

Smoking may pose a lower risk for infection with high risk oral and oropharyngeal HPV than it was previously believed probably because the oral mucosa keratinization makes it stronger against minor traumas and consequently HPV infection. On the other hand, high levels of alcohol consumption have been linked to a higher risk of HPV positivity, but this association needs further research in order to be more fully established [68].

Normally, people acquire HPV during their adolescent years, or when they approach their twenties, when they start their sexual life. An immune competent person can suppress HPV or even eliminate it, and suppressed HPV may be kept subclinical for years [8].

Among the leading protective factors, saliva stands out. It is composed of lysozymes, lactoferrin, IgA and cytokines which seems to be the reason behind low HPV transmission through self-inoculation, oral sex, and the virtually inexistence of transmission through kissing. It has been suggested that regular consumption of carotenoids would contribute to make HPV persistence less likely, and a high consumption of folic acid would reduce the risk of HPV infection [4].

5. HPV associated oral injuries

HPV infection range from asymptomatic to visible lesions, which can be benign or malignant [6]. The most common oral manifestations are described below:

5.1. Condyloma acuminatum

The lesion is caused by the abnormal proliferation of a squamous stratified epithelium [23]. Formerly it was believed that the only transmission route was by sexual contact, but now it is known that there are other routes, such as self-inoculation and mother-fetus transmission [15]. However, sexual contact remains the main route of transmission (20%) [23], and people who carry these lesions and practice oral sex have a 50% chance to acquiring oral condyloma. The incubation period range from 3 weeks to an undetermined period of time; after that, clinic progression will depend on cell permissiveness, virus type and host immune situation [24].

Condyloma acuminatum has tropism to tongue, lips, palate and mouth floor. Clinically, it is described as little pinkish or whitish nodules which proliferate in papillary projections that might be either pedicle or sessile. Outline surfaces present even more evident cauliflower shapes than papilloma, mainly when they converge (Figure 1 – A, B).

Histologically, oral condylomata are typically papillary proliferations of squamous epithelium with prominent acanthosis and parakeratin that line deep crypts, similar to their counterparts in the lower genital tract. Koilocytosis is the classic diagnostic feature, consisting of cells with perinuclear halos of various sizes and accompanied by variability in nuclear size and chromaticity, as well as nuclear membrane irregularity. These features are most prominent toward the surface of the lesion (Figure 1 – C, D) [25].

HPV presence was first determined by immunohistochemistry and later by hybridization with 75 to 85% of positivity [15]. The most involved types are 6 and 11 [5, 15, 18].

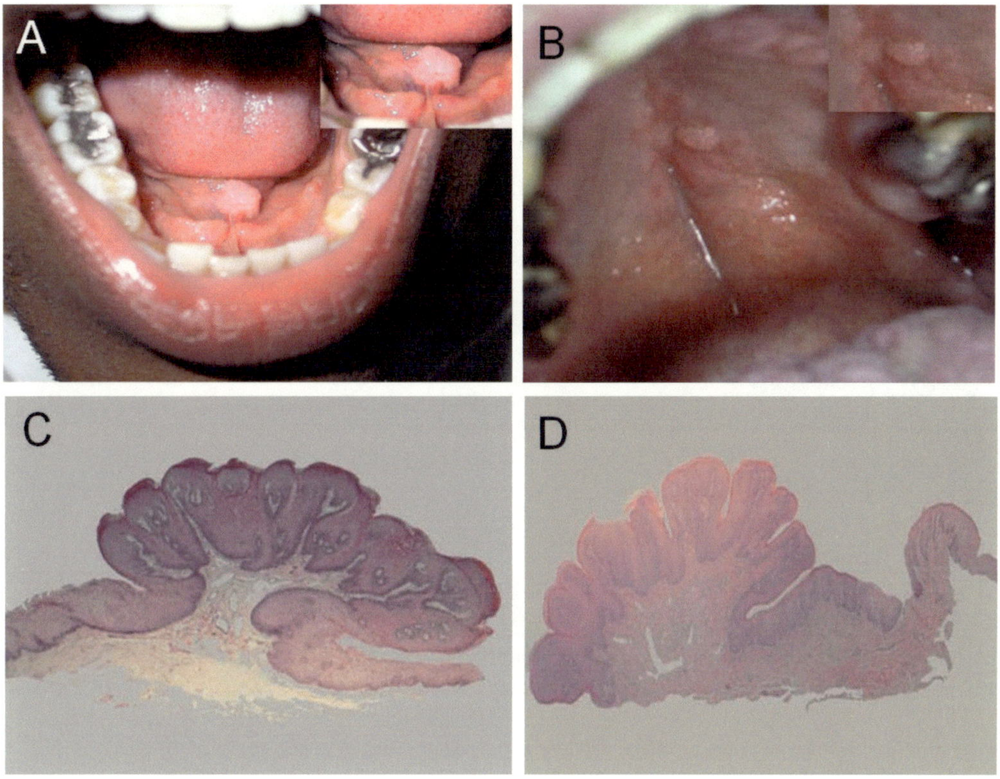

Figure 1. Condyloma acuminatum. Rose-colored nodule with a cauliflower-like surface in the floor of the mouth (**A**; inset – closer view). Lesion on the hard palate (B; inset – closer view). Microscopically, panoramic view of acanthosis with papillary folds, parakeratosis and elongation of rete ridges (**C**, **D**) (HE, Objective 2.5x). *Clinical images obtained from the archives of the Stomatology Specialization at Odontoclínica Central do Exército (OCEx).*

Differential diagnoses include oral squamous papilloma, verruca vulgaris, molluscum contagiosum, seborrheic keratosis, lichen planus and oral squamous cell carcinoma (OSCC) [15].

Condyloma acuminatum treatment is not always necessary. For 20-30% of HPV patients, lesions are self-limited and resolve spontaneously within six months, while for 60% of them, lesions may regress in a year. Relapses affect 20-30% of patients undergoing treatment, and they may reappear on the same sites or on different locations [24]. The choice of therapy is based on a range of factors, such as lesions size, aspect, number and sites. Other factors of equal significance include patient preference, costs, and adverse effects [23]. Commonly, lesions have been treated by excisional surgery, but in the last years a wider choice of treatments have become available, e.g., cryotherapy, electro cauterization and CO_2 laser. Other options include caustic agents, such as trichloroacetic acid, podophyllin and 5-flourouacil which may cause tissue destruction [23].

5.2. Verruca vulgaris (Common wart)

Verruca vulgaris, also known as common wart is one of the most common lesions affecting mainly children [15], but seldom on oral mucosa [6].

It is usually found on lips, hard palate, gingival, and tongue dorsal surface [15], but especially on lips and tongue [18] (Figure 2 - A, B). Differential diagnoses is made with oral squamous papilloma and condyloma acuminatum [15, 18].

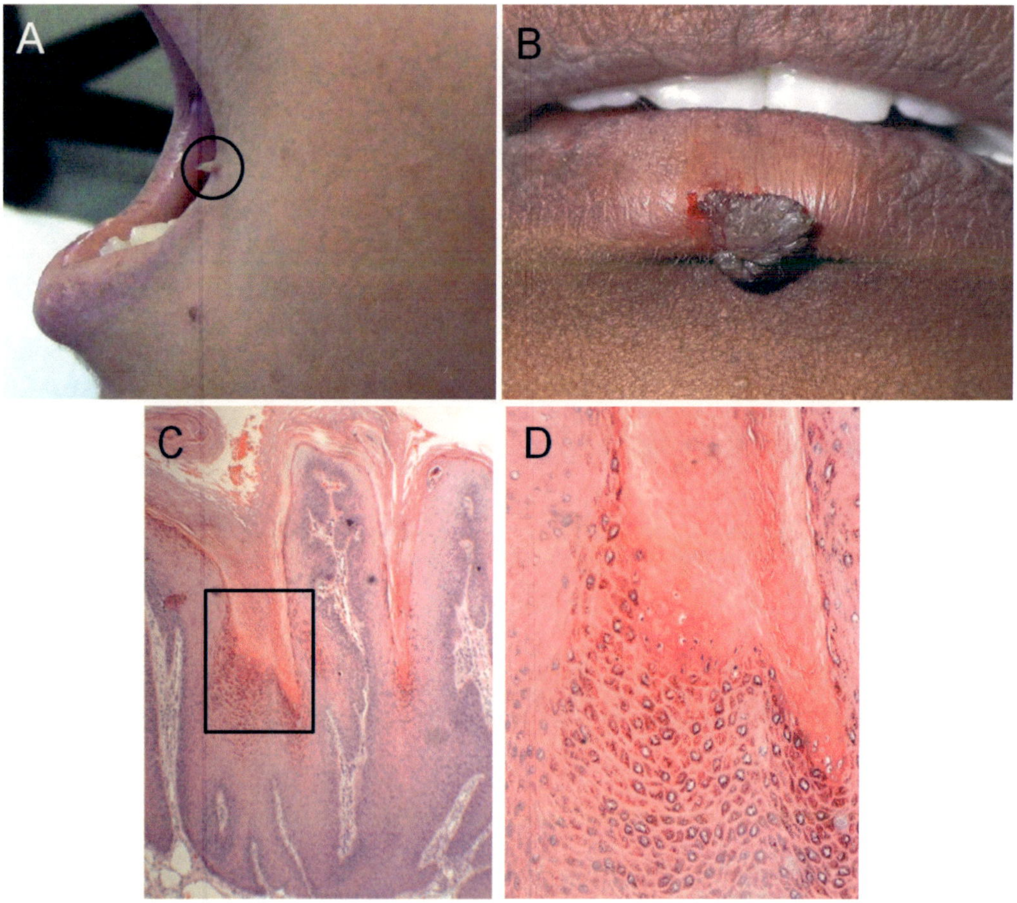

Figure 2. Verruca vulgaris. Exophytic lesion with hyperkeratotic surface, forming finger projections in the left commissure of the lip (**A**, circle). Lesion on the lower lip (**B**). Microscopically, panoramic view of acanthosis with papillary folds, hyperortoparakeratosis and elongation of rete ridges (**C**; HE, Objective 4x). Koilocitosis (**D**; HE, Objective 20x). *Clinical images obtained from the archives of the Stomatology Specialization at Odontoclínica Central do Exército (OCEx).*

Histologically, verruca vulgaris show an almost symmetrical structure, with elongated rete ridges that are shorter at the periphery than in central area. Thin elongated connective tissue papillae form papillomatosis. The cryptoform surface shows a conspicuous hyperkeratinization, predominantly composed of orthokeratin. The stratum granulosum is often pronounced, particularly in the grooves between the elongated connective tissue papillae. Koilocytes may be seen. In the connective tissue, some dilated capillaries and a slight infiltration with lymphocytes are usually seen (Figure 2 C, D) [26]

Immunohistochemical methods and hybridization tests showed HPV presence in 43 to 100% of the studied lesions [15].

Most oral warts are self-limited, and resolve within 2 years. Aesthetic discomfort or bite injuries induce patients to look for treatment. Some treatment techniques are cauterization, surgical removal, liquid nitrogen cryotherapy, local hyperthermia, topic 5-fluoracil, CO_2 laser, salicylic acid, squaric acid, interferon and wart material implantation [18].

5.3. Oral squamous papilloma

Oral squamous papilloma (OSP) is a benign tumor that may occur in all ages, but it more commonly affects adults between 30 and 50 years old [15]. It is mainly related to HPV 6 and 11 [15, 18]. In adults, the lesion is usually located in the oral mucosa, mostly on palate and tongue, while in children the laryngotracheobronchial complex is a more common site [27].

OSP affects the soft palate, the lingual frenulum as well as the lower lip [15] and the uvula [27], most often presenting as a single, small lesion smaller than 1 cm, with exophytic growth and a wide basis or pedicle. On histopathology the pattern of epithelial proliferation repeats features described in the previous lesions, with squamous cell acanthosis, hyperkeratosis and a centrally disposed fibrovascular core.(Figure 3 – A, E). Koilocytosis may be present or not.

Oral squamous papilloma may be isolated or multiple-recurring, which is more likely to affect immunosuppressed patients, such as HIV-positive patients. Multiple-recurring papilloma is also more likely to be malignant [27] and tends to relapse more often [28]. Differential diagnoses include exophytic carcinoma, verrucous carcinoma and condyloma acuminatum [27]. Surgical removal is the first choice of treatment, but electrocauterization, cryosurgery and interferon injections are other effective treatment courses [8].

5.4. Focal epithelial hyperplasia (Heck disease)

Focal epithelial hyperplasia (FEH) or Heck disease was first described in 1965 [15] and can affect all age groups [29], but it is more common in children and adolescents (3 to 18 years) [30]. Malnutrition, poor hygiene and low social condition as well as genetic background also play an important role [31] in lesion development.

FEH shows a benign epithelial growth and commonly affects oral mucosa, lips, tongue [18], particularly the lower lip and more rarely the palate, floor of the mouth and oropharynx [30]. Clinically it presents as multiple papules (3 – 10 mm) [30] that tend to converge. They are characteristically nodular, sessile, circumscribed, painless and soft masses on oral mucosa. Color may range from pale pink to normal mucosa [15, 29- 31]. (Figure 4 – A, B). The diagnosis is both clinical and histological [30, 32].

Microscopically it shows epithelial hyperplasia, acanthosis, mild parakeratosis and anastomosing rete ridges. Superficial layers of the epithelial tissue contain cytophatic changes

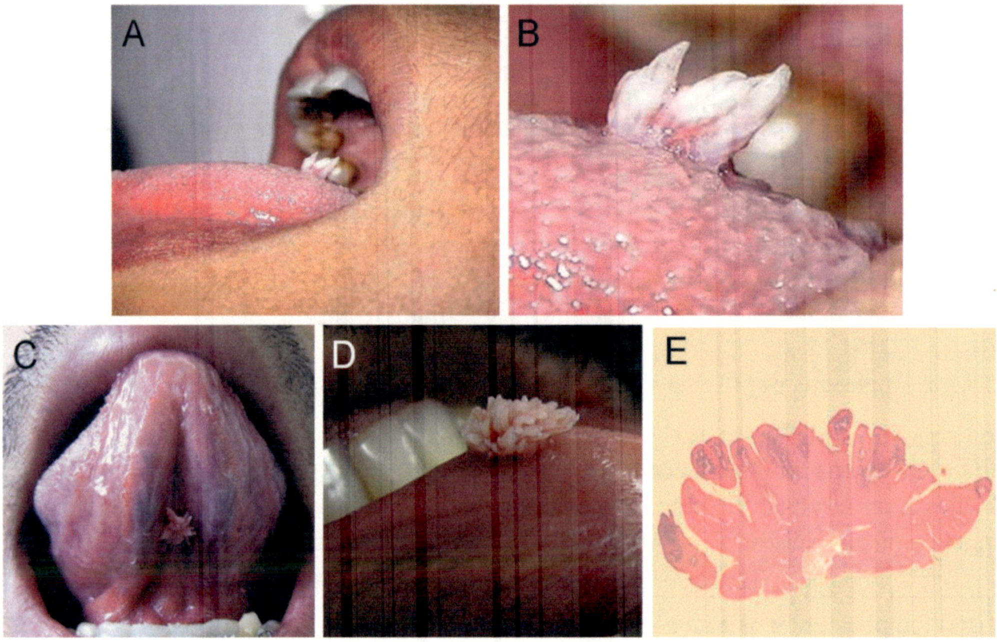

Figure 3. Oral squamous papilloma. Exophytic lesion with hyperkeratotic whitish surface, forming finger projections on the dorsum of the tongue (**A-B**). Lesion on the inferior surface of the tongue (**C**). Lesion on the lower lip (**D**). Microscopically, panoramic view of acanthosis with papillary folds, hyperortoparakeratosis, elongation of rete ridges and a centrally disposed fibrovascular core (**E**; HE, Objective 2.5x). *Clinical images obtained from the archives of the Stomatology Specialization at Odontoclínica Central do Exército (OCEx).*

(koilocytosis) and apoptotic or dyskeratotic cells with an apparent mitotic appearance (mitosoid cells) (Figure 4 – C, D) [30].

FEH has a steady association with HPV infection, and the most common types are 13 and 32 [15, 29]; they account for approximately 90% of infections [30, 32]. HPV-32 might be found in other type of lesions, but never out of the oral region [15]. Both HPV-1 and 11 are rare and show potential for malignancy. So far, the only malignant transformation reported has been found with HPV-24 [32].

Differential diagnoses include condyloma, viral warts, neuroma, white sponge nevus, oral papillomatosis, [30] and inflammatory fibrous hyperplasia.

FEH normally regresses spontaneously in a few months or years, but it can take longer [30]. Thus, treatment is often chosen to mitigate aesthetic problems or repeated bite injuries [31]. The most effective methods are surgical excision, electrocoagulation, cryotherapy [31], CO_2 laser and interferon [30].

5.5. Oral lichen planus

Oral lichen planus (OLP) is a common chronic immunomediated disease [18, 33, 34] of unknown etiology seemingly related to HPV in some lesions [18], affecting the skin and the

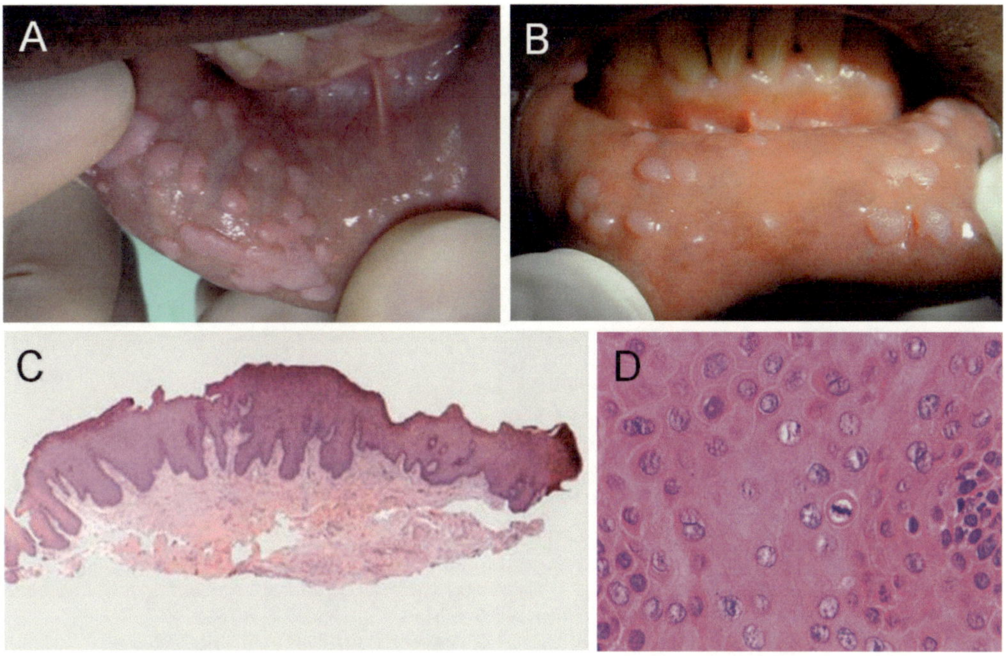

Figure 4. Focal Epithelial Hyperplasia. Multiple flat and coalescent papules on the lower lip mucosa (**A-B**). Microscopically, panoramic view showing acanthosis and irregular elongation and anastomosis of rete ridges (**C;** HE, Objective 2.5x). Classic "mitosoid" figure (**D**; HE, Objective 40x). *Clinical images obtained from the archives of the Stomatology Specialization at Odontoclínica Central do Exército (OCEx).*

mucosa [33-, 35]. OLP prevalence ranges from 0, 5% to 4% [35] and mainly affects the female population [33-35]. The most prevalent age is between 30 to 60 years old, although occurrence in children and adolescents seems to be on the rise [35]. In around 15% of the cases the skin is affected and this number increases to around 85% of cases affecting the mucosa, particularly the oral and genital mucosa. The oral mucosa is affected in 20% to 30% of the cases. Besides being more common, OLP is more resistant to treatment than skin OLP [34]. A possible relationship between OLP to Hepatitis C has been hypothesized, but it has not been clearly established.

Diagnoses depend on clinic manifestation as well as histopathology results [35]. OLP lesions are usually bilateral and symmetric affecting areas the oral mucosa, gingiva as well as the dorsum of the tongue and the lip mucosa (Figure 5 – A, F).

The lesions may be single or multiple and may present in a wide range of forms- cauliflower-like, striated or annular. Long-time evolution of a lesion is usually atrophic, and when the lesion is located on the tongue it may cause papillae loss and modify gustation (Figure 5 – G, F). Extensive lesions are also more painful [35].

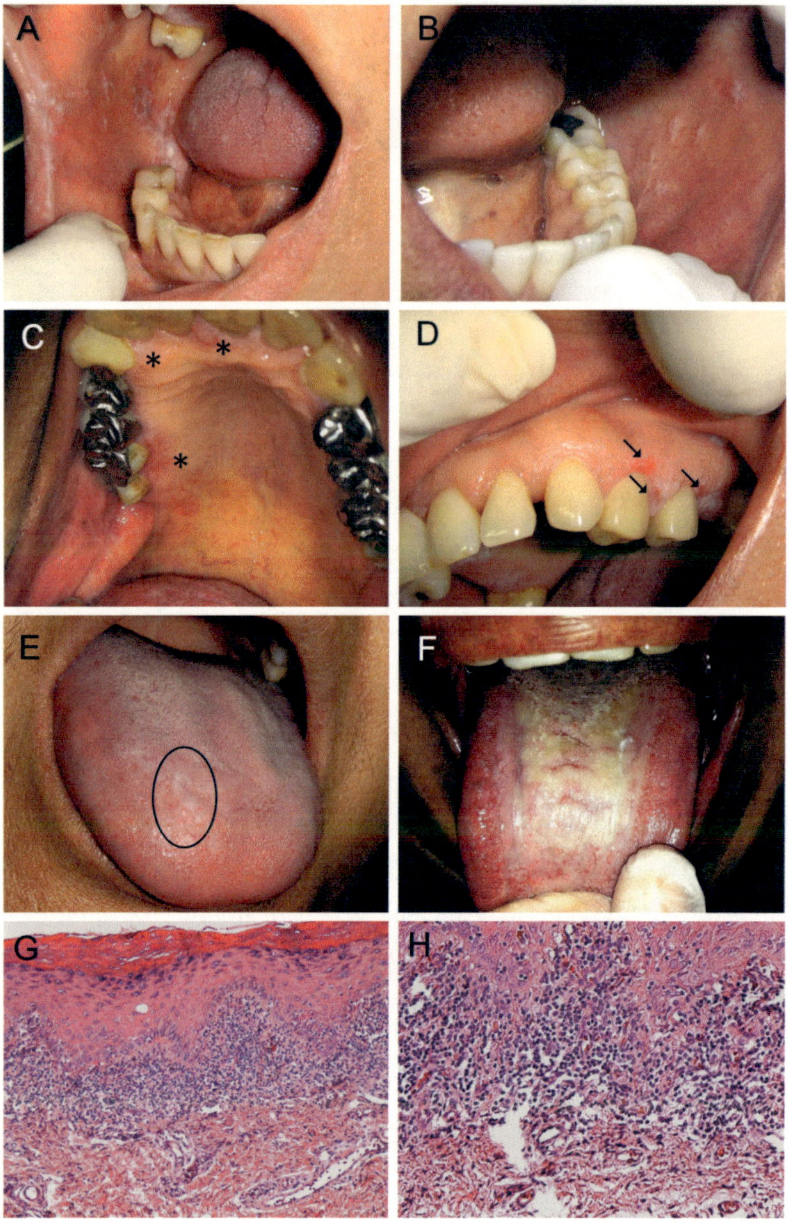

Figure 5. Oral lichen planus. Most prominent features are bilateral white striae in buccal mucosa, with certain symmetry (**A-B**). Gingiva may also be affected (**C-D**) (*) and it may show atrophic symptomatic spots surrounded by Wickham striae (arrows). When it affects the tongue, it is not as typical (**E-F**) and may be confused with oral leukoplakia or smoker's tongue. Microscopically a strong sub epithelial lymphocytic infiltrate should be present (**C**; HE, Objective 10x), in association with degeneration of the basal layer (**D**; HE, Objective 20x) and absence of epithelial dysplasia..*Clinical images obtained from the archives of the Stomatology Specialization at Odontoclínica Central do Exército (OCEx).*

According to Silverman's classification OLP may be presented as reticular, erosive and atrophic forms [33]. Each form has its different clinic evolution and determines different intensity and duration, with the possibility of evolving from one form into another [35].

On histopathology, we may find acanthosis in keratotic lesions, and atrophy in older lesions. Two important findings are hydropic degeneration of the basal layer, as well as a strong subepithelial lymphocytic infiltrate (Figure 5 – G, H). Those lesions that present dysplasia should not be classified as OLP [36, 37]. Biopsy should be preferably performed on keratotic areas, however this might be a complicated intervention when the patient has extensive oral candidiasis [34, 35]. Some other pathologic entities may present similar histopathologic features, such as lichenoid reaction, which is similar to lichen planus, but usually is related to amalgam fillings or certain medicines [33, 34].

The most prevalent and commonly found HPV types are 11 and 16 [18].

The conditions that may be considered as differential diagnosis of OLP include the reticular form which should be distinguished from systemic lupus erythematosus, candidiasis, traumatic lesions, secondary syphilis, hairy leukoplakia and incipient OSCC. The erosive form should be distinguished from aphthae, mucous membrane pemphigoid, pemphigus vulgaris, drug reaction, polymorphic erythema and systemic lupus erythematosus acute lesions [35].

Malignant transformation is reported for OLP, however, a current tendency is to consider those lesions that do not fulfill established clinical and pathologic criteria for OLP as oral lichenoid lesions. These lesions mimic OLP and would be the ones truly at risk of becoming a OSCC [36, 37].

Treatment does not assure cure, for unknown reasons, but it does reduce symptoms, particular when they are severe, atrophic and widespread. Unlike the asymptomatic reticular form, erosive lesions need prompt symptomatic treatment. Oral hygiene reduces inflammatory lesions and topic corticosteroids may be used in the form of mouth wash. Calcineurin inhibitor, a topic immunosuppressive agent, and topic retinoid, such as imiquimod, are other treatment options, with the latter being used together with topic corticosteroids [33-35].

5.6. Oral leukoplakia

Leukoplakia is considered a premalignant lesion or potentially malignant disorder on oral cavity, and reported rates of development into malignancy vary widely depending on the method of diagnosis and definition criteria used for oral leukoplakia [38]. The most common malignant transformation is into oral squamous cell carcinoma (OSCC) [38, 39], with percentages ranging from 3 to 37% [38].

Oral leukoplakia prevalence ranges from 0, 4 to 0, 7%, and there is no variability related to gender. However, some researchers believe that prevalence among women is higher [38].

Etiology is uncertain; however smoking along with alcohol consumption is pointed as the main risk factors. There are possible cofactors, such as candidiasis, HPV and more recently Epstain-Barr virus (EBV) has been associated with these lesions in imunossupressed patients [38]. EBV rarely affects immunocompetent people and it does not need a specific treatment [40]. Treatment should address the underlying cause of immunosuppression.

Oral leukoplakia may be located on lip vermillion, gingival, tongue and floor of mouth, and it is on these latter regions that there is a higher risk of malignancy (around 43%) [38, 40]. Oral leukoplakia distribution may be local or disseminated [41] (Figure 6 – A, F).

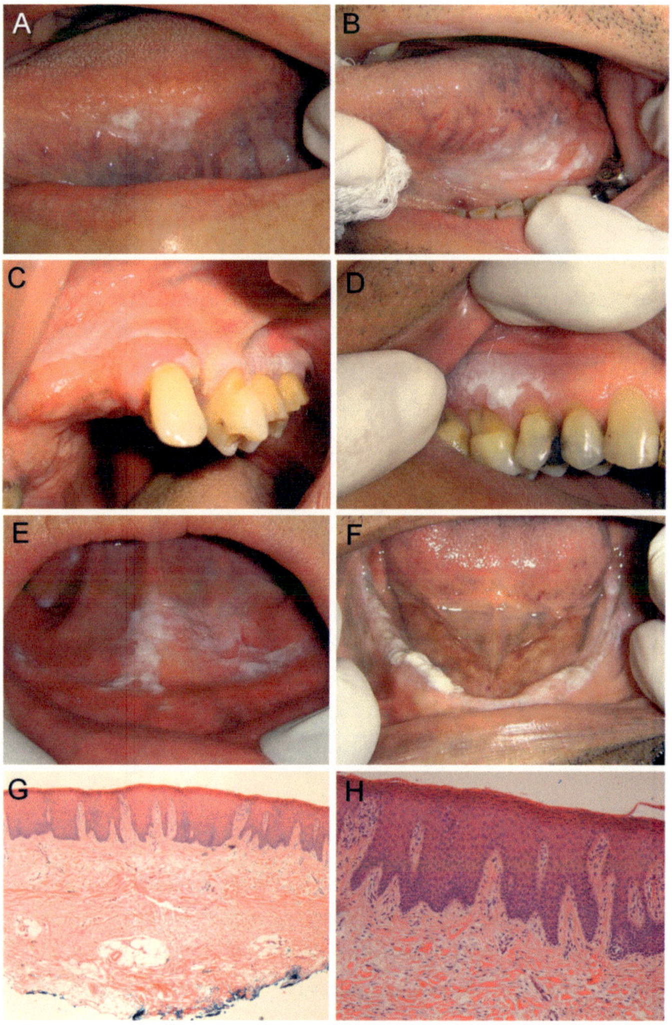

Figure 6. OL: Oral leukoplakia. OL located at lateral (**A-B**) and ventral tongue show higher risk for malignant transformation. These lesions may be homogenously white (**A**), or associated with ulcers (**B**). Other common location is gingiva (**C-D**), floor of mouth (**E**) and alveolar ridge (**F**) and a traumatic cause or association with candidiasis should be ruled out before biopsy. Microscopically leukoplakia can demonstrate only epithelial hyperplasia with acanthosis and hyperparakeratosis (**G**; HE, Objective 4x), without dysplasia (**H**; HE, Objective 20x). In this case inflammatory infiltrate was scarce. *Clinical images obtained from the archives of the Stomatology Specialization at Odontoclínica Central do Exército (OCEx).*

Histological examination reveals a range of epithelium changes varying from innocuous hyperplasia to dysplasia of varying degrees [18]. However, more commonly, OL presents hyperkeratosis and epithelial hyperplasia without dysplasia [38] (Figure 6 – G, H). Depending on the dysplasia degree, it may be classified as low, intermediate and high risk of malignancy [38], so that severity of the dysplasia is the key standard in malignancy prediction [39]. However, diagnosis of dysplasia is rather subjective and as such it is highly dependent on the pathologist/researcher [38, 39]. Another controversial issue is that it is virtually impossible to accurately predict which lesion, even among those with dysplasia, will develop into a malignant one [39]. Rather, we might get to know which lesion is more likely to become malignant, if clinic and histological characteristics are analyzed in association [38.37]

Viral etiology is unclear. Although HPV 6, 11 and 16 have been predominantly found, and also HPV 18, 31, 33, 35 [18, 38] in lesions, the viral etiology remains controversial. It seems that lesions which contain HPV are less malignant than oral leukoplakia in smokers, similar to what happens in OSCC. HPV-16 is present in 80% of the lesions, regardless of malignancy [5], and it has already been established that type 16 is related to OSCC in nonsmoker or nondrinkers. EBV seems to be an etiologic factor of oral leukoplakia because it appears in a great number of malignant lesions in imunossupressed patients [38]

Differential diagnoses are leukoedema, white sponge nevus (*Cannon's disease*), contact dermatitis lesions, chronic biting, nicotinic stomatitis, OSCC, oral hairy leukoplakia, verrucous carcinoma, OLP and secondary syphilis.

There has not been any agreement as to the best treatment course, and prevention (smoking and drinking avoidance and a diet rich in fruits and vegetables) remains the best approach. A topical treatment based on topical bleomicyn and systemic retinoid is used as an effective short term treatment, however there are doubts as to its long term efficacy. Invasive treatments include cryosurgery, CO_2 laser, and surgical resection. They are effective in the short run, but lesions may relapse in the long run [38, 42]

5.7. Oral verrucous carcinoma

Oral verrucous carcinoma (OVC) is a squamous cell carcinoma (SCC) subtype [15, 43, 44], but it shows a much more benign behavior, with well distinguished morphology and clinical presentation. It is located on the head, neck and genitals, and more notably on the oral mucosa, and it has low probability of metastasis [43, 44].

OVC is a rare tumor and had been described by Ackerman [15, 43, 44] in 1948 as a cancer that involves the lips, oropharynx and laryngeal mucosa. It is also known as Ackerman's tumor. However, the condition has also been referred as florid oral papilomatosis, epithelioma cuniculatum, carcinoma cuniculatum and also as Buschke-Loewestein tumor [43]. Nowadays carcinoma cuniculatum is considered as a separated pathologic entity [45].

The etiopathogenesis of OVC is unknown, but some studies have found associations mostly with smoking, some alcohol ingestion and infection by HPV [15, 44]. OVC related co-factors are poor oral hygiene, OLP or the presence of leukoplakia lesions. HPV may have an important role in tumor development and progression, but further research is necessary [44].

HPV has been widely described as one of the causes of OVC, and the most commonly found types are 6, 11, 16 and 18, which were identified by polymerase chain reaction (PCR), restriction fragments analyses and DNA slot hybridization [44].

Oral verrucous carcinoma is a male disease and affects predominantly the 50-80 age group [44]. OVC is characteristically situated on the oral mucosa, gingiva, mandible alveolus crest, tongue and lips [44].

It appears with slow exophytic growth, resulting in verrucous cauliflower lesions, with white plaques, normally extensive and with well demarcated hyperkeratotic lesions [15, 43, 44]. It is well circumscribed, invasive only on surface, with low probability of metastasis [43] (Figure7 – A, C). People usually look for doctors because of the extensive rapid growth, which scares them.

OVC histology is characterized by the presence of acanthosis and keratinization with keratin plugging and clefting [43, 44]. They are irregular and may extend into cleft. Atypia is minimal and usually there is inflammatory infiltrate on the subepthelial layer around epithelial invaginations which seem to compress the underlying tissue ("elephant feet") [44] (Figure 7 – D, E).

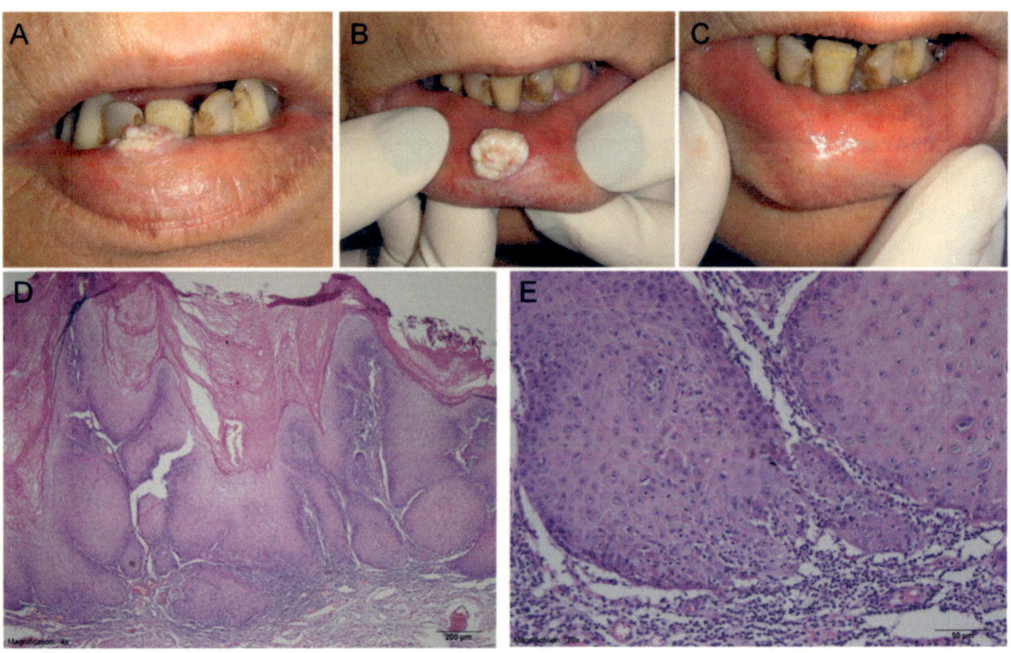

Figure 7. Oral verrucous carcinoma of the lip mucosa. Typical clinical presentation showing an indolor sessile nodule with a white verrucous surface (**A,B**). Surgical excision was performed resulting in an excellent esthetic and functional outcome (**C**). Microscopically, evident hyperkeratosis is observed, with epithelial acanthosis and invasion as pushing borders towards the stroma (**D**). Minimal epithelial atypia is seen along with a strong lymphocytic infiltrate (**E**). *Images obtained from the archives of the Stomatology Specialization at Odontoclínica Central do Exército (OCEx).*

Main OVC differential diagnosis is verrucous hyperplasia, which is very similar, clinically and histologicallly. Verrucous hyperplasia has in fact been regarded as an OVC precursor [43]. Other differential diagnoses are OLP, benign keratosis, chronic candidiasis, verruca vulgaris, oral leukoplakia, reactive keratosis epithelial hyperplasia, pseudoepitheliomatous hyperplasia. It is difficult to distinguish OSCC from OVC, because they may share a similar clinical picture and incisional biopsy excerpts may not contain atypias [44].

Besides that, tumors mainly composed of OVC may contain small areas of OSCC and behave as one. Ideally, for definitive diagnosis the entire tumor mass with its surrounding tissue should be excised and sent for histopathologic analysis [43].

The treatment main option is surgical resection [15, 46] that may be associated with radiotherapy particularly on larger lesions. Relapse rate is high when surgical resection or radiotherapy is performed in isolation. Prognosis of OVC is better than for other types of tumor. Cytostatic drugs, such as α- interferon (IFN), should be considered for patients who cannot undergo surgery, but results are not superior from those obtained with surgery [46].

5.8. Oral Squamous Cell Carcinoma (OSCC)

OSCC is a worldwide problem [47], representing approximately 3% of all malignant neoplasms; which means more than five thousand diagnosed cases a day [48], and more than 90% of all oral cancers [49].

It is a condition primarily related to environmental factors [8] and lifestyle as heavy smoking (more than a pack a day) and drinking (more than 100g a day) [47]. These two are the main risk factors for malignant epithelial transformation. Other risk factors include compromised immune system, poor buccal hygiene and inadequate eating habits [47, 49]. However, OSCC may affect 15 to 20% of patients with no known risk for the condition [8].

Friedrich et al. reported a 20% to 30% HPV association with OSCC [50]. A meta-analysis indicates that oral infection with HPV is an independent risk factor for OSCC. [51] Typically, elderly people [47, 49] are more affected than young people. However, the incidence in young adults is increasing. Some studies have shown that OSCC in young adults follow a different clinical course, being more aggressive and affecting more males [47]. On the other side, other authors have shown no difference in survival among elderly and young adults with OSCC [52].

The most commonly affected site for OSCC is the tongue, especially on inferior and lateral surfaces (40%) [53](Figure 8 – A, F), but it can also affect buccal mucosa, lips, posterior mandibular ridge, gingiva, hard palate and retromolar trigone [47, 49, 53, 54].

The clinical picture may vary among OSCC types. Typically they are nodular or ulcerative lesions [15, 18], with exophytic or ulceroproliferative features [47]. At more advanced stages lesions present an ulcerated center, not well defined with hard borders. At this point, symptoms such as loss of teeth, bleeding, dysarthria, dysphagia, odynophagia and otalgy may develop [54].Some of them, for unknown reasons, do not progress into metastasis, while others infiltrate quickly, invading the lymph nodes [55]. Tongue and floor of the mouth tumors invade cervical lymph nodes in up to 25% of initial stage cases [56, 57] and are often submitted to elective neck dissection. Cervical metastasis at diagnosis is the main indicator of a bad prognosis [45].

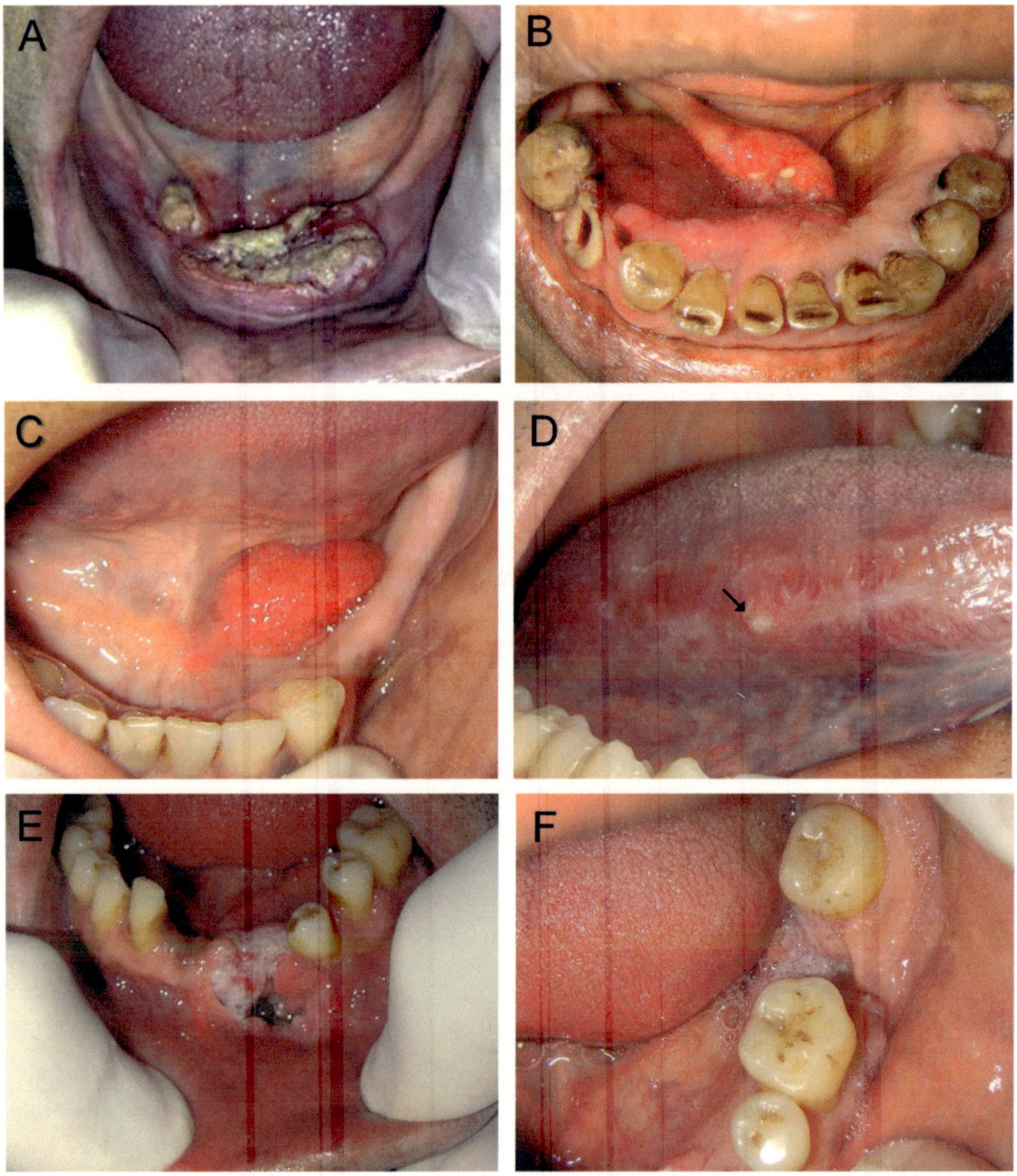

Figure 8. Clinical aspect of OSCC. It may present as an exophityc nodule, ulcerated (**A-B**) or not (**C**). It can also be detected as a small induration interspersed in a white plaque (**D** - arrow). It may show intra osseous invasion (**E**), with a strong white component, and reach distant sites (**F**) from the initial spot. *Images obtained from the archives of the Stomatology Specialization at Odontoclínica Central do Exército (OCEx).*

Histologically a range of features may be present, but it is important to detect epithelial invasion in the stroma, that may occur as islands, cords, sheets and isolated epithelial malignant cells. Keratin may be present, mostly in well and moderately differentiated tumors. There are varying degrees of atypia, nuclear and cellular pleomorphism with aberrant and regular mitosis (Figure 9 – A, D). Usually poorly differentiated tumors are related to recurrence [58]. Clinic and histological features are important to determine treatment, prognostic factors and survival rates [58, 59]. There is a TNM staging scheme, for OSCC and salivary gland tumors [60]. At the initial stages survival rates reach 80%, while at more advanced stages they decrease to 21% [54].

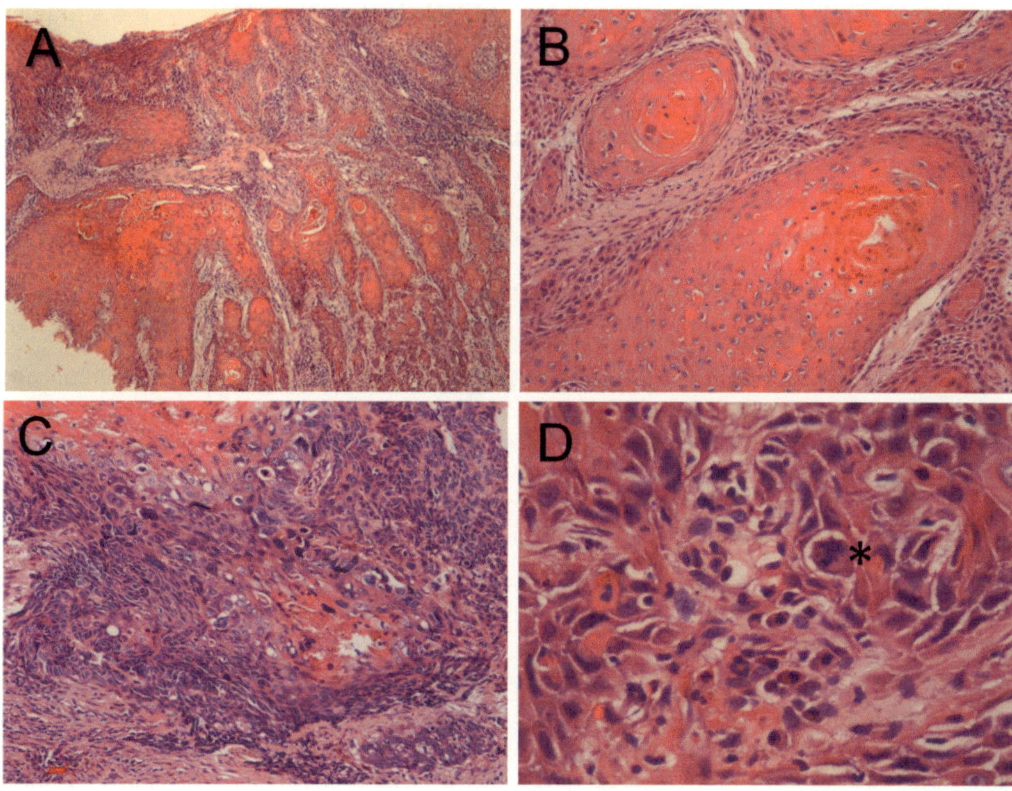

Figure 9. OSCC histopathology. It is possible to observe superficial non affected oral epithelia and tumoral islands in the stroma (**A**; HE, Objective 4x). A closer view of the tumoral islands with central keratin (**B**; HE, Objective 10x). Pleomorphism and atypia are observed (**C**; HE, Objective 10x), as well as mitosis (*) and intercellular bridges (**D**; HE, Objective 20x).

A correlation between HPV and cervical SCC of the utherus has been identified, but despite the strong evidence of HPV presence, there is no clear-cut proof that would point to HPV as an isolate SCC cause on oral cavity. Some studies argue that HPV is a mere supporting causer [1, 61] while another study indicates that tumors positive for oncogenic types of HPV may show better survival [62], mainly in oropharynx, where HPV positive tumors are associated with a specific morphology (basaloid squamous cell carcinoma, a subtype of conventional carcinoma) and positivity for p16 using immunohistochemistry [63].

HPV-16 has been found in 90% of head and neck cancers and in 50% of oropharynx [1, 18, 53, 64]. However, some authors have not found such association [64].

Potentially malignant disorders such as leukoplakia, erytroplakia, proliferative verrucous leukoplakia and lichen planus may progress to OSCC [1] and upon biopsy, there may be already areas of an actual OSCC [65].

Surgical resection is the treatment of choice when the lesion is placed on oral cavity while chemoradiotherapy is used when the oropharynx is the afflicted site [22] or if it is a tumor in a very advanced stage [66].

Surgery may impair some functions as speech, swallowing, and chewing and abruptly change quality of life. To maintain swallowing and speech, an alternative course is ablative surgery (microvascular free tissue), but this is not regarded to be as effective as surgical resection. In advanced stage when metastasis is located on upper aerodigestive tract, treatment should be multimodal, combining surgery and chemoradiotherapy [46].

Recurrent OSCC is challenging as the risk of complication is increased due to fibrosis and tissue hipovascularization [51].

Radiotherapy may be primary, adjuvant or neoadjuvant. It is regarded as primary for unresectable tumor or for patients who cannot undergo surgery, adjuvant as a post-surgery complementary method, and neoadjuvant when performed before surgery to facilitate tumor resection [54].

6. HPV oncogenic potential

HPV infection may lead to cell immortalization by means of infection of the mucosa and skin basal epithelial cells, which are the only ones that keep in the cell cycle [8, 61]. It may be by itself a causative agent of malignant transformation or when associated with other unclear cofactors [61]. However, some researchers have argued that HPV is not able to cause malignant transformation, despite the studies which point to the contrary [12].

Some factors should come into play to immortalize cells: virus type, synergetic action among physics, biological and chemical agents and genetic constitution, which are able to modify the natural course of the disease. But if the exposed person has a favorable condition and acquires high risk HPV it becomes easier to integrate viral DNA into human genome [61].

Oral HPV has been diagnosed in OSCC and it is believed that it has been involved in oral carcinogenesis by transforming the keratinocytes through a mechanism involving E6 and E7 proteins. However, the mechanisms behind immune response against high risk HPV remain unclear [67-69].

7. HPV detection methods

The identification of various types of HPV is a recent technological advance due to the growth impossibility in tissue cultures and research animals.

Diagnoses methods vary from simple to sophisticated ones, ranging from light microscopy to DNA expression, with low to high sensitivity. Light microscopy and in situ hybridization are considered low sensitivity methods because it only tests positive when there are more than 10 viral DNA copies per cell. Among the intermediate sensitivity methods we find southern blot, do blot and reverse hybridization with a positive detection result when there is from 1 to 10 DNA copies per cell. High sensitivity methods, such as PCR, needs less than 1 viral DNA copy per cell for microorganism detection [70].

7.1. Light microscopy

This method provides some data, even though it has low sensibility and it does not inform the HPV type. The most common HPV induced changes are epithelial thickening, prominent keratohyalin granules, hyperkeratosis, nuclear dysplasia, hyperchromasia, double nucleation of superficial and intermediated cell, perinuclear cytoplasmic halos, and atypical immature metaplasia [9].

7.2. Electron microscopy

HPV particles may be identified by electron microscopy (EM), but not the HPV type. EM can detect the presence of virion on koilocytic and dyskeratotic cell nuclei, but it is a limited method to investigate infection, because high risk HPV do not reproduce and as such cannot be identified through EM [5].

7.3. Molecular methods

Molecular methods can be divided into two types: non-hybridization, such as in situ amplification, southern and dot blot hybridization and the amplified, such as target amplification, signal amplification and probe amplification. Target amplification is best exemplified by PCR. Signal amplification may be represented by hybrid technique sample. Probe amplification which is a compound-probe is added to a probe generating signal (Ligase Chain Reaction) according to literature [5].

7.4. *In Situ* Hybridization (ISH)

In situ hybridization using biotinylated probes is a common method for detecting HPV in oral epithelium. It is practical and economical for screening for HPV in clinical pathology laboratories. In situ hybridization also permits direct comparison of viral DNA location with histologic morphology [9, 71]. Although this technique is highly sensitive in cases in which individual nuclei contain a high copy number of the target DNA, as is likely to occur in most active infections, the method of ISH often fails to detect cases in which subgenomic fragments of the viral DNA have been incorporated into the host genome and the infection is nonproductive of intact viral particles. So when there is low viral DNA amount, it leads to low sensitivity [71, 72]

7.5. Southern blot and dot blot hybridization

Southern Blot classifies and identifies new viral types. It is a labor-intensive process that requires well trained skills and depends on a new generation of equipments. This technique requires the total length of a DNA molecule, and offers additional information about viral integration and subtype [70].

Dot blot is a simplified southern blot, requiring less sophisticated facilities, but it is rarely performed because of its low sensitivity. It is often used as detection kits available on the market [70].

7.6. Target amplification

The classic example of target amplification is PCR. This is the best subtype detection method due to the high sensitivity [9]. It is commonly used as diagnostic tool for HPV DNA epidemiological investigation, but because of the high cost this method cannot be used in a routine clinical practice. PCR has a high sensitivity and it is very effective for both malignant and pre malignant lesions identification, and material can be collected with oral swab or wash [7, 9].

7.7. Hybrid Capture technology (HC)

Using signal amplification with microplate chemiluminescent detection, this method identifies nucleic acid due to its high sensitivity [9]. HC is a very important tool to detect high risk HPV, and the method has identified HPV 16, 18, 31, 33, 35, 39, 45, 51, 52, 56, 58, 59, 68 types [9]. This technique is able to identify 5000 viral copies per sample [73].

7.8. Probe amplification

Probe amplification methods differ from target amplification in that the amplification products contain a sequence only present in the initial probes. It is used currently as an important diagnostic application, the detection of high-risk genotypes of human papilloma viruses (HPV) [74].

7.9. Education and vaccine prophylaxis

One simple and effective prophylactic measure is patient education. It must be clear to patients that even after treatment the virus remains on the oral mucosa, so it is imperative to maintain good oral hygiene, condom use in all sexual relations and refrain from promiscuous sexual behavior. Clinical examinations have to be done periodically and smoking and chronic alcoholism must be abolished.

It is crucial that the population in general be informed about HPV prevention as a control strategy and early diagnosis promotion. Raising awareness of HPV through education is essential to develop population perception about risk factors, mainly those related to sexual activity[18]. It is also important to discourage early sexual initiation [69].

In view of the increasing figures of cervix cancer, the US Food and Drugs Administration (FDA) approved in 2006 a vaccine against HPV [75]. There is a bivalent vaccine that contains L_1 HPV-16/18 protein which generates a huge number of genotype specific antibody [75]. For HPV 16/18 vaccine efficiency is round 96% on cervix cancer [69]. There is also a tetravalent vaccine that works in the same way as the bivalent, but provides further immunity enclosing HPV types 6, 11, 16, 18 [75]. Both of them use virus- like particles in their composition [9].

The vaccine(s) stimulates humoral response, but it also stimulates B cell immune memory response, which persists for five years [69]. After a 5 years follow up, it has demonstrated 100% of efficacy on persistent infection prevention [8].

As HPV's physiopathology is very similar on the affected sites, whether they are the skin, cervix, penile, anus or oral mucosa, there is no reason to doubt that the vaccine which works well on the cervix would also prove effective for the prevention of oral mucosa lesions [75].

As HPV-16 seems to be an important risk factor for the progress of malignant lesions (because it is found in most OSCCs), it might be possible that the vaccine would prevent or even treat them [8].

HPV vaccine seems to be less effective on women who have already been exposed to the virus, hence the public health focus on vaccinating girls before their first sexual relation to prevent warts and more disaster lesions in the future [8, 9]. Some countries have promoted vaccination for any females from 9 to 26 years who have never had sexual experience before [76]. Other countries promote vaccination for females up to 45 years old [77]. Vaccines for men aged 11 up to 26 years old in order to prevent genital warts and anal cancer was approved in 2011 by the US Advisory Committee on Immunization Practices [78].

HPV is as frequent in men as in women; however, it is often asymptomatic in males, what makes them a HPV reservoir to cervix and non- cervical lesions in females, transmitted mainly by sexual activity [69]. Current studies have been done in order to further assess the natural history of the HPV infection in men [79, 80].

A therapeutic vaccine is under study, one which could be used as adjuvant on surgery or radiotherapy, to clean up microscopic waste of the lesion, thus generating immune response.

In view of the potential risks of HPV and the potential benefits of the vaccine (some not yet fully established) some researchers favor the extended use of the vaccine to all age groups of both sexes, regardless of previous sexual practice, as a form to interrupt the transmission cycle and as a preventive strategy in controlling and avoiding the risks posed by HPV, including various types of cancer in different locations in the human body.

Acknowledgements

We would like to thank Professor Simone Lourenço and Márcia Sother who were active in building clinical images archives for the Stomatology Specialization Course at Odontoclinica Central do Exército (OCEx – Rio de Janeiro, Brasil).

Author details

Helena Lucia Barroso dos Reis[1,4], Silvia Paula de Oliveira[2,3], Danielle Resende Camisasca[1,4], Juliana Bittencourt Pessoa[5], Ana Beatriz Azevedo Queiroz[2], Mauro Romero Leal Passos[4], Philippe Godefroy[4], Dennis de Carvalho Ferreira[2], Thais Camporez Pimentel[5] and Antonio Chambo Filho[5]

1 Federal University of Espirito Santo, Brazil

2 Federal University of Rio de Janeiro, Brazil

3 Odontoclinica Central do Exercito of Rio de Janeiro, Brazil

4 Fluminense Federal University, Brazil

5 Santa Casa de Misericórdia School of Science, Brazil

References

[1] Feller L, Khammissa RAG, Wood NH et al. Epithelial maturation and molecular biology of oral HPV. Infect Agent Cancer 2009;4:16.

[2] Syrjänen S, Lodi G, von Bültzingslöwen I, Jontell M et al. Human papillomaviruses in oral carcinoma and oral potentially malignant disorders: a systematic review. Oral Dis 2011 Apr;17 Suppl 1:58-72.

[3] Durzynska J, Pacholska-Bogalska J, Kaczmarek M et al. HPV genotypes in the oral cavity/oropharynx of children and adolescents: cross-sectional survey in Poland. Eur J Pediatr 2011;170:757–61.

[4] Ezquenazi D, Filho IB, Carvalho MGC et al. The frequency of human papillomavirus findings in normal oral mucosa of healthy people. Braz J Otorhinolaryngol 2010;76(1):78-84.

[5] Kumaraswamy KL, Vidhya M. Human Papilloma virus and oral infections: an update. J Cancer Res Ther 2011;7(2):120-7.

[6] Syrjänen, S. The role of human papillomavirus infection in head and neck cancers. Ann Oncol 2010;21(7) 243-5.

[7] Michl P, Pazdera J, Prochazka M et al. Human Papillomavirus in the etiology of head and neck carcinomas. Biomed Pap Med Fac Univ Palacky Olomouc Czech Repub 2010;154(1):9–12.

[8] Mannarini L, Kratochivil V, Calabrese L et al. Human Papilloma Virus (HPV) in head and neck region: review of literature. Acta Otorhinolaryngol Ital 2009;29:119-26.

[9] Chlaudhary AK, Singh M, Sundaram S et al. Role of human papillomavirus and its detection in potentially malignant and malignant head and neck lesions: updated review. Head Neck Oncol 2009;1:22.

[10] Castro TMPPG, Filho IB, Nascimento VX et al. HPV detection in the oral and genital mucosa of women with positive histopathological exam for genital HPV, by means of the PCR. Braz J Otorhinolaryngol 2009;75(2):167-71.

[11] Fakhry C, Sugar E, D'Souza G et al. Two-Week versus Six-Month Sampling Interval in a Short-Term Natural History Study of Oral HPV Infection in an HIV-Positive Cohort. PLoS One 2010;5(7):e11918.

[12] Panonne G, Santoro A, Papagerakis S et al. The role of human papillomavirus in the pathogenesis of head & neck squamous cell carcinoma: an overview. Infect Agent Cancer 2011;6:4.

[13] Rombaldi RL, Serafini EP, Mandelli J et al. Transplacental transmission of Human Papillomavirus. Virol J 2008;5:106.

[14] Zwenger SR. Bogarting that joint might decrease oral HPV among cannabis users. Curr Oncol 2009;16(6):5-7.

[15] Castro TMPPG, Filho IB. Prevalence of human papillomavirus (HPV) in oral cavity and oropharynx. Braz J Otorhinolaryngol 2006;72(2):272-82.

[16] Sánches–Vargas LO, Díaz-Hernández C, Martinez-Martinez A. Detection of Human Papilloma Virus (HPV) in oral mucosa of women with cervical lesions and their relation to oral sex practices. Infect Agent Cancer 2010;4;5(1):25.

[17] Pereira CM, Melo LG, Correa MM et al. Oral HPV infection in a boné marrow transplantation patient: a case report with atypical clinical presentation and unexoected outcome. Braz J Infect Dis 2010;14(1):89-91.

[18] Castro TMPPG; Neto CER, Scala KA et al. Oral manifestations related to papillomavirus. Braz J Otorhinolaryngol 2004;70(4):546-50.

[19] Rombaldi RL, Serafini EP, Mandelli J et al. Perinatal transmission of human papillomavirus DNA. Virol J 2009;6:83.

[20] Filho JAX, Simoceli L, Imamura R et al. Recurrent laryngeal papillomatosis: a 10-year experience. Braz J Otorhinolaryngol. 2003;69(5): 599-604.

[21] Rintala MAM, Grénman SE, Järvenkyla ME et al. High-risk types of humam papillomavirus (HPV) DNA in oral and genital mucosa of infants during their first 3 year of life: experience from the finnish HPV family study. Clin Infect Dis 2005;15;41(12): 1728-33.

[22] Reis HLB, Ferreira DC, Forattini AG, Souza PG, Curvelo JAR, Passos MRL. Genital and oral human papillomavirus infection in a patient from the group of women who have sex with women. Clinics 2010; 65(12): 1383-1385.

[23] Syrjänen K, Syrjänen S. HPV infection of the oral Mucose. Papillomavirus infections in human pathology. Chichester, England: John Wiley & Sons Ltd, 2000:380.

[24] Scheurer ME, Tortolero-Luna G, Adler-Storthz K. Human papillomavirus infection: biology, epidemiology, and prevention. Int J Gynecol Cancer 2005; 15: 727–746.

[25] Anderson K M, Perez-Montiel D, Miles L et al. The histologic differentiation of oral condyloma acuminatum from its mimics. Oral Surg Oral Med Oral Pathol Oral Radiol Endod 2003; 96:420-8.

[26] Praetorius F. HPV-Associated diseases of oral mucosa. Clinics in Dermatology 1997;15:399-413.

[27] Jaju PP, Suvarna PV, Desai RS. Squamous papilloma: case report and review of literature. Int J Oral Sci 2010;2(4),222-5.

[28] Carneiro TE, Marinho SA, Verli, FD et al. Oral squamous papilloma: clinical, histologic and immunohistocheamecal analyses. J Oral Sci 2009;51(3):367–72.

[29] Bassioukas K, Danielides V, Georgiou I et al. Oral focal epithelial hyperplasia. Eur J of Dermat 2000;10(5):395-7.

[30] Vera-Iglesias E, García-Arpa M, Sanchéz-Caminero P et al. Focal epithelial hyperplasia. Actas Dermosifiliogr 2007;98(9):621-3.

[31] Hashemipour MA, Shoryabi A, Adhami S et al. Extensive Focal Epithelial Hyperplasia. Arch Iran Med 2010;13(1):48-52.

[32] Delgado Y, Torrelo A, Colmenero I et al. Hiplerplasia epitelial focal. Actas Dermosifiliogr 2005;96(10):697-9.

[33] Fernández-González F, Vázquez-Ávarez R, Reboiras-López D et al. Histopathological findings in oral lichen planus and their correlation with the clinical manifestations. Med Oral Patol Oral Cir Bucal 2011;1;16(5):e641-6.

[34] Edwards PC, Kelsch R. Oral Lichen Planus: Clinical Presentation and Management. J Can Dent Assoc 2002;68(8):494-9.

[35] Nico MMS, Lourenço SM, Fernandes JD. Oral lichen planus. An Bras Dermatol 2011;86(4):633-43.

[36] van der Meij EH, van der Waal I. Lack of clinicopathologic correlation in the diagnosis of oral lichen planus based on the presently available diagnostic criteria and suggestions for modifications. J Oral Pathol Med 2003; Oct;32(9):507-12.

[37] van der Waal I. Potentially malignant disorders of the oral and oropharyngeal mucosa; terminology, classification and present concepts of management. Oral Oncol 2009; Apr-May;45(4-5):317-23.

[38] Martorell Calatayud A, Botella-Estrada R, Bagán-Sebastián et al. Oral Leukoplakia: Clinical, Histopathologic, and Molecular Features and Therapeutic Approach. Actas Dermosifiliogr 2009;100:669-84.

[39] Smitha T, Sharada P, Girish HC. A white patch or plaque that cannot be characterized clinically or histologically as any other disease. J Oral Maxillofac Pathol 2011;15(1):26-33.

[40] Kreuter A, Wieland U. Oral hairy leukoplakia: a clinical indicator of immunosuppression. CMAJ 2011;183(8):932.

[41] Sapna N, Vandana KL. Idiopathic linear leukoplakia of gingiva: a rare case report. J Indian Soc Periodontol 2010;14(3):198-200.

[42] Lodi G, Sardella A, Bez C, et al. Interventions for treating oral leukoplakia. Cochrane Database Syst Rev 2006; Oct 18;(4):CD001829.

[43] Alkan A, Bulut E, Gunhan O et al. Oral Verrucous Carcinoma: A Study of 12 Cases. Eur J Dent 2010;4(2):202-7.

[44] Santoro A, Pannone G, Contaldo M el al. A Troubling Diagnosis of Verrucous Squamous Cell Carcinoma ("the Bad Kind" of Keratosis) and the Need of Clinical and Pathological Correlations: A Review of the Literature with a Case Report. J Skin Cancer 2011;2011:370605.

[45] Barnes L, Eveson J.W., Reichert P., Sidransky D. World Health Organization Classification of Tumours. Pathology and Genetics of Head and Neck Tumours. Lyon: IARC Press; 2005.

[46] Kang CJ, Chang JT, Chen IH et al. Surgical Treatment of Oral Verrucous Carcinoma.Chang Gung Med J 2003;26(11):807-12.

[47] Falaki F, Dalirsani Z, Pakfetrat A et al. Clinical and histopathological analysis of oral squamous cell carcinoma of young patients in Mashhad, Iran: a retrospective study and review of literature. Med Oral Patol Oral Cir Bucal 2011;16(4):e473-7.

[48] Fan S, Tang QL, Chen WL et al. A review of clinical and histological parameters associated with contralateral neck metastases in oral squamous cell carcinoma. Int J of Oral Sci 2011;3(4):180-191.

[49] Arkbulut N, Oztas B, Kursun S et al. Delayed diagnosis of oral squamous cell carcinoma: a case series. J Med Case Reports 2011;5(1):291.

[50] Friedrich RE, Sperber C, Jakel T, Roser K, Loning T. Basaloid lesions of oral squamous epithelial cells and their association with HPV infection and P16 expression. Anticancer Res 2010;30:1605–1612.

[51] Miller CS, Johnstone BM. Human papillomavirus as a risk factor for oral squamous cell carcinoma: a meta-analysis, 1982-1997. Oral Surg Oral Med Oral Pathol Oral Radiol Endod 2001; Jun 91(6):622-35.

[52] Warnakulasuriya S. Global epidemiology of oral and oropharyngeal cancer. Oral Oncol 2009;45(4-5):309-316.

[53] Termine N, Panzarella V, Falaschini S et al. HPV in oral squamous cell carcinoma vs head and neck squamous cell carcinoma biopsies: a meta-analysis. Ann Oncol 2008;19(10):1681-90.

[54] Kademani D. Oral Cancer. Mayo Clin Proc 2007;82(7):878-87.

[55] Cordella C, Lubbers HT, Rivelli V et al. An evaluation of the preoperative hemoglobin level as a prognostic factor for oral squamous cell carcinoma. Head Neck Oncol 2011;15;3:35.

[56] Dias FL, Kligerman J, Matos de Sa G, et al. Elective neck dissection versus observation in stage I squamous cell carcinomas of the tongue and floor of the mouth. Otolaryngol Head Neck Surg 2001;125(1):23-9.

[57] Kligerman J, Lima RA, Soares JR, et al. Supraomohyoid neck dissection in the treatment of T1/T2 squamous cell carcinoma of oral cavity. Am J Surg 1994;168(5):391-4.

[58] Camisasca DR, Silami MA, Honorato J, Dias FL, de Faria PA, Lourenco SQC. Oral squamous cell carcinoma: clinicopathological features in patients with and without recurrence. ORL J Otorhinolaryngol Relat Spec 2011;73(3):170-6.

[59] Camisasca DR, Honorato J, Bernardo V, et al. Expression of Bcl-2 family proteins and associated clinicopathologic factors predict survival outcome in patients with oral squamous cell carcinoma. Oral Oncol 2009;45(3):225-33.

[60] Nguyen NP, Chi A, Nguyen LM et al. Human papillomavirus-associated oropharyngeal cancer: a new clinic entity. QJM 2010;103(4):229–36.

[61] Ritchie JM, Smith EM, Summersgill KF, Hoffman HT, Wang D, Klussmann JP, Turek LP, Haugen TH. Human papillomavirus infection as a prognostic factor in carcinomas of the oral cavity and oropharynx. Int J Cancer 2003; 104(3): 336-44.

[62] Syrjanen S. Human papillomaviruses in head and neck carcinomas. N Engl J Med 2007;356(19):1993-5.

[63] Ha PK, Pai SI, Westra WH et al. Real-time quantitative PCR demonstrates low prevalence of human papillomavirustype 16 in premalignant and malignant lesions of the oral cavity. Clin Cancer Res 2002; 8(5):1203-9.

[64] Warnakulasuriya S, Johnson NW, van der Waal I. Nomenclature and classification of potentially malignant disorders of the oral mucosa. J Oral Pathol Med 2007;36(10): 575-80.

[65] Hassel AJ, Danner D, Freier K et al. Oral health-related quality of life and depression/ anxiety in long-term recurrence-free patients after treatment for advanced oral squamous cell cancer. J Craniomaxillofac Surg 2012;40(4):e99-102.

[66] Ji X, Neumann AS, Sturgis EM et al. p53 codon 72 polymorphism associated with risk of human papillomavirus-associated squamous cell carcinoma of the oropharynx in never smokers. Carcinogenesis 2008;29(4):875-9.

[67] Westra, W.H. The changing face of head and neck cancer in the 21st century: the impact of HPV on the epidemiology and pathology of oral cancer. Head Neck Pathol 2009;3(1):78-81.

[68] Feller F, Wood NH, Khammissa RA et al. Human papillomavirus-mediated carcinogenesis and HPV-associated oral and oropharyngeal squamous cell carcinoma. Part 2:Human papillomavirus associated oral and orapharyngeal squamous cell carcinoma. Head Face Med 2010;6:15.

[69] Oliveira MC, Soares RC, Pinto LP et al. HPV and oral carcinogenesis: a bibliographic review. Braz J Otorhinolaryngol 2003;69(4):553-9.

[70] Shroyer KR, Greer Jr RO. Detection of human papillomavirus DNA by in situ hybridization and polymerase chain reaction in premalignant and malignant oral lesions. Oral Surg Oral Med Oral Pathol 1991;71:708-13.

[71] Coutlee F, Danielle R, Alex F, Eduardo F. The laboratory diagnosis of genital human-papilloma virus infections. Can J Infect Dis Med Microbiol 2005;16:83-91.

[72] Tang WK. Oncogenic human papillomavirus infection: Epidemiology in local high-risk women. Hong Kong Dermatol Venereol Bull 2002;10:160-63.

[73] Ginocchio CC, Barth D, Zhang F. Comparison of the Third Wave Invader human papillomavirus assay and the Digene HPV hybrid capture assay for detection of high-risk HPV. J Clin Microbiol 2008; 46:1641-1646.

[74] Gillson ML, Chaturvedi AK, Lowy DL. HPV prophylactic vaccines and potential prevention of noncervical cancers in both men and women. Cancer 2008;15;113(10): 3036-46.

[75] Einstein MH, Baron M, Levin MJ,et al. Comparative immunogenicity and safety of human papillomavirus (HPV)-16/18 vaccine and HPV-6/11/16/18 vaccine: follow-up from months 12–24 in a Phase III randomized study of healthy women aged 18–45 years. Hum Vaccin 2011; 7: 1343–1358.

[76] Centers for Disease Control and Prevention. Recommendations on the use of quadrivalent human papillomavirus vaccine in males–Advisory Committee on Immunization Practices (ACIP), 2011. http://www.cdc.gov/mmwr/preview/mmwrhtml/mm6050a3.htm (accessed 26 Jul 2013).

[77] Daron GF, Waller JL, Miller J et al. Variables associated with human papillomavirus (HPV) vaccine acceptance by men. J Am Board Fam Med 2009; 22 (1):34-42.

[78] Kreimer AR, Pierce Campbell CM, Lin HY et al. Incidence and clearance of oral human papillomavirus infection in men: the HIM cohort study. Lancet 2013; Sep 7;382(9895):877-87.

[79] Kreimer AR, Villa A, Nyitray AG et al. The epidemiology of oral HPV infection among a multinational sample of healthy men. Cancer Epidemiol Biomarkers Prev 2011; Jan;20(1):172-82.

Section 2

Bacterial Infectious Diseases

Chapter 3

Newer β-Lactamases and *E.coli* — A Cause of Concern

Silpi Basak and Monali N. Rajurkar

Additional information is available at the end of the chapter

http://dx.doi.org/10.5772/57578

1. Introduction

In 1941, the Magic Bullet Penicillin was first used clinically in an Oxfordshire constable, Albert Alexander, but within one year Rammelkamp reported the identification of isolates of *Stphylococcus aureus,* resistant to this miracle drug [1]. Within a short span of 70 years, from discovery of Penicillin to Tigecycline, some hospital strains have developed which are resistant to almost all available antimicrobials and the mankind is busy in writing obituary for antimicrobials [2].

Infact, the rising trend of developing resistance to multiple antibiotics in microbes, leads to therapeutic failure. Presently, antimicrobial resistance (AMR) is a major threat to patient care and disease control throughout the world.

The World Health Day theme on 7th April 2011 was 'Antimicrobial resistance and its global spread'. World Health Organisation has raised the issue in 2011 that "Combat drug Resistance - No action today, No cure tomorrow" [3]. Not only the Gram positive bacteria like Methicillin Resistant *Staphylococcus aureus* (MRSA), Vancomycin Resistant Enterococci (VRE) etc. even the several Gram negative bacteria of Enterobacteriaceae family e.g. *E.coli, Klebsiella pneumoniae, Enterobacter sp. etc,* and *Pseudomonas aeruginosa, Acinetobacter baumani, Burkholderia species* etc. also develop resistance to most of the antibiotics now a days.

Actually, the pace in which bacteria develop resistance is much higher than the rate of development of newer antimicrobials. The antibiotic resistance is mainly developed due to inappropriate and irrational use of antibiotics. In 2011, two new terms were coined i.e. multidrug resistant (MDR) and Extreme drug resistant (XDR) organisms. MDR is defined as non-susceptibility to one or more antibiotics in three or more antibiotic classes and XDR is defined as non-susceptibility to all potentially effective antimicrobials respectively [4]. β – lactamases are the important mechanism of drug resistance among the Gram negative bacteria.

Though *E.coli* is a commensal of human or animal intestine, *E.coli* is the most commonly isolated bacterial species in clinical laboratories and is incriminated in infectious diseases involving every human tissue and organ system [5]. Theodare Escherich, a German pediatrician identified *Escherichia coli* in 1885 and named it *'Bacterium coli commune'* [6]. He also established the pathogenic role of *E.coli* through his studies. The nomenclature *'Bacterium coli'* was widely used until 1919 when Castellani and Chalmers described the genus Escherichia [7]. The type species is *Escherichia coli*. Some species like *E.fergusonii, E.hermanii* and *E.vulneris* are considered opportunistic pathogens and are associated with wound infection in humans [8]. *Escherichia albertii,* the sixth species associated with cases of diarrhoea in children of Bangladesh, has been proposed by Huys et al in 2003 [9].

About 80% cases of urinary tract infection are due to *E.coli* [8]. It is commonly involved in Gram negative sepsis and endotoxic shock. *E.coli* can cause diarrhoea, wound infections, pneumonia in hospitalized patients and meningitis in neonates.

E.coli is the organism that is most widely studied in its various aspects. *E.coli* is the model organism for studies on cell structure, growth and metabolism. It is considered to be good vehicle for the cloning of genes from prokaryotic and eukaryotic cells and for expression of gene products [8].

E.coli is susceptible to 97% ethylene trioxide (ETO) and 95% Hydrochlorofluorocarbon-ETO (HCFC-ETO) respectively [10]. Chlorine 1 ppm is capable of eliminating approximately 4 $\log_{10}$ of *E.coli* O157:H7 within a minute [11]. E.coli strains causing intestinal and extra intestinal infections, exhibits many virulence factors such as: Adhesins, O antigens, Hemolysin, Siderophore production / Iron sequestration / Aerobactin production, Cell surface hydrophobicity, Outer membrane proteins e.g. Porins etc. Haemagglutinin, Verotoxin, Cytotoxic necrotizing factor (CNF), Enterotoxin, Colicins, Gelatinase production, Serum resistance are other major virulence factors of *E.coli*. Complete serotyping of *E.coli* is based on three antigen detection as O, K & H i.e. O:K:H. If fimbrial virulence factor is present then serotype should be expressed in terms of O:K:H:F.

A. *E.coli* — Role as a pathogen

They are classified into two types [12] – (a) Enterovirulent *E.coli,* (b) Uropathogenic *E.coli*

a. **ENTEROVIRULENT***E.coli***:** Adherence is one of the most important virulence mechanisms of enterovirulent *E.coli.*

Enterovirulent *E.coli* strains are classified into

Enteropathogenic *E.coli* (EPEC), Enterotoxigenic *E.coli* (ETEC), Enteroinvasive *E.coli* (EIEC), Verocytotoxin – producing *E.coli* (VTEC), Enteroaggregative *E.coli* (EAEC), Diffusely adherent *E.coli* (DAEC) etc.

b. **UROPATHOGENIC***E.Coli* (UPEC)

E.coli is the predominant uropathogen isolated from acute community acquired urinary tract infections and is responsible for 85% of asymptomatic bacteriuria and more than 60%

of recurrent cystitis [13]. *E.coli* strains involved in urinary tract infections includes O groups 1, 2, 4, 6, 7 etc.

B. Laboratory diagnosis

E.coli can be detected in the laboratory by conventional tests [5]. *E.coli* are Gram negative rod, motile and on Mac Conkey's agar form lactose fermenting nonmucoid colonies. Routine biochemical tests done for E.coli are : Catalase test: Positive, Oxidase test: Negative, Triple sugar iron agar test: Acid slant/Acid butt with gas, Indole test: Positive, Methyl red test: Positive, Voges-Proskauer (VP) test: Negative, Citrate utilization test: Negative, Nitrate reduction test: Positive, Oxidative / Fermentative test (Hugh & Leifson): Fermentative metabolism, Lysine Decarboxylase test: Positive.

1.1. Antibiotibiotic sensitivity pattern

Intrinsic resistance is rarely seen in genus Escherichia. Susceptibility of individual strain to different antimicrobials varies greatly, thus antibiogram is used as an epidemiological marker. This resistance pattern is plasmid mediated. *E.coli* shows transferable resistance to one or multiple drugs [14]. Recently *E.coli* isolated from intestinal as well as extraintestinal specimens has become resistant to most of the routinely used antibiotics.

A. Beta - lactamases

Beta lactamases are enzymes produced by wide range of Gram negative and Gram positive bacteria. This enzyme is responsible for resistance to β-lactam antibiotics like Penicillins, Cephalosporins, Cephamycins and Carbapenems. The β-lactamase enzymes break the beta-lactam ring and thus inactivate the antibacterial properties. Abraham and Chain (1940) discovered penicillinase, first β-lactamase to be identified in *E.coli* before Penicillin was introduced for clinical use [15]. The name β-lactamase was given by Pollock in 1960 [16]. First plasmid mediated β-lactamase was "TEM" named after the name of first patient Temoniera in whom the enzyme was first detected [17].

Classification of β-Lactamases can be done by -

a. Functional or Bush Jacoby Mederios classification [18]

b. Molecular or Ambler classification [19]

Ambler in 1980s classified β – lactamases into various groups and according to him, there are three main classes as A, C and D [19]. Metallobetalactamases belong to class B which exhibits potent hydrolyzing activity not only against Carbapenems but also to other β – lactam antibiotics. *E.coli* is one of those Gram negative bacteria that has potential to develop all the major classes of β – lactamases including Metallobetalactamases.

Determination of β-lactamase production could be done by acidometric method, iodometric method and Chromogenic cephalosporin method using nitrocephin [20].

B. Extended spectrum beta – lactamase (ESBL)

Extended spectrum beta – lactamase (ESBL) producing strains are emerging pathogens causing Health care associated infections (HAI) and pose great therapeutic challenge in recent years.

ESBLs were first detected in *Klebsiella pneumoniae* in 1983 [21, 22]. ESBL are classified under molecular AMBLer class A penicillinase having serine residue at their active site. ESBLs are responsible for resistance to one or more β-lactam antibiotics including third generation cephalosporins. Typically ESBLs are derived from genes for TEM-1, TEM-2 or SHV-1 by mutations that alter the amino acid sequence around the active site of β-lactamases [23,24]. ESBLs are inhibited by β-lactam inhibitors like Clavulanic acid, Sulbactam and Tazobactam. ESBLs are produced by Enterobacteriaceae family, *Pseudomonas aeruginosa, Acinetobacter species* etc.

Detection of Extended Spectrum β-lactamase (ESBL) production:

The ESBL in *E.coli* is detected by two approaches: 1.Screening tests and 2.Confirmatory tests. Screening test detect reduced susceptibility to indicator drugs. According to Clinical Laboratory Standard Institute (CLSI) guidelines indicator drugs used for *E.coli* & Klebsiella spp. are Cefotaxime, Ceftazidime, Ceftriaxone or Aztreonam [25]. Screening tests are not specific because mechanism other than ESBLs may also give positive results. Therefore, positive screening test should be followed by confirmatory tests.

Different confirmatory tests include Double disk approximation test, [26,27]. Comparison of Minimum inhibitory concentratin (MIC) or inhibitory zone around disk in presence or absence of β-lactamase inhibitor [28], Vitek ESBL test [29], Etest [30], three-dimentional test [31] etc. For identification of specific ESBL different molecular detection methods can be applied like DNA probes, PCR with oligonucleotide primers oligotyping, PCR followed by restriction fragment length polymorphism analysis, ligase chain reaction and nucleotide sequencing etc [32]. Commonly primers used for detecting bla genes are [33]:

CTX Forward – CGCTTTGCGATGTGCAG

Reverse - ACCGCGATATCGTTGGT

These techniques are available only in research centers and are beyond the scope of routine Clinical Microbiology Laboratories in India considering the presence of too many different types of ESBLs and the high cost.

C. Amp C beta-lactamase [34]

Amp C β-lactamases were first reported in 1988. Amp C β-lactamases are found either on chromosome (inducible) or on plasmid (non-inducible). Amp C β-lactamase producing bacteria show resistance to most of Cephalosporins including Cephamycin (Cefoxitin, Cefotetan) except Carbapenems. But they also hydrolyze Penicillins and Aztreonem. These are not inhibited by beta-lactam inhibitors such as Clavulanic acid, Tazobactam and Sulbactam.

Detection of AMPC β-Lactamase production: Presently, all plasmid mediated Amp C β-lactamases have similar substrate profile to chromosomal Amp C β-lactamases. But the only difference is chromosomal Amp C β -lactamases are inducile where as plasmid mediated Amp C β –lactamases are uninducible [35]. Amp C β-lactamase producing strains could be detected by disc antagonism test [36], modified three dimensional test (MTDT) [37], Amp C disc test [38], double disk synergy test and disc potentiation test using 3-amino-phenyl-boronic acid (APB) etc [39].

http://dx.doi.org/10.5772/57578

D. Carbapenemases

These include β – lactamases which cause Carbapenem hydrolysis, with elevated Carbapenem MICs and they belonged to molecular classes A, B and D. Molecular classes A, C and D include the β – lactamases with serine at their active site, whereas class B β – lactamases are all metalloenzymes which require Zn++ for their activation [40].

Molecular class A carbapenemase – Class A serine carbapenemases belong to functional group 2f include chromosomally encoded NMC(Not Metalloenzyme Carbapenemase), IMI (Imipenem hydrolyzing β-lactamase) and SME(*Serratia marcenscens* enzyme) and plasmid mediated KPC (*Klebsiella pneumoniae* carbapenemase) and GES / IBC(integron borne cephalosporinase), etc [40]. All have the ability to hydrolyse Carbapenems, Cephalosporins, Penicillins and Aztreonem and all are inhibited by Clavulanic acid and Tazobactam. The chromosomal class A carbapenemase are infrequently found and can be induced by Imipenem and Cefoxitin. The KPC (*Klebsiella pneumoniae* carbapenemase) producing strains are found in *Klebsiella pneumoniae*, Enterobacter species, Salmonella species and other Enterobacteriaceae [41,42].

Class D Serine carbapenemases - The OXA (Oxacillin hydrolysing) β-lactamase with carbapenemase activity was detected by Patow et al in 1993 and the enzyme was purified from *Acinetobacter baumani [40].* They have been also found in Enterobacteriaceae and *P.aeruginosa* and were described as penicillinase capable of hydrolyzing Oxacillin and Cloxacillin [43,44]. They are not inhibited by Clavulanic acid and EDTA and were designated as ARI-1 (Acinetobacter Resistant to Imipenem) and reside on large plasmid.

Metallobetalactamases (MBL)

They belong to molecular class B β – lactamases, requiring one or more divalent cations (Zn^{++}) for their activation [45] and have 3 characteristics [2] –

1. Hydrolyze carbapenems
2. Resistant to clinically used β – lactamase inhibitors and
3. Inhibited by EDTA, a metal ion chelator.

The first MBL detected was chromosomally encoded and was detected in *Bacillus cereus* [46]. They possess a high level of resistance to all Carbapenems, Penicillins, Cephamycins, Cephalosporins and beta-lactamase inhibitor combinations.

Classification of MBLs

On the basis of Imipenem and other β-lactam hydrolysis, MBLs are classified into different subgroups as [47] –

Subgroup3a- possess broad spectrum activity; Subgroup3b – preferential avidity for carbapenem; Subgroup 3c – hydrolyze carbapenems poorly compared to other β-lactam substrate.

At molecular level MBLs are classified into [48] –

Class B1 – possess key Zn co-ordinating residues of three histidines and one cystein eg. IMP, VIM, GIM and SPM – 1,

Class B2 – possess asparagine instead of histidine at first position of principal Zn binding motif, NXHXD. e.g. Aeromonas species and *Serratia fonticola* enzyme SFH – 1.

Class B3 – MBL L_1 unique among all β-lactamases in being functionally represented as a tetramer.

The numbering scheme has been recently updated to accommodate newly discovered MBLs.

MBLs are inhibited by EDTA (Ethylene diamino tetraacetic acid), 2 Mercaptoethanol, 5-Mercaptoacetic acid, 2 Mercapto propionic acid, Copper Chloride and Ferric Chloride. MBLs are classified mainly into two types – Chromosomally encoded and Plasmid encoded or Acquired or Transmissible type. Usually metallobetalactamase producing strains are susceptible to Colistin or Polymyxin B. MBLs do not hydrolyze aztreonam very well, which characteristic is different than ESBLs or Class A β-lactamases [48].

The acquired MBLs are further classified into different types depending on their place of origin as VIM (Italy or Greece), SPM (Brazil), GIM (Germany), SIM (Korea), DIM (Dutch), NDM/PCM (New Delhi metallobetalactamases/Plasmid coded metallobetalactamases).

NDM – 1: NDM – 1 was named after New Delhi, capital of India as NDM – 1 and was first described by Young et al in December 2009 in an individual who acquired infection in a Hospital in India due to Carbapenam resistant *Klebsiella pneumoniae* strain [49].

In March 2010, researchers from Mumbai found that most of Carbapenam resistant bacteria carried bla_{NDM-1} gene. The gene is carried on plasmids and is readily transferred between different strains of bacteria by horizontal gene transfer. All these strains were resistant to most of routinely used antibiotics like Aminoglycosides, β-lactams, Quinolones but sensitive to Tigecycline and Colistin [50]. Recently, Espinal et al identified a new variant of NDM-1 in *Acinetobacter baumannii* and designated it as NDM-2. They reported that, the clonal dissemination of a NDM-2 producing *A. baumannii* was isolated in an Israeli rehabilitation ward [51]. Recently, a new variant of the New Delhi metallo-enzyme (NDM) carbapenemase, NDM-4 and NDM-5, was identified in *E.coli* from two patients both of them had a history of hospitalization in India [52,53].

Detection of Metallo β-lactamase production

Carbapenems often used as an antibiotic of last resort for treating serious infections caused by multi-drug resistant (MDR) organism. Reduced susceptibility to any Carbapenem can be used as a screen for carbapenemases. Positive screening tests are to be followed by a confirmatory test for MBL production.

Although a variety of phenotypic methods have been proposed for the detection of carbapenemases, none have been recommended by CLSI. The classical Hodge [54], Modified Hodge test (MHT) [55] are economical approach for detection and confirmation of carbapenemase activity and Re – Modified Hodge test [56] for detection of MBL. However, the first two tests cannot differentiate between a class A carbapenemase and MBL, making a further confirmatory test necessary. Imipenem is more sensitive but less specific Carbapenem for this test allowing detection of even OXA carbapenemases.

MBL detection tests involving inhibitors such as ethylene diamine tetraacetic acids (EDTA) and 2-Mercaptopropionic acids (2-MPA) have been recommended by various workers [57]. Tris/EDTA disks can also be used in combination with a Carbapenem disk to detect Carbapenem - hydrolyzing enzymes and to differentiate between class A enzymes and MBLs. MBLs are inhibited by the Tris/EDTA disk. The inhibition of MBL can be enhanced by the addition of chelators. Double disk synergy test (DDST) [55] and Disk potentiation tests [58] are based on this principle. For detection of MBL many other methods used are MBL E-test using imipenem/imipenem-EDTA [59], reduction of MIC in presence of EDTA and polymerase chain reaction (PCR) [60].

Commonly primers used for detecting Class B metalloenzyme genes are [40]:

VIM-1 Forward – TTATGGAGCAGCAACCGATGT

Reverse - CAAAAGTCCCGCTCCAACGA

PCR is specific for gene family IMP, VIM, etc. and hence, many other specific primers can be used for different MBL genes. The main disadvantage of PCR is that it requires tailor-made DNA primers and cannot differentiate between variants and may not detect new variants.

E. Detection of Klebsiella pneumoniae carbapenamases (KPCs) [61]

KPCs can be mainly detected by Combined disk method using Imipenem and Imipenem with Phenyl boronic acid, Molecular methods like PCR etc.

Recently, Carbapenem Resistant Enterobacteriaceae (CRE) pose a real threat to Medical fraternity as the increased frequency with which Enterobacteriaceae cause infection and the mortality associated with infection caused by CRE. Most of the studies reported newer β-lactamases including MBL production in nonfermenters like *Pseudomonas aeruginosa, Acinetobacter species* etc. There are very few studies that report MBL production in Enterobacteriaceae [19]. Hence, we have conducted the study to detect newer β - lactamases producing *E.coli* strains by phenotypic methods, isolated from different clinical specimens.

2. Material & methods

A total Number of 450 *E.coli* strains isolated from different clinical specimens like urine, stool, blood, pus etc. were studied. The strains were characterized as *E.coli* according to conventional identification tests [5]. *E.coli* ATCC 25922 was used as positive control for all the conventional tests. Few recent tests were also included to identify *E.coli* which could reduce the number of biochemical tests and there by cost also e.g. Motility- Indole- Lysine (MIL) medium [62], Methylumbelliferyl- β-D- Glucuronide(MUG) MacConkey's medium [63]. All the *E.coli* strains isolated from urine samples were subcultured on Hi chrome UTI agar for direct detection of *E.coli*.

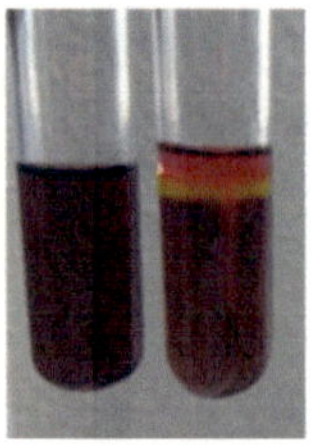

Photo 1 : Motility – Indole – Lysine medium
Motility +VE,
Indole production test +ve,
Lysine decarboxylase test +ve.

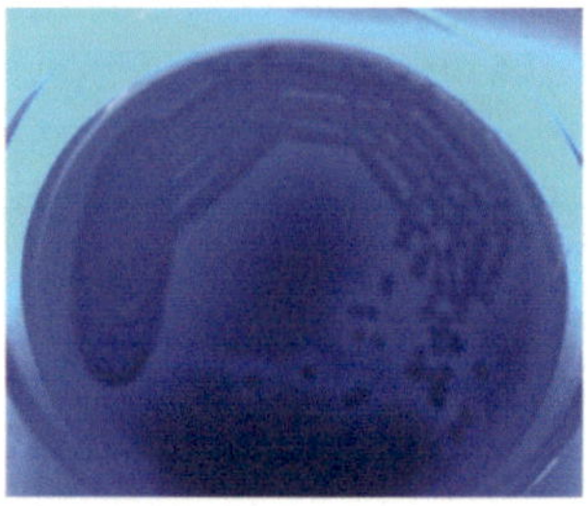

Photo 2: MUG Mac Conkey's agar Typical bluish fluorescence

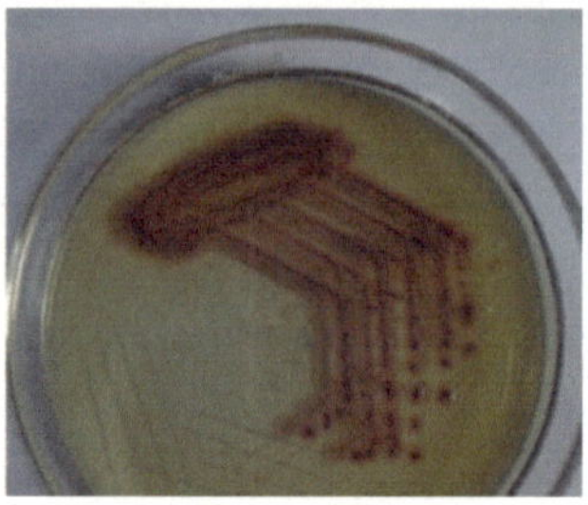

Photo 3 : Hi Chrome UTI agar : *E.coli*

2.1. Antibiotic susceptibility test

Antibiotic susceptibility test for all 450 strains of *E.coli* were done using Mueller Hinton(MH) agar plate with commercially available antibiotic discs (Himedia Pvt Ltd, India) by Kirby Bauer disc diffusion method [64] according to CLSI guidelines [65]. *E.coli* ATCC 25922 was used as control.

Lawn culture of test strain (turbidity adjusted to 0.5 Mc Farland standard) was put on MH Agar plate. The antibiotic disks were put on inoculated plate with all aseptic precaution. Antibiotic susceptibility test was done for Aminoglycosides like Amikacin (AK-30μg), Gentamicin (GEN-10μg), Cephalosporins like Ceftazidime (CAZ-30μg), Cefotaxime (CTX-30μg), Fluoroquinolones like Ciprofloxacin (CIP–5μg), Monobactams like Aztreonam (AT-30μg), Carbapenems such as Imipenem (IPM-10μg), Etrapenem (ETP-10μg) etc. For urine sample an additional disk of Nitrofurantoin (NIT-300μg) and only for MBL producing strains, Colistin (CL-10μg) disk were used

All 450 *E.coli* strains were tested for newer β-lactamases e.g. Extended Spectrum β-lactamases(ESBLs), AMPC β-lactamases Metallobetalactamases(MBLs) and Klebsiella pneumoniae producing Carbapenemases (KPCs) [28, 30, 39, 58, 59, 61]. As Metallobetalactamases are also found in carbapenem susceptible organisms., we have screened carbapenem sensitive strains also for MBL production.

2.2. Detection of newer β-lactamases

2.2.1. Detection of ESBL production [28]

Combined disk method as per CLSI guideline and ESBL E-test were used for ESBL detection.

In Combined disk method, lawn cultures of test strains (turbidity adjusted to McFarland 0.5 standard) were put on MH agar plates. Ceftazidime (CAZ) 30 μg disc and Ceftazidime plus Clavulanate (CAC) 30μg plus 10μg discs were put widely apart on that MH plate. After overnight incubation at 37^0C increase in zone diameter of ≥5 mm with CAC disk as compared to CAZ disk alone was considered positive for ESBL detection.

In ESBL E-test, lawn culture of test strain (turbidity adjusted to McFarland 0.5 standard) was done on a MH agar plate & ESBL E-test strip (AB Biomeriux) was placed. After overnight incubation at 37^0C, MIC ratio of ceftazidime/Ceftazidime Clavulanic acid (TZ/TZL) ≥ 8 or deformation of ellipse or phantom zone present was considered positive for ESBL production.

2.2.2. Detection of AmpC β- lactamases [39]

For, detection of Amp C β –lactamase producing strains substrate inducer combination of Imipenem (10μg) / Ceftazidime(30 μg) disks and for confirmation disk potentiation test using 3 aminophenyl boronic acid (100 mg/ml) was used.

In Disk potentiation test, lawn culture of test strain (turbidity adjusted to McFarland 0.5 standard) was done on MH agar plate. Two ceftazidime(30μg) disks with centre to centre distance of 30mm were placed on that MH plate. 3-aminophenylboronic acid (APB) was dissolved in DMSO at a concentration of 100mg/ml. 10μl of this APB solution was added to one of the ceftazidime disk. After overnight incubation at 37^0C, an increase in zone size of ≥5mm around the Ceftazidime - APB disc compared to Ceftazidime disc only was recorded as a positive result for Amp C β-lactamase production.

2.2.3. Detection of both ESBL & AmpC β -lactamase producing strains [66]

As ESBL and AMPC β – lactamase can be produced by a single strain and ESBL production is suppressed if the same strain also produces Amp C β –lactamases ,we followed the following methods.

Lawn culture of test strain (turbidity adjusted to McFarland 0.5 standard) was done on MH agar plate. To detect the strains producing both ESBL and AMPC β – lactamases, we used one disk containing Ceftazidime and Clavulanic acid (CAC) and the other 02 disks containing Ceftazidime (CAZ) only, placed widely apart. On CAC disk 10μl of 3-aminophenyl boronic acid (3 – APB) (100mg/ml) solution was put. 3 – APB inhibit the growth of AmpC β – lactamases and ESBL genes can be expressed whereas 10 μl of 3 – APB solution was also put on one of the CAZ disk. The plates were incubated 37^0C overnight. The zone diameter of ≥ 5 mm around CAC disk with 3 - APB compared to CAZ only was recorded as ESBL positive and increase in zone diameter of ≥5 mm around CAZ and 3 – APB disc compared to zone diameter of CAZ only was considered positive for AmpC β – lactamase production.

2.2.4. Detection of metallobetalactamases (MBL)

All 450 *E.coli* strains were screened for Carbapenemase activity by Classical Hodge test [54] and for MBL production by Re-Modified Hodge test [56],DDST [55], DP test [58] and MBL ETest.

Re-Modified Hodge Test (Re–MHT) [56]: All 450 *E.coli* strains were subjected to Re-modified Hodge test for detection of carbapenemase activity. The broth culture of *Escherichia Coli* ATCC 25922 was adjusted to a turbidity of 0.5 McFarland standards and was used to put lawn culture on MH agar plates with sterile swab. After drying, a 10μg Imipenem disc (HiMedia) was placed at the centre and10 µl of 50mM zinc sulfate solution was added to Imipenem disk. Then, a test strain of E.coli was streaked from the edge of the disk to the periphery in four different directions. The plate was incubated overnight at 37°C. The presence of a cloverleaf shaped zone of inhibition due to MBL production by the test strain was considered as positive Re - Modified Hodge test (Re - MHT).

Imipenem-EDTA double disk synergy test (DDST) [55]: The IMP-EDTA double disk synergy test was performed for detection of Metallobetalactamases. Test strains i.e. *E.coli* (turbidity adjusted to 0.5 McFarland standard) were inoculated on to Mueller Hinton agar plate. After drying, a 10µg Imipenem disk and a blank sterile filter paper disk (6mm in diameter, Whatman filter paper no.2) were placed 10mm apart from edge to edge. 10 µl of 50mM zinc sulfate solution was added to the 10 µg Imipenem disk. Then, 10µl of 0.5 M EDTA (Sigma, USA) solution was applied to the blank filter paper disk. As disodium-EDTA is difficult to be solubilised in sterile water, we had used dipotassium-EDTA which is easily soluble in sterile water. Enhancement of the zone of inhibition towards the EDTA disk was interpreted as a positive result.

Disk Potentiation Test (DP) [58]: The IMP-EDTA combined disk test was performed for detection of metallobetalactamases. Test strains (turbidity adjusted to 0.5 McFarland standard) were inoculated on to MH agar plate. Two imipenem disk (10 µg) were placed on the plate wide apart and 10 µl of 50mM zinc sulphate solution was added to each of the imipenem disks. Then 10µl of 0.5M EDTA solution was added to one of the disk and the plates were incubated at 35^0 C for 16-18 hrs. If the increase in inhibition zone with the Imipenem and EDTA disk was ≥7 mm than the imipenem disk alone, it was considered as MBL positive.

MBL E-Test — Confirmatory test

The MBL E-test was done and interpreted using test strains and Quality control strains according to manufacturer's instructions. Overnight broth culture of test strain (turbidity adjusted to 0.5 McFarland standard) was used to inoculate MH agar plate. The MBL E-test strip was put on that inoculated MH plate with a sterile forceps and plates were incubated at 37^0C for 18-20 hrs. After incubation, MIC ratio of Imipenem /Imipenem-EDTA (IP/IPI) of ≥8 or deformations of ellipse or phantom zone indicate MBL production.

Colistin E test: All MBL producing *E.coli* strains were tested with Colistin E test (AB bioMerieux, Solana, Sweden). The Colistin E-test was done and interpreted using test strains and Quality control strains according to manufacturer's instructions.

2.2.5. Detection of Klebsiella pneumoniae carbapenemases (KPCS)

It was done by Combined disk method [61]. Lawn culture of test strain (turbidity adjusted to 0.5 Mc Farland) was put on MH agar plate and 2 Imipenem (10 µg) disks were put widely apart. To one Imipenem disk 10 µl Phenyl boronic acid solution (400µg/disk) was put. Then the MH agar plates were incubated at 37^0C overnight. After incubation, the test should be considered positive when growth inhibitory zone around the disk containing Imipenem and Phenyl boronic acid was ≥ 5 mm compared to zone diameter of Imipenem alone.

http://dx.doi.org/10.5772/57578

2.2.6. Detection of class D enzymes

Several workers have reported that Class D enzymes i.e. OXA – 48 type are the most difficult carbapenemase producers to be identified phenotypically [42,43]. Hence, we did not include detection of Class D carbapenemase in our study.

3. Observation

Figure 1: Incidence of MBL, ESBL & Amp C β –lactamase producing *E.coli* strains (n = 450)

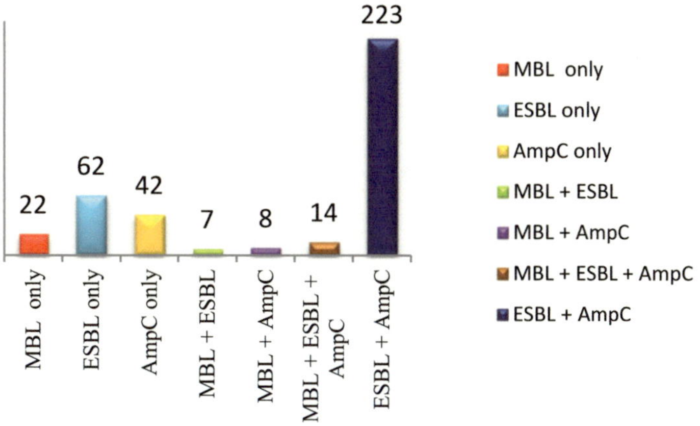

Figure 1. Shows incidence of different β – lactamases e.g. MBL, ESBL, AMPC β – lactamases producing *E.coli* strains. Out of 450 *E.coli* strains studied, 378 (84%) strains produced any of the 3 types of β – lactamases i.e. MBL, ESBL and Amp C β –lactamases, either alone or in combinations. Photographs of different methods used to detect newer β-lactamases phenotypically is given below (photo 4,5,6,7,8,9,10,11,12)

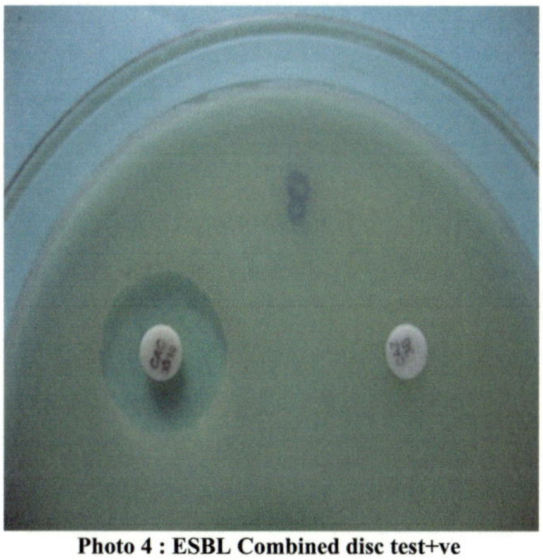

Photo 4 : ESBL Combined disc test+ve

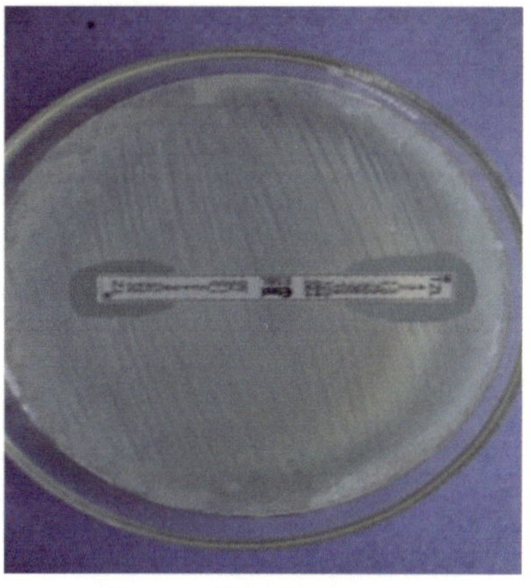

Photo 5 : ESBL Etest :positive

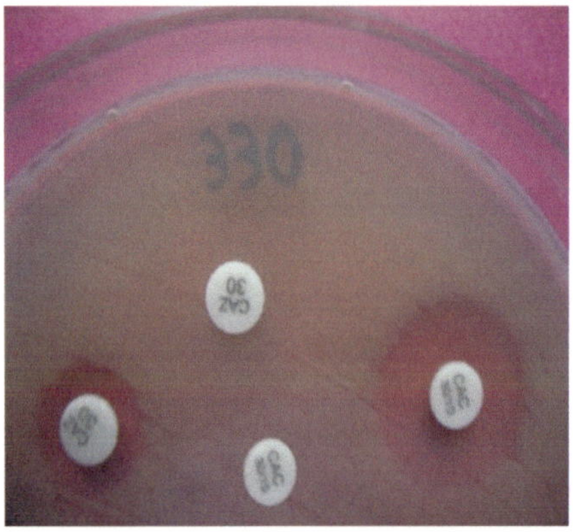

Photo 6 : Both ESBL & AmpC β- lactamase +ve

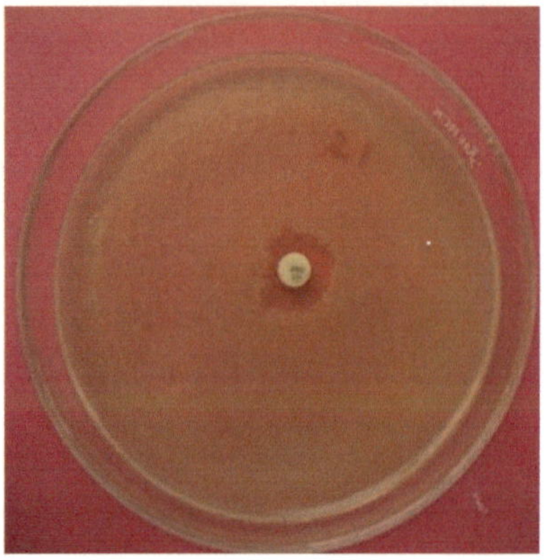

Photo 7 : Classical Hodge test +ve

3.1. Detection of MBL

In photo 5 ESBL E Test positive shows MIC of Ceftazidime (TZ) 6 μg/ml and Ceftazidime Clavulanic acid (TZL) 0.25μg/ml respectively i.e. MIC ratio of TZ/TZL is 24. Out of 378 β - lactamase producing E.coli strains 223(59%) produced both ESBL andAmp C β –lactamases. Out of total 51 MBL producing *E.coli* strains 14 (27.5%) strains produced all the three types of β – lactamases i.e. MBL, ESBL and AMPC β – lactamases. In Photo 11 MBL E Test positive shows MIC of Imipenem (IP) 24 μg/ml and Imipenem-EDTA (IPI) < 1μg/ml respectively i.e. MIC ratio of IP/IPI is > 24 and also presence of Phantom zone.

All 51MBL positive *E.coli* strains were sensitive to Colistin with MIC range from 0.032 to 0.25μg/ml and were detected by E test for Colistin (bioMe'rieux) (Photo 12).

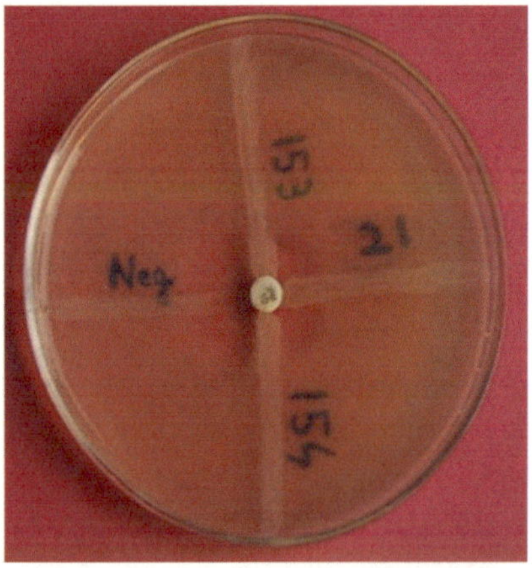

Photo 8 : Remodified Hodge test +ve

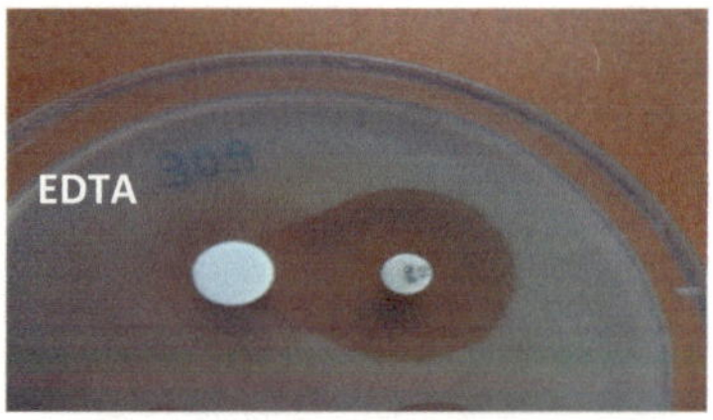

Photo 9 : DDST test +ve

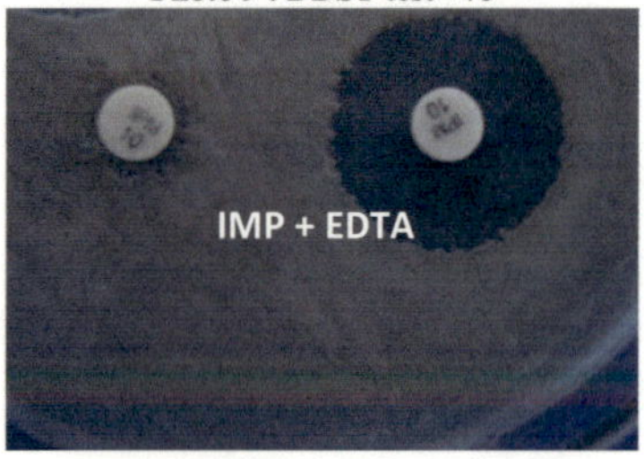

Photo 10 : Disc potentiation test +ve

http://dx.doi.org/10.5772/57578

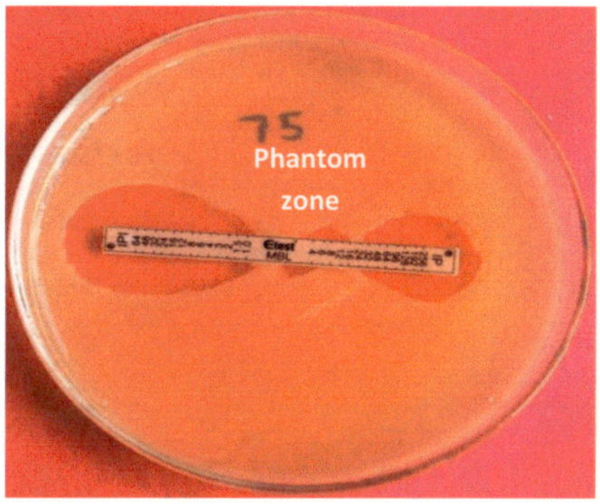

Photo 11 : MBL E test +ve

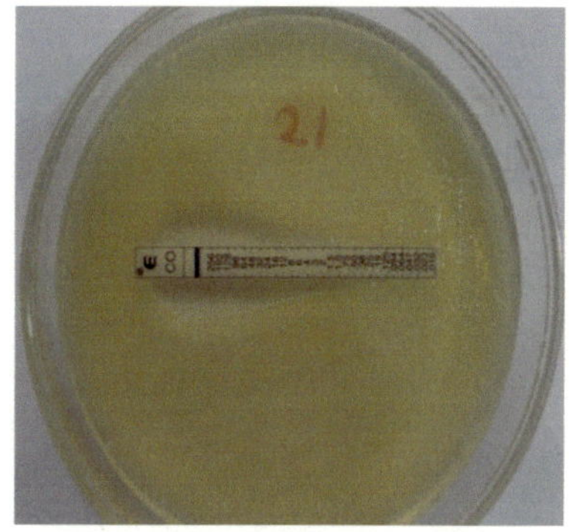

Photo 12: Colistin E test : MIC 0.125 µg/ml

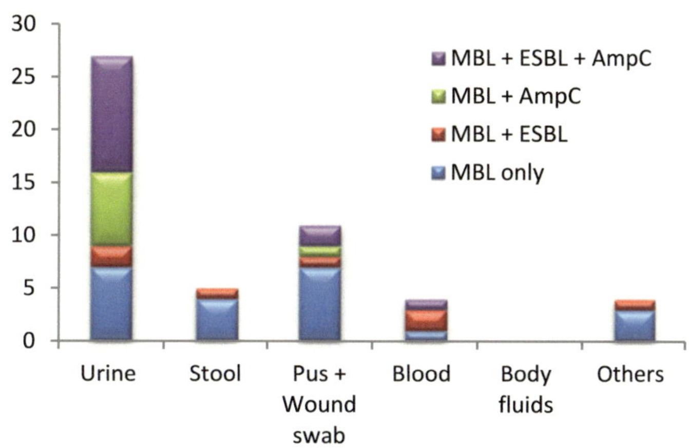

Figure 2. Isolation of MBL producing *E.coli* strains from different clinical specimens (n = 51)

Out of total 450 *E.coli* strains 218 (48.4%) were isolated from urine, 92 (20.4%) from stool, 61 from pus and wound swab, 30 from blood, 10 from body fluids and 39 from other specimens e.g. e.g. Endotracheal (ET) tube secretions, broncho-alveolar lavage etc.

Figure 2 shows out of total 51 MBL positive *E.coli* strains maximum 27(53%) strains were isolated from urine followed by 11(21.6%) strains from pus and wound swab. Out of 27 MBL positive *E.coli* strains isolated from urine 12(44.4%) had history of catheterization and 2(7.4%) had history of instrumentation in urethra (e.g.dilatation, etc). Only 01 urine sample received from High Dependency Unit and that *E.coli* strain produced all 3 types of β – lactamases i.e. MBL, ESBL and Amp C β –lactamases In our study, total 14 *E.coli* strains were positive for all 3 types of β – lactamases i.e. MBL, ESBL and AMPC β – lactamases,and out of which 11 (78.6%) strains were isolated from urine samples which was quite alarming. No MBL producing *E.coli* strain was isolated from body fluids. Out of 92 stool samples, 5 (5.4%) were MBL producers, 15 (16.3%) were only ESBL producer and 13 (14.1%) were only AMPC β – lactamase producer.

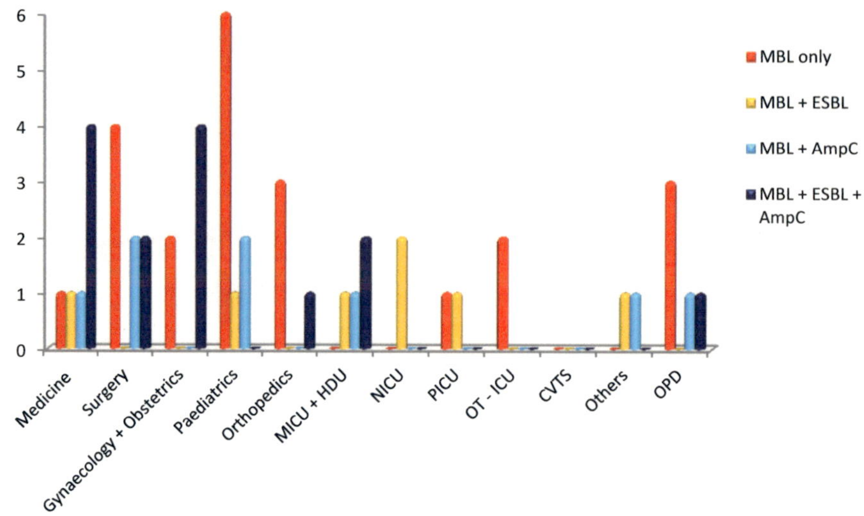

Figure 3. Isolation of only MBL and MBL with other β - lactamase producing *E.coli* strains from different clinical specialities (n = 51)

Figure 3 shows maximum 9/51 (17.7%) MBL producing *E.coli* strains were isolated from Pediatrics ward. No MBL producing strain was isolated from Cardiovascular & Thoracic Surgery (CVTS) ward. From Medicine ward, 16 *E.coli* strains were only ESBL producers and 10 were only Amp C β – lactamase producers.

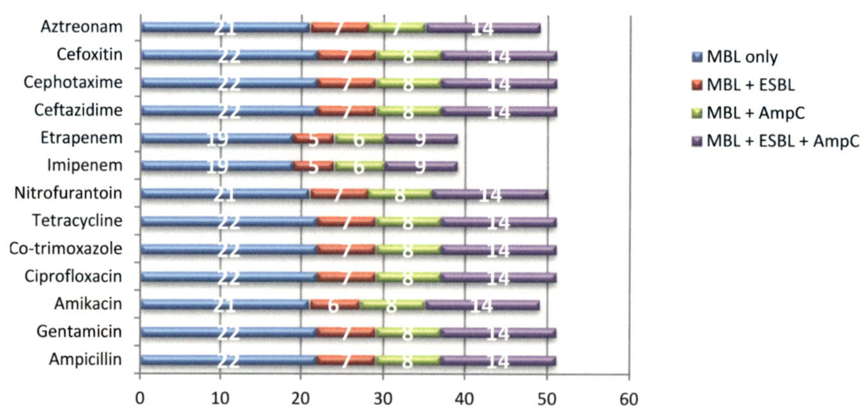

Figure 4. Antibiotic resistance pattern of MBL producing *E.coli* strains (n = 51)

Figure 4 shows out of total 51 MBL producing *E.coli* strains, 39 (76.5%) strains were resistant to Imipenem and Etrapenem by disc diffusion method. The MBL producing strains of *E.coli* showed total resistance to Ampicillin, Gentamicin, Ciprofloxacin, Co – trimoxazole, Tetracycline, Ceftazidime, Cephotaxime and Cefoxitin. But all MBL positive *E.coli* strains (100%) were sensitive to Colistin. Out of total 450 *E.coli* strains, only 58.9% strains were sensitive to

http://dx.doi.org/10.5772/57578

Amikacin and only 28.2% strains were sensitive to Ciprofloxacin. Nitrofurantoin was used for urine specimen only (n = 218) and 67.9% strains were sensitive to Nitrofurantoin. Amongst the 51 MBL producing *E.coli* strain, 12 (23.5%) strains were sensitive to Imipenem and Etrapenem by disk diffusion test. Out of 12 Imipenem sensitive MBL producing *E.coli* strain, 5 (41.7%) strains produced all 3 types of β – lactamases.

Strains	**Phenotypic methods**		
	Re - MHT	**DDST**	**DP**
MBL + ve (n = 51) By MBL – E test	**45**	**46**	**51**
MBL – ve (n = 399) By MBL – E test	**401**	**402**	**399**
False negative	**6**	**5**	**0**
False positive	**4**	**2**	**0**
Sensitivity %	**88.2**	**90.2**	**100**
Specificity %	**99**	**99.5**	**100**
Positive predictive value	**91.8**	**95.8**	**100**
Negative predictive value	**98.5**	**98.8**	**100**
Efficiency	**97.8**	**98.5**	**100**

Table 1. Performance of different phenotypic methods compared to MBL – E test in identifying MBL + ve *E.coli*

Table 1 shows Sensitivity, Specificity, Positive predictive value, Negative predictive value and Efficiency calculated for Re – Modified Hodge test (Re – MHT), Double disk synergy test (DDST) and Disk potentiation (DP) test, compared to MBL – E test in identifying MBL positive E.coli strains. MBL – E test is considered as standard phenotypic reference method for detection of MBL positive strains. The sensitivity of Re - MHT was 88.2% and specificity was 99% whereas sensitivity of DDST was 90.2% and specificity was 99.5%. DP test was having sensitivity and specificity of 100%. The efficiency of Re – MHT was 97.8%, DDST was 98.5% and DP was 100%, when compared to MBL - E test as standard reference method.

4. Discussion

The emergence of antibiotic resistance occurs by a) spontaneous mutation and vertical gene transfer and b) horizontal gene transfer through transformation, transduction, conjugation, transposons (jumping genes) etc. The rapidity of development of antimicrobial resistance in organisms, leads to selection pressure of antibiotics like 3rd generation of cephalosporin- ESBL inhibitor combination, Monobactams and Carbapenems. Recently, Carbapenem resistant Enterobacteriaceae (CRE) pose a real threat to Medical fraternity as the increased frequency with which Enterobacteriaceae cause infection and the mortality associated with infection caused by CRE and ESBL producing bacteria. In mid1990, CTX-M 15 was first reported as ESBL in India. Now, CTX-M 15 is established as globally dominant ESBL and primary cause of acquired resistance to 3rd generation Cephalosporins in Enterobacteriaceae. Walsh TR et al in year 2005 noted that MBL genes have spread from *Pseudomonas aeruginosa* to Enterobacteriaceae and a clinical scenario for MBL appears to simulate the global spread of ESBL in recent future. bla $_{NDM-1}$ gene on plasmid can be readily transferred between different strains of bacteria by horizontal genre transfer [47].

In the present study, 52(11.6%), 56(12.4%) and 342 (76%) *E.coli* strains were isolated from Outpatient Departments(OPDs), Intensive Care units (ICUs) and Inpatient Departments(IPDs) respectively. Maximum 25 (44.6%) *E.coli* strains were isolated from Medicine ICU (MICU) and High dependency unit (HDU). In a previous study conducted in our laboratory in 2008, Basak et al have already reported the incidence of ESBL producing *E.coli* in our hospital as 41.3% [67] whereas 5 years after, in the present study, the incidence of ESBL producing *E.coli* were 68%, out of which only 13.8% strains produced ESBL alone and other strains produced ESBL, Amp C β-lactamases and MBL in combination. Pakzad I et al in 2011 have reported 28% of their *E.coli* strains as ESBL producers [68]. Sinha et al in 2008 had reported that 40.8% of *E.coli* strains were ESBL producers and 24% were AMPC β-lactamase producers [69]. 37.5% and 47.8% of *E.coli* strains were reported to be Amp C β –lactamases producers in the study conducted in Chennai, India and Kolkata,India respectively, whereas in our study 65.3% *E.coli* were Amp C β-lactamase producers.

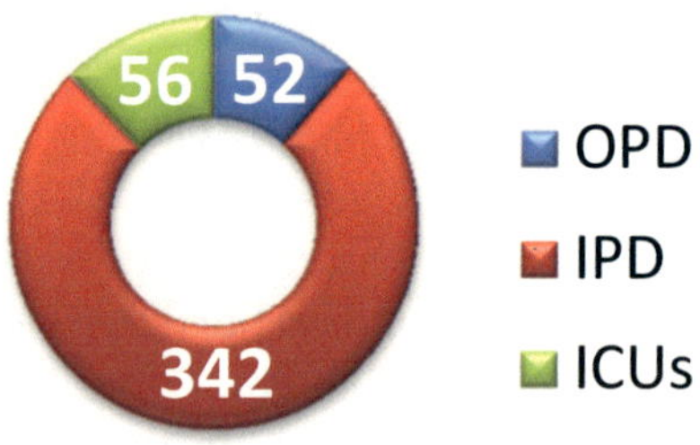

Figure 5. Isolation of *E.coli* strains from OPD, IPD and ICUs

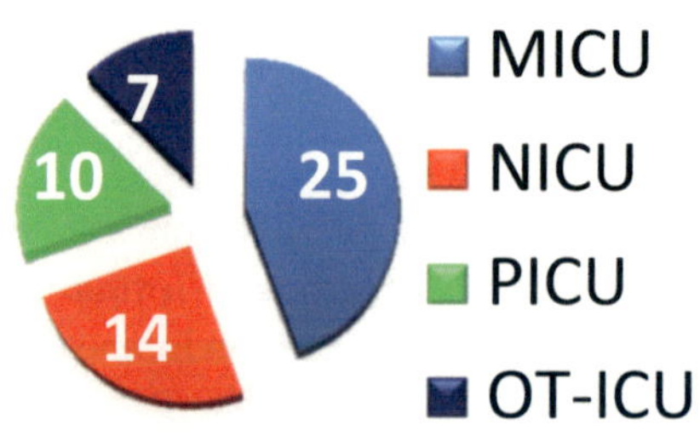

Figure 6. Isolation of *E.coli* strains from different ICUs (n = 56)

Various authors have reported MBL producing *E.coli* strains from 2.9% (Pandya et al from Gujrat, India) [70], to 6.8% (Tsakris et al from Greece) [61] to 25% (Enwuru NV et al from Nigeria) [13]. In the present study 51(11.3%) MBL producing *E.coli* strains were isolated. MBL production was detected in both Imipenem resistant (39/41 i.e. 95.1%) and Imipenem sensitive 12/409 i.e. 2.9% strains also. It indicates that if only Imipenem resistant strains would have been screened, 2.9% MBL producing strains would have been missed. But no Klebsiella pneumoniae producing carbapenemases were detected in our present study. In 2011, Tsakris et al reported 15.9% KPC producing *E.coli* in their study. Tsakris et al have also reported that 19(43.2%) *E.coli* strains produced Amp C β –lactamases and ESBL and 15(34%) *E.coli* strains produced ESBL [61]. In another study in 2012, Gupta V et al have reported 17(68%) *E.coli* strains to be ESBL positive [71].

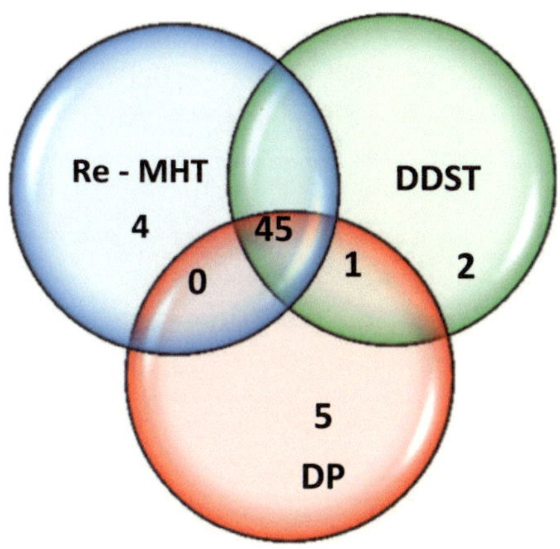

Disk Potentiation test (DP)
True + ve : 51
Re – modified Hodge test (Re – MHT) Double Disk Synergy test(DDST)
True + ve : 45 True + ve : 46
False + ve : 4 False + ve : 2

Figure 7. Phenotypic detection of metallobetalactamase (MBL) producing *E.coli* strains by various methods. (n = 450)

Walsh et al in 2002 have reported that the MBL – E test results were in 100% agreement with the results from the genotypic Polymerase chain reaction (PCR) and biochemical methods [59]. They have also reported that the E test MBL strip IP/IPI has the ability to detect MBLs both chromosomally and plasmid mediated, in aerobic and anaerobic bacteria. This novel method could be used by Clinical Laboratories to monitor the emergence of the MBL [59].

Omair et al in 2012, have reported that MBL – E test have been taken as a gold standard method for MBL detection [72]. Manoharan et al have reported that MBL - E test has taken as a phenotypic standard method for MBL detection though the test is expensive. Double disk synergy test (DDST) and Disk potentiation (DP) tests are economical and simple to perform but DDST is observer dependent while DP test is measurable with lesser chance of subjective error [45].

In the present study, we studied MBL positive *E.coli* strains by MBL E – test and compared the results of other phenotypic methods for MBL detection i.e. Re – Modified Hodge test (Re-MHT), Double disk synergy test (DDST) and Disk potentiation (DP) test.

In figure 7, the venndiagram showing interrelationship of Re – modified Hodge test (Re – MHT), Double disk synergy test (DDST) and Disk potentiation test (DP) for detection of MBL producing *E.coli.*

In the present study when results of all three phenotypic methods were compared with MBL – E test results, it was found that 45/51 (88.2%) MBL positive strains were positive by all three phenotypic method i.e. Re – Modified Hodge test (Re- MHT), Double disk synergy test (DDST) and Disk potentiation (DP) tests. 04 and 02 were false positive by Re – MHT and DDST methods respectively, whereas6/51 (11.8%) and 5/51(9.8%) were false negative by Re – MHT and DDST method respectively. Amongst all three phenotypic methods, DP was best correlated with MBL – E test. By DP test 51 MBL positive E.coli strains were detected and no false positive and false negative result was found (Sensitivity 100% and specificity 100%).

5. Epidemiology

E.coli are responsible for various infections like urinary tract infection, diarrhoea, pneumonia, bacteremia, upper respiratory tract infections, wound infections, osteomyelitis and neonatal meningitis [73,74].

The successful outcome of clinical use of 3rd generation cephalosporines unfortunately led to the increased use and emergence of ESBL producing Enterobacteriaceae. With the emergence of ESBL and Amp C β – lactamase production in *E.coli, Klebsiella pneumoniae* and other Enterobacteriaceae, Carbapenems were used as last resort to treat those infections. Because of selective pressure of Carbapenems, even carbapenemases producing Enterobacteriaceae (CRE) has emerged.

Most common MBL found worldwide in Enterobacteriaceae were VIM (Verona integron encoded MBL) and IMP (active on imipenem). Multidrug resistant *E.coli* harboring New Delhi metallobetalactamase - 1 (NDM-1) isolated from a patient returned to Canada from India [75], was reported first in 2009. NDM -1 was also recognized among Enterobacteriaceae 32 from Mumbai, 13 from Varanasi and 3 from Guwahati in India and 25 isolates from eight different cities in Pakistan. These isolates were from cases of bacteraemia, ventilator associated pneumonia and community acquired urinary tract infections [76].

NDM - 1 spread largely to different countries like Australia, Japan, Brazil, Belgium, Canada, Germany etc [77]. The gene encoding NDM – 1is called bla_{NDM-1}, located on transmissible plasmid which may include other antibiotic resistance genes also leading to extensive drug resistant phenotypes (so called 'superbugs'). A recent report from ICU and wards of Sir Gangaram hospital Delhi, India showed 8.1% NDM – 1 positive E.coli [78]. In January 2011, the name of NDM–1 was changed to PCM (Plasmid encoding Carbapenem resistant metallo-betalactamases) [79].

Metallobatalactamases are also found in Carbapenem susceptible organisms. This hidden MBL gene can spread unnoticed in hospitals if isolates are reported sensitive without screening for presence of MBL [48].

The prevalence of ESBL and Amp C beta lactamases in a single isolate reduces effectiveness of beta – lactam and beta - lactamase inhibitor combinations while MBLs and Amp C beta–lactamases confer resistance to carbapenems and Cephamycin. Unfortunatenly thses enzymes usually co-exist in same isolate.

6. Prevention and control

As *E.coli* are one of the commonest cause of both health care and community acquired infections, rapid identification of beta lactamase producing *E.coli* is crucial for appropriate treatment and timely implementation of infection control measures in Health care set-up. Indeed, delayed detection of ESBLs, Amp C β – lactamase and MBL producing strains, raise the possibility of spread of these strains into the community. These issues combined with the limited therapeutic options available to treat patient infected with these organisms, have made CRE of epidemiological importance globally [80]. ESBLs and Carbapenem resistant strains may lead to outbreaks of infection in HealthCare Set-up also.

Phenotypic methods can be useful for routine detection of ESBLs and carbapenemase production, among Gram negative bacteria particularly when PCR is not available.

Screening of colonisation with multidrug-resistant organisms (MDROs) upon admission to hospitals has been advocated in patients who have already received healthcare in endemic countries. The CDC recommends, if previously unrecognized cases are identified of being infected with β-lactamase producing strains, a round of surveillance culture from high risk areas i.e. ICUs or wards from where detected, should be considered in any Health Care Setup. In addition prompt notification, must be made to infection control team members when CRE are identified in Clinical Microbiology Laboratories.

Antimicrobial stewardship has been suggested as the most important efforts to control multidrug resistant organisms (MDROs) [81]. It has been found to be most effective, if efforts are directed towards an overall decrease in antimicrobial use rather than targeting a specific antimicrobial class. Limiting use of invasive devices is another potentially important preventive mechanism for MDROs including β- lactamase producing organisms. Health care workers (HCW) should follow hand hygiene practices while giving patient care preferably using an alcohol based hand rubs or antimicrobial soap and water if hands are visibly soiled, and also follow Standard precautions and Additional precautions as per the indications.

7. Conclusion

In the present study, all MBL – E test positive *E.coli* strains (100%) were detected by Disk potentiation test also. MBL producing *E.coli* strains must be tested in both carbapenem resistant as well as sensitive strains by Disk potentiation method using Imipenem – EDTA. Disk potentiation method is simple to perform and materials used are cheap, non-toxic, and easily accessible and allowed for objective interpretation of results. It is also quite good in detecting carbapenem sensitive MBL producing strains.

Beta-lactamase producing organisms are detected by E test, which is standard phenotypic method and also by Polymerase chain reaction (PCR) which is a gold standard, but both are costly and require expertise. Failure to detect these enzymes has contributed to their uncontrolled spread and commonly to therapeutic failures.

Hence to conclude, for detection of ESBL, combined disk method using Ceftazidime / Ceftazidime Clavulanic acid(CAZ/CAC), for detection of Amp C β-lactamases confirmatorty Disk potentiation test using Ceftazidime / Ceftazidime - 3-aminophenylboronic acid and for detection of Metallo β-lactamases(MBL) producing *E.coli*, disk potentiation test using Imipenem/Imipenem - EDTA should be done in both carbapenem sensitive as well as resistant isolates by all Clinical Microbiology Laboratories to prevent its dissemination and also for a good therapeutic outcome.

Author details

Silpi Basak and Monali N. Rajurkar

Department of Microbiology, J.N.Medical College, Wardha, India

References

[1] Rammelkamp M. Resistance of Staphylococcus aureus to the action of penicillin. Proc Roy Soc Exper Biol Med 1942;51:386-9.

[2] Basak S, Attal RO, Rajurkar MN. Pseudomonas Aeruginosa And Newer β -Lactamases:An Emerging Resistance Threat. In: Infection Control – Update, edited by Christopher Sudhakar, Intech publication, February 2012:181-198. (Online open access book) http://www.intechopen.com/articles/show/title/ pseudomonas-aeruginosa-and-newer-lactamases-an-emerging-resistance-threat

[3] Sharma A. Antimicrobial resistance: No action today, no cure tomorrow. Indian Jr. of Med. Microl. 2011;29(2):91-2.

[4] Falagas ME, Karageorgopoulos DE. Pandrug resistance (PDR), Extensive drug resistance (XDR) and Multidrug resistance (MDR) among Gram Negative Bacilli: Need for international Harmonization in Terminology. Clin.Inf.Diseases. 2008;48:1121-22.

[5] Washington CW Jr, Stephen DA, William MJ, Elmer WK, Gary WP, Paul CS, Gail LW. Ch.6 The Enterobacteriaceae In; Koneman's color atlas and textbook of Diagnos-

tic Microbiology, 6th ed. Lippincott Williams & Wilkins, Philadelphia PA, USA, 2006:211-302.

[6] Escherich T. Die Darmbakterrien des Neugeborenen and suglings Fortschr Med 3, 1885;512-22, 547-54.

[7] Castellani A and Chalmers AJ. Manual of tropical medicine. 3rd ed. New York: Wiliams Wood & Co. 1919.

[8] Cheasty T, Smith HR. Escherichia Ch. 52 In: Topley and Wilson's Microbiology and Microbial infections 10th ed. Bacteriology Vol.2 Borriello SP, Murray P, Funke G Hodder Arnold 1360-85.

[9] Huys G, Cnockaert GM et al. Escherichia albertii species nov a diarrhoegenic species isolated from stool specimens of Bangladeshi children. Int. J. Syst. Evol. Microbiol. 2003;53:807-10.

[10] Rutala WA, WebeR DJ. Clinical effectiveness of low temperature sterilization technologies Infect. Control Hosp. Epidemiol 1998;19:798-804.

[11] Rice EW, Clark RM, Johnson CH. Chlorine inactivation of Escherichia coli O157;H7. Emerg. Infect. Dis 1999;5:461-3.

[12] Shoorashetty RM, Nagarathnamma T, Prathibha J. Comparison of the boronic acid disk potentiation test and cefepime – clavulanic acid method for the detection of ESBL among AMPC – producing Enterobacteriaceae. Indian Jr.Med.Microbiol 2011;29(3):297-301.

[13] Enwuru NV, Enwuru CA, Ogbonnia SO et al. Metallo-betalactamase production by Escherichia coli and Klebsiella species isolated from Hospital and Community subjects in Lagos, Nigeria. Nature and Science. 2011;9(11):1-5.

[14] Holmes B and Gross RJ. Coliform bacteria: various other members of the Enterobacteriaceae In Parker MT and Collier LH (eds) Topley and Wilson's Principles of bacteriology, virology and immunity 8th edn. London Edward Arnold, 1990;415-41.

[15] Abraham EP, Chain E. An enzyme from bacteria able to destroy penicillin. *Nature* 1940; *146* : 837.

[16] Pollock MR. Personal communication. 1965.

[17] Datta N, Kontomichalou P. Penicillinase synthesis controlled by infectious R Factors in *Enterobacteriaceae*. *Nature* 1965; *208* : 239-44.

[18] Bush K, Jacoby GA, Medeiros A. A functional classification scheme for beta lactamase and its correlation with molecular structure. *Antimicrob Agents Chemother* 1995; *39* : 1211-33.

[19] Ambler RP. The structure of *β*-lactamases. Phil. Trans. R. Soc. Lond. B. Biol. Sci. 1980; 289:321–31.

[20] Miles RS, Amyes SGB. Laboratory control of antimicrobial therapy in chapter :8. Mackie & McCartney's Practical Medical Microbiology 14th ed: JG Collee, AG Fraser, BP Marmion, A Simmons, Editors. Churchil Livingston. Indian Reprints, 2008; 151-78.

[21] Livermore DM et al. Multicentre evaluation of the VITEK 2 advanced expert system for interpretive reading of antimicrobial resistance tests. J.Antimicrob.Chemother. 2002;49:289-300.

[22] Tenover FC et al. Detection and reporting of organisms producing extended spectrum β – lactamases : Survey of laboratories in continent. J. Clin. Microbiol. 1999;37:4065-4070.

[23] Thompson KS. Controversies about Extended spectrum and Amp C β-lactamases. Emerging Infectious Diseases 2001;7(2):333-6.

[24] Steward CD, Rasheed JK, Hubert SK, Biddle JW, Raney PM, Anderson GJ, Williams PP, Brittain KL, Oliver A, McGowan JE Jr, Tenover FC. Characterization of clinical isolates of Klebsiella pneumoniae from 19 laboratories using National Committee for Clinical Laboratories Standards Extended spectrum β-lactamase detection methods. J Clin Microbiol 2001; 39 (8):2864-72.

[25] Moubareck C.et al. Countrywide spread of community and hospital acquired extended spectrum beta-lactamase (CTX-M-15) producing Enterobacteriaceae in Lebanon. J Clin Microbiol 2005; 43: 3309-13.

[26] Aggarwal R, Chaudhary U, Bala K. Detection of extended spectrum β-lactamase in Pseudomonas aeruginosa. Indian J Pathology & Microbiol 2008; 51 (2):222-4.

[27] Jarlier V et al. Extended spectrum beta-lactamase conferring transferable resistance to newer β-lactam agents in Enterobacteriaceae: hospital prevalence and susceptibility patterns. Rev Infect Dis 1988; 10:867-78.

[28] Carter MW, Oakton KJ, Warner M, Livermore DM. Detection of extended spectrum beta lactamases in Klebsiellae with the Oxoid combination disk method. *J Clin Microbiol* 2000; *38* : 4228-32.

[29] Tzepeli E, Giakkoupi P, Sofianou D, Loukova V, Kemeroglou A, Tsakris A. Detection of extended-spectrum beta-lactamases in clinical isolates of *Enterobacter cloacae* and *Enterobacter aerogenes*. *J Clin Microbiol* 2000; *38* : 542-6.

[30] Washington CW Jr, Stephen DA, Williams MJ, Elmer WK, Gary WP, Paul CS, Gail LW. Antimicrobial Susceptibility Testing in chapter 17. Koneman;s Colour Atlas and Textbook of Diagnostic Microbiology, 6th ed, Lippincott Williams & Wilkins, Philadelphia PA, USA, 2006; p:945-1021.

[31] Thomson KS, Sanders CC. Detection of expanded-spectrum beta-lactamases in members of the family *Enterobacteriaceae*: comparison of the double disk and three-dimensional tests. *Antimicrobial Agents Chemother* 1992; *36* : 1877-82.

[32] Steward CD, Rasheed JK, Hubert SK, Biddle JW, Raney PM, Anderson GJ, Williams PP, Brittain KL, Oliver A, McGowan JE Jr, Tenover FC. Characterization of clinical isolates of Klebsiella pneumoniae from 19 laboratories using National Committee for Clinical Laboratories Standards Extended spectrum β-lactamase detection methods. J Clin Microbiol 2001; 39 (8):2864-72.

[33] Shahcheraghi F, Nasiri S, Noveiri H The survey of genes encoding beta – lactamases, in Escherichia coli resistant to beta – lactam and non beta – lactam antibiotics Iranian Jr. of Basic Medical Sciences 2010;13(1):230-237.

[34] Moland ES, Kim SY, Hong SG et al. Newer β – lactamases : Clinical and Laboratory Implications, Part II. Clin.Microbiol.Newsletter 2008;30(11):79-84.

[35] Barnaud G, Arlet G, Verdet C, Gaillot O, Lagrange PH, Phillipon A. Salmonella enteritidis: Amp C plasmid mediated inducible β-lactamases (DHA-1)with an amp R gene from Morgagnella morgagnii. Antimicrob Agents Chemother 1998; 42: 2352-8.

[36] Sander CC, Sanders WE, Goering HV. In vitro antagonism of β-lactam antibiotics by cefoxitin. J Antimicrob Chemother 1982;21: 968-75.

[37] Manchanda V, Singh NP. Occurrence and detection of AMPC b-lactamases among Gram negative clinical isolates using a modified three-dimensional test at Guru Tegh Bahadur Hospital, Delhi, India. J Antimicrob Chemother 2008; 51: 415-18.

[38] Black, J. A., E. S. Moland, and K. S. Thomson. AMPC disk test for detection of plasmid-mediated AMPC β-lactamases in *Enterobacteriaceae* lacking chromosomal AMPC β-lactamases. J. Clin. Microbiol. 2005; 43:3110–13.

[39] Yagi T, Wachino J,Kurokawa H, Suzuki S, et al. Practical methods using boronic acid compounds for identification of class C β-lactamase producing Klebsiella pneumonia and Escherichia coli. J of Clin Microbiol. 2005;43(6): 2551-8.

[40] Queenan AM, Bush K. Carbapenemases: the versatile β-lactamases. Clinical Microbiology Review 2007;20(3):440-58.

[41] Hossain, A., Ferraro MJ., Pino RM., Dew III RB., Moland ES et al. Plasmid mediated carbapenem-hydrolyzing enzyme KPC-2 in an Enterobacter sp. Antimicrob. Agents Chemother. 2004;48:4438–40.

[42] MiriagouV, Tzouvelekis LS, Rossiter S., Tzelepi E., Angulo FJ, Whichard J.M. Imipenem resistance in a *Salmonella* clinical strain due to plasmid-mediated class A Carbapenemase KPC-2. *Antimicrob.Agents Chemother*. 2003;47: 1297–1300.

[43] Bush, K., and R. B. Sykes. Characterization and epidemiology of β-lactamases Elsevier Science Publishers BV, Philadelphia, PA 1987.

[44] Naas, T., P. Nordmann. OXA-type β-lactamases. *Curr. Pharm.Des*. 1999; 5: 865–879.

[45] Manoharan A, Chatterjee S, Mathai D, SARI Study Group. Detection and Characterization of metallobetalactamases producing Pseudomonas aeruginosa. Indian J Med Microbiol 2010; 28(3):241-3.

[46] Lim HM., Pene J.J., Shaw RW. Cloning, nucleotide sequence and expression of the Bacillus cereus 5/B/6 β-lactamase II structural gene. *J. Bacteriol.* 1988;170:2873-2878.

[47] Walsh TR, Toleman MA, Poirel L, Hordmann P. Metallo-betalactamases : the quiet before the storm?. Clin.Microbiol.Rev. 2005;18:306-325.

[48] Franklin C, Liolios L, Peleg AY. Phenotypic Detection of carbapenem susceptible Metallobetalactamase producing Gram-negative bacilli in the clinical laboratory. J of Clin Microbiol. 2006;44 (9): 3139-44.

[49] Yong D, Toleman MA, Giske CG, Cho HS, Sundman K, Lee K, Walsh TR Characterization of a new metallo-beta-lactamase gene, bla(NDM-1), and a novel erythromycin esterase gene carried on a unique genetic structure in Klebsiella pneumoniae sequence type 14 from India. Antimicrob Agents Chemother 2009;53(12):5046-54.

[50] Deshpade P, Rodrigues C, Shetty A, Kapadia F, Hedge A, Soman R. New Delhi Metallo-β lactamase (NDM-1) in Enterobacteriaceae: Treatment options with Carbapenems Compromised. J.of Asso. Of Physicians of India 2010;58:147-150.

[51] Espinal P, Fugazza G, Lopez Y, Kasma M, Lerman Y, et al. Dissemination of NDM-2 producing Acinetobacter baumannii clone in an Israeli Rehabilitation Centre. 2011. doi:10.1128/AAC.00679-11.

[52] Nordmann P, Boulanger A, Poirel L. NDM – 4 Metallo-betalactamase with increased carbapenemase activity from Escherichia coli. Antimicrob.Agents Chemother. 2012;56:2184-86.

[53] Hornsey M, Phee L, Wareham DW. A noval variant, NDM – 5 of the New Delhi metallo-betalactamase in a multidrug – resistant Escherichia coli ST 648 isolate recovered from a patient in the United Kingdom. Antimicrob. Agents Chemother. 2011;55:5952-54.

[54] Lee K, Lim Y S, Yong D, Yum J H, Chong Y. Evaluation of Hodge test and imipenem-EDTA double disk synergy test for differentiation of metallobetalactamases producing clinical isolates of Pseudomonas spp and Acinetobacter spp. J Clin Microbiol 2003; 41: 4623 – 9.

[55] Lee K, Chong Y, Shin H B, Kim Y A, Yong D, Yum J H.., Modified Hodge and EDTA disk synergy test to screen metallobetalactamases producing strains of Pseudomonas spp and Acinetobacter spp.Clin Microbiol Infect.2001;7: 88 – 91.

[56] Rai S, Manchanda V, Singh NP, Kaur IR. Zinc dependent carbapenemases in Clinical isolates of family Enterobacteriaceae. Indian Jr. of Med.Microbiol. 2011;29(3):275-9.

[57] Arkawa Y, Shibata N, Shibayama K, Kurokawa H, Yogi T, Fusiwara H, et al. Convinient test for screening metallobetalactamases producing gram-negative bacteria using thiol compounds. J Clin Microbiol 2000; 38: 40 – 3.

[58] Yong D, Lee K, Yum J H, Shin H B, Rossolinism, Chong Y. Imipenem – EDTA disk method for differentiation of metallobetalactamases producing clinical isolates of Pseudomonas spp and Acinetobacter spp. J Clin Microbiol 2002; 40: 3798 – 801.

[59] Walsh, T. R., Bolmstrom A, Qwarnstrom A, and Gales A. Evaluation of a new Etest for detecting metallolactamases in routine clinical testing. J. Clin. Microbiol. 2002; 40:2755–9.

[60] Marchiaro P, Mussi MA, Ballerini V, Pasteran F, Viale AM, Vila AJ, et al. Sensitive EDTA-based microbiological assays for detection of metallobetalactamases in nonfermentive Gram-negative bacteria. J Clin Microbiol 2005; 43: 5648-52.

[61] Tsakris A, Digalaki KT, Poulou A, Vrioni G et al. Comparative evaluation of combined disk tests using different boronic acid compounds for detection of Klebsiella pneumoniae carbapenemase – producing Enterobacteriaceae clinical isolates. J.Clin.Microbiol. 2011;49(8):2804-09.

[62] Reller LB and Mirrett S. Motility – Indole – Lysine medium for presumptive identification of enteric pathogens of Enterobacteriaceae. J.Clin.Microbiol.1975;2(3):247.

[63] Trepeta RW and Edberg SC. Methylumbelliferyl – beta-D-glucuronide – based medium for rapid isolation and identification of Escherichia coli. J.Clin.Microbiol. 1984;19(2):172.

[64] Bauer AW, Kirby WMM, Sherris JC, Jurek M. Antibiotic susceptibility testing by standardised single method. Am.J.Clin.Pathol.1966;45:493-96.

[65] Clinical and Laboratory Standards Institute. *Performance standards for antimicrobial disk tests*; Approved Standards, 9th ed. CLSI Document M2- A9, Vol. 26 No 1. Wayne PA 2006.

[66] Coudron PE. Inhibitor – based methods for detection of plasmid mediated AMPC β – lactamases in Klebsiella species, Escherichia coli and Proteus mirabilis. J.Clin.Microbiol. 2005;43:4163-7.

[67] Basak S, Mallick SK, Bose S. Extended spectrum beta – lactamase producing Escherichia coli and Klebsiella pneumoniae isolated in a rural hospital. Jr.Indian Med.Assoc. 2009;107(2):855-58.

[68] Pakzad I, Ghafourian S, Taherikalani, M et al. qnr Prevalence in Extended Spectrum Beta-lactamases (ESBLs) and NoneESBLs Producing Escherichia coli Isolated from Urinary Tract Infections in Central of Iran. Iranian Jr Basic Mel Sci. 2011;14(5):458-64.

[69] Sinha P, Sharma R, Rishi S et al. Prevalence of extended spectrum beta lactamase and Amp C beta lactamases producers among Escherichia coli isolates in a tertiary care hospital in Jaipur. Indian J Pathology & Microbiology 2008;51(3):367-369.

[70] Pandya NP, Prajapati SB, Mehta SJ, Kikani KM et al. Evaluation of various methods for detection of metallo-betalactamase(MBL) production in Gram negative bacilli. Int J Biol Med Res 2011;2(3):775-77.

[71] Gupta V, Bansal N, Singla N et al. Occurance and phenotypic detection of class A carbapenemases among Escherichia coli and Klebsiella pneumoniae blood isolates at a tertiary care center. J Microbiol, Immuno and Infect 2012;xx: 1-5.

[72] Omair M, Usman J, Kaleem F et al. Evaluation of Combined disk method for detection of metallo-betalactamase producing Gram negative bacilli. Malaysian Jr. of Microbiol. 2012;8(1):21-5.

[73] Melzer M and Peterson I. Mortality following bacteraemic infection caused by extended spectrum beta-lactamase (ESBL) producing E.coli compared to non-ESBL producing E.coli. Jr. Infect. 2007;55(3):254-59.

[74] Nordmann P, Cuzan G, Naas T. The real threat of Klebsiella pneumoniae carbapenemase producing bacteria. Lancet Infect. Dis. 2009;9(4):228-36.

[75] Mulvey MR, Grant JM, Plewes K, Roscoe D, Boyd DA. New Delhi Metallo-beta- lactamase in Klebsiella pneumoniae and Escherichia coli, Canada. Emerg Infect Dis 2011; 17(1):103-6. Doi10.3201/eid701.101358.

[76] Kumaraswamy KK, Toleman MA, Walsh TR, Bagaria J et al Emergence of a new antibiotic resistance mechanism in India, Pakistan and the UK : A molecular, biological and epidemiological study. Lancet Infect.Dis. 2010;10:597-602.

[77] Hammerum A, Toleman MA, Hansen F, Kristensen B et al. Global spread of New Delhi metallo-betalactamase – 1 The Lancet 2010;10:829-30.

[78] Ganga Ram study finds high levels of superbug NDM – 1. Available from: http://www.articles.timesofindia.indiatimes.com/2011-10-05/delhi/30246456_1_ndm1-antibiotic-resistant-superbug-mark-toleman. [Last accessed on 2012 Apr 12].

[79] Science, names giving and names calling: Change NDM-1 to PCM, Mens Sana Monographs. http://www.msmonographs.org/article?issn=0973-1229; year=2011; volume=9;issue=1;spage=294;epage=319;aulast=Singh. Retrieved 2011-03-11.

[80] Gupta N, Limbago BM, Patel JB et al. Carbapenem resistant Enterobacteriaceae : Epidemiology and Prevention. Health care Epidemiology 2011; 53: 60-7.

[81] Siegel JD, Rhinehart E, Jackson M, Chiarello L. and Healthcare Infection control practices Advisory committee. Management of multidrug resistant organisms in health care settings, 2006 Am J Infect Control 2007;35:S165-93.

Chapter 4

Convergence of host immune mechanisms in *Mycobacterium tuberculosis* pathogenesis

Ramesh Chandra Rai

Additional information is available at the end of the chapter

http://dx.doi.org/10.5772/58319

1. Introduction

Although the millennium development goal to stop tuberculosis (Tb) epidemic is almost achieved, still in 2012 there were 8.6 million new cases and 1.3 million deaths worldwide [of which 3, 20,000 people were co-infected with HIV too (WHO 2013)]. The rate of new Tb cases has been falling but decline rate at 2 percent per annum is still slow. Progress to handle multidrug resistant tuberculosis (MDR Tb)-defined by resistance to rifampicin and isoniazid (often accompanied by additional resistance), which accounts for 3.6 percent of the new and 20.2 percent of the previously treated Tb cases-is also slow (WHO 2013). Emergence of extremely drug resistant (XDR) strains of *Mycobacterium tuberculosis* (M tb) which is about 9.6 percent of the MDR Tb cases (WHO 2013) is a looming threat to the programmes aimed to stop tuberculosis. The XDR strains are resistant to isoniazid and rifampicin (first line drugs); at least to one of the three injectable second line drugs (amikasin, kanamycin or capreomycin) and also to any of the fluoroquinolone drugs to tuberculosis. The MDR and XDR Tb account for much higher death rates among the incident cases.

Induction of autophagy, Vitamin D and arachidonic acid metabolites play a decisive role in determining the susceptibility or resistance to the *Mycobacterium tuberculosis* infections. Additionally, cytokine responses play a major role. Among the cytokines, important ones are type I/ type II interferons, TNF-α and IL-1β in combination with other cytokines such as IL-4, IL-6, IL-8, IL-10, IL-12, IL-17, IL-22 etc. (Ottenhoff TH, 2012). M tb has evolved strategies to suppress the immune response mounted against it and even exploits host molecular pathways for its survival benefits. Regulation of apoptosis versus necrosis by M tb or its host has emerged as a major player in determining the survival or clearance of the pathogen. Many of these pathways have components with opposite roles favouring either host or the pathogen. They also are interconnected and the final outcome of the infection depends on the result of their converging effects.

1.1. Tb epidemiology

Tb incidence is generally considered as notifications of the cases with correction for underreporting and non-diagnosis. The total incidence of Tb cases in 2012 was in the range of 8.3-9.0 million globally (WHO 2013). Out of these, children account for 0.5 million cases and 3.1 million cases were among women. According to the WHO report on tuberculosis, most of the cases were from Asia and African regions-India (2.0-2.4 million), China (0.9-1.1 million), South Africa (0.4-0.6 million), Indonesia and Pakistan with 0.45 million and 0.4 million cases respectively, which is dangerously high. The report suggests that it is developing countries and specifically, the poor who are gripped tightly by the disease and who account for the maximum number of new cases and deaths worldwide. Awareness and access to diagnostic labs in developing countries is still low in addition to the lack of availability of affordable treatment. The combination of factors results in the spread of the pathogen to many people before being diagnosed. Diagnostic methods to distinguish latent tuberculosis from active disease and treatment options for latent Tb also are urgently required otherwise tuberculosis cannot be eradicated completely. There is some progress in this area and newer methods to diagnose latent Tb are being developed (Singh SB et al., 2013). In a recent study, Harari A et al. 2011, showed the possibility of discriminating latent Tb from active disease which could not be differentiated by a tuberculin skin test (TST) or interferon gamma release assay (IGRA). They utilized a flow-cytometry based method and analysed the functionality of M tb specific CD4 T cells from cohorts. Their results suggests that CD4 T cells are multifunctional and able to produce IL-2, TNF-α and IFN-γ in latent Tb cases while they dominantly produce TNF-α (single positive) in active disease conditions (Harari A. et al. 2011). Also since BCG is almost 100 years old with varied efficacy, new pre-and post-exposure vaccines are needed to prevent tuberculosis.

1.2. M tb pathogenesis

The genus Mycobacterium originated millions of years ago, but the members of the M tb complex evolved about 15,000-35,000 years back (Gutierrez MC et al., 2005). The noted occurrence of tuberculosis in humans is from their prehistoric remains and from Egyptian mummies dated back to 3000-2400 years (Zink AR et al., 2003). Respiratory tract is the main route of entry of the pathogen as airborne droplets containing the bacterium reaches the lung-a suitable site for this aerobic organism to establish infection. However other tissues and organs viz. lymphatic system, central nervous system, pleura, liver, spleen, bones and joints are also susceptible to infection by M tb and manifestation of the disease (Bloom BR and Small PM, 1998; Golden MP and Vikram HR, 2005). Once in the lung, alveolar macrophages engulf the bacterium, a process facilitated by binding of the lipo-arabinomannan on the bacterial cell wall to the mannose receptors on macrophages. Complement receptors on the macrophage surface also take part in the process of endocytosis of opsonised M tb (Ernst JD, 1998; Kang PB et al., 2005; Kerrigan AM and Brown GD, 2009). These interactions culminate in the release of cytokines which stimulate the adaptive arm of the immune system and eventually leads to

http://dx.doi.org/10.5772/58319

inflammatory response at the site of infection. Other cells of the innate and adaptive immune system migrate to the infection site and try to contain the bacterium by forming a specialized structure called granuloma.

The granuloma plays a major role in preventing the escape of the bacterium to other sites and also creates a localized immune response. If the immune response directed against the pathogen is capable of successfully containing it, granulomas shrink with the formation of the caseous centres, which is the case in immune-competent individuals (Dannenberg AM Jr. and Rook JA, 1994; Doherty TM and Andersen P, 2005). M tb is unable to replicate within the caseous centres due to hypoxia, acidic pH and presence of the fatty acids which are toxic to the bacterium but some organisms become dormant and persist for many years (Smith I, 2003). However, if the bacterium is able to survive by utilizing various immune evasion tactics and is able to replicate, necrosis of the infected macrophages takes place. It leads to the degradation of cells composing the granuloma and lipids (especially cholesterol) from the dying cells serve as a rich source of nutrient for the bacterium (Orme IM, 2013). Subsequent destruction of the cells leads to liquefaction within the interior of the granuloma where bacteria lives an apparently extracellular life, probably in the form of a pellicle or biofilms (Ojha AK et al., 2008; Orme IM, 2013) – a part of the bacterial life cycle not well perceived in the scientific arena. At this stage, the pathogen is far from the reach of current drugs available for treating tuberculosis and the components of the immune system modulated by the vaccine to tackle the infection (Orme IM, 2013). The calcification process initiated inside the granuloma after necrosis push the bacterium to the periphery and probable rupture of the membrane leads to dissemination of the bacterium. At this point, M tb is capable of dissemination to other organs of the body and is also released to the external environment as aerosol droplets when the host coughs, sneezes, shouts or sings and thus is able to start a new cycle of infection.

Though a high number of people fall prey to the bacterium very often but remain asymptomatic unless there are perturbations in the immune status of the person. The probability of developing active disease after getting infected is high in the initial two years but at least 5-10 percent of the people develop disease during their lifetime (Harada N, 2006; O'Garra A et al., 2013). In this chapter some of the host molecular pathways or their components and the signalling axes which play crucial roles in the inhibition or survival of the M tb and some of the recent research in the area has been highlighted.

2. Interferon signalling

Type I interferons e.g. interferon-α and interferon-β are implicated in progression of the tuberculosis. Mice with impaired type I interferon signalling are better protected from the pathogen (Manca C et al., 2001). *In-vitro* studies also show that M tb infection leads to up regulation of the genes of type I interferon signalling pathways and genes induced by them (Remoli ME et al., 2002). On the other hand interferon-γ, a type II interferon is critically important in protection against tuberculosis (Flynn JL et al., 1993; Trinchiari G, 2010). It plays its role by various mechanisms including activation of macrophages, enhances functioning of

CD8 T cells and through reactive nitrogen species (Flynn JL et al., 1993; Green AM et al., 2013). Thus both types of interferons have important and opposite roles in determining the mycobacterial pathogenesis (Teles RM et al., 2013). Berry et al., 2010, found a Tb-specific transcriptional signature in blood which could help in discrimination between latent and active disease and also distinguishes Tb from other infectious and inflammatory diseases. They reported 86 gene signatures which are specific to tuberculosis. These genes are mostly interferon inducible and consists of both type I and type II interferon signalling pathways and could be novel targets for Tb treatment.

3. IL-1β signalling pathway in tuberculosis

IL-1β imparts immunity to tuberculosis and mice lacking in IL-1β or its receptors are susceptible to M tb infection (Mayer-Barber KD, 2010). It is an important factor in host immunity and virulent mycobacteria suppress the IL-1β production which is regulated by type I interferons in macrophages (Novikov A et al., 2011). IL-1β has been shown to possess bactericidal activity in the macrophages derived from murine and humans (Jayaraman P et al., 2013). It upregulates secretion of tumor necrosis factor (TNF) and cell surface expression of TNFR1, thus facilitates TNF signalling which culminates in caspase-3 activation leading to growth inhibition of M tb through apoptosis of the infected macrophage (Jayaraman P et al., 2013). They also showed that this effect of TNF on the M tb infected macrophage is due to autocrine mode of action. In synergy with vitamin D, IL-1β drives transcriptional expression of the antimicrobial peptide genes such as defensin beta 4 (DEFB4), cathepsins, cathelicidins and ubiquitin derived peptides which have M tb killing ability (Alonso S, 2007; Liu PT et al, 2009; Ottenhoff TH, 2012). Results from the work of Liu PT et al. 2009, also suggest that the coherent action of IL-1β and vitamin D is an integral part of the TLR2/1 signalling mediated antimicrobial activity.

IL-1β being a pro-inflammatory cytokine is under tight regulation to prevent the immune-pathology and subsequent tissue damage during chronic infections. Mishra et al., 2013, showed that level of this cytokine is regulated by IFN-γ induced release of nitric oxide (NO) which in turn regulate the inflammasome NLRP3 (nucleotide binding and oligomerization domain-like receptor family pyrin domain containing 3) during M tb infections. This regulation happens at the stage of caspase1 mediated processing of pro-IL-1β to IL-1β and is specifically NLRP3 dependent (Mishra BB. et al., 2013).

4. Inflammasomes in tuberculosis

As briefly discussed above inflammasomes play a regulatory role in tuberculosis and imparts protection if activated. For its survival M tb prevents the activation of inflammasomes, caspase-1 dependent processing of pro-IL-1β and phagosome maturation through its gene zmp1 (Master SS et al., 2008; Lazarevic V and Martinon F, 2008). It has been shown that the production of IL-1β is dependent on the recognition of M tb by pattern recognition receptors

(PRR) TLR2/TLR6 and NOD2 (Kleinnijenhuis J et al., 2009). TLR4, the other PRR which is important in M tb recognition does not play major role in production of IL-1β. The immune adaptor molecule MyD88 has a central role in the transcription of the IL-1β mRNA during M tb infection (Kleinnijenhuis J et al., 2009).

Absence in melanoma 2 (AIM2) inflammasome is a cytosolic sensor of the DNA and recognises DNA viruses and intracellular bacteria. Co-localisation of M tb DNA with AIM2 inflammasome has been observed suggesting their direct interaction (Saiga H et al., 2012). AIM2 inflammasomes are involved in activation of macrophages and secretion of IL-1β during infection with pathogenic strain of *Mycobacterium bovis* suggesting its co-operative role in host immunity (Yang Y, 2013). AIM2 deficient mice are more susceptible to M tb infection and are defective in production of IL-1β and IL-18 and mount poor Th1 response (Saiga H et al., 2012). These authors also speculated on the role of AIM2 inflammasome in suppressing type I interferons in M tb infections. NLRP3 inflammasome is implicated in the protective immune response to M tb infection by facilitating the maturation process of IL-1β (Rathinam VA et al., 2012). However, M tb suppresses the activation of the NLRP3 inflammasome by inducing IFN-β, while IFN-β induces the AIM2 inflammasome which is detrimental to the pathogen (Fernandes-Alnemri T et al., 2010; Tsuchiya K et al. 2010; Briken V et al., 2013). Thus M tb balances the level of IFN-β such that NLRP3 inflammasome is kept suppressed and the AIM2 inflammasome is not allowed to be activated. This is done by the ESX-1 secretion system which is dependent on the ESAT6-an RD1 region encoded protein of M tb (Shah S et al., 2013).

Activating inflammasomes, although critical for protection from M tb infection and tuberculosis, also need to be regulated to prevent the tissue damage and rampant inflammation. Host regulation of NLRP3 inflammasome is done by nitric oxide which acts as its negative regulator during M tb infection and consequently controls the level of IL-1β (Mishra BB. et al., 2013).

5. Arachidonic acid metabolites

M tb on engulfment by macrophages tries to prevent the apoptosis of the harbouring macrophage so that it can establish a niche for itself. It also promotes necrosis of the macrophages in which it resides which help its spread to the neighbouring cells before establishment of the adaptive immune response of the host (Divangahi M et al., 2013). Several lines of research suggest that metabolic products of arachidonic acids such as leukotrienes, lipoxins and eicosanoids play decisive roles by regulating innate and adaptive immunity in the mycobacterial pathogenesis (Divangahi M et al., 2010). The prostaglandins and lipoxins, metabolites of arachidonic acid, have opposite roles. While prostaglandins such as prostaglandin E2 (PGE2) is pro-inflammatory in nature and promotes apoptosis, lipoxins inhibit it and promotes necrosis which results in the spreading of the bacterium (Tobin DM et al., 2010). Lipoxins e.g. Lipoxin A4 and its metabolites are anti-inflammatory in nature, repress TNF-α and stops neutrophil recruitment to the site of infection (Tobin DM et al., 2010). The other metabolite leukotriene B4 (LTB4) enhances level of TNF-α and thus creating a state of hyper-inflammation which is also not a healthy state for the host. Thus, TNF-α is regulated by metabolic products of arachidonic acid to keep its optimum level so that M tb infection is controlled while hyper-inflammation is also prevented.

6. Role of vitamin D

Deficiency of vitamin D is associated with higher incidence and manifestation of tuberculosis (Nnoaham KE, 2008; Verway M et al., 2013) and its supplementation helps to overcome this disease. Vitamin D is also able to restore the impaired secretion of TNF-α from macrophages of HIV-positive people (Anandaiah A et al., 2013). It acts as a mediator of innate immune response against M tb by mediating signals from toll like receptors to the activation of antimicrobial peptides (Liu PT et al., 2006). Liu PT et al. 2006, demonstrated that TLR stimulation by M tb or lipo-polysaccharide activates vitamin D receptors and subsequent downstream signalling activates transcription and translation of cathelicidin, a peptide with antimicrobial properties and thus creating an antimicrobial state in the human macrophages. Vitamin D has a modulatory role on the levels of cytokines specifically IL-1β and thus aid in immunity to the pathogen (Verway M et al., 2013). It also regulates the role of NLRP3/ caspase1 inflammasome leading to regulation of the levels of IL-1β and cross talk between alveolar epithelial cells and macrophages which is required for the synthesis and release of antimicrobial peptides (Verway M et al., 2013).

1, 25-dihydroxyvitamin D3, the active component of vitamin D, plays a major role in induction of autophagy during M tb infections (Yuk JM et al., 2009). This function of vitamin D3 is performed by activation of transcription of Beclin-1 and Atg5 genes and is mediated by cathelicidins (Yuk JM et al., 2009). Vitamin D3 also helps in the formation of autophagosomes, autophagolysosomes and co-localization of M tb cells with them, an important step in the killing of the bacterium (Yuk JM et al., 2009).

7. Role of foamy macrophages

After being engulfed by macrophages M tb dys-regulates its lipid metabolism which leads to lipid accumulation within a subset of these macrophages giving them a characteristic foamy phenotype. The lipid packed foamy macrophages have been associated with several chronic disease conditions such as atherosclerosis and during infections with persistent intracellular pathogens e.g. M Tb, Chlamydia and Toxoplasma (Kalayoglu MV and Byrne GI, 1998; Portugal LR et al., 2008; Galkina E and Ley K, 2009). Triglycerides, phospholipids and cholesterol constitute the low density lipo-proteins (LDL) and in foamy macrophages the influx and efflux of LDLs is dys-regulated (Russell DG, et al., 2009). Cholesterol gets esterified when the macrophage attains foamy phenotype and is retained as lipid droplets (Russell DG et al., 2009). Recently it has been shown that triacylglycerols (TAG) of M Tb are derived from host TAG and are imported by the bacterium for its lipid synthesis (Daniel J et al., 2011). M tb incorporates host derived lipids directly into its own pool and the accumulation of neutral lipids by the M tb leads to its lipid fastness (Daniel J et al., 2011).

It is shown that pathogenic mycobacteria synthesize oxygenated mycolic acids which induce foamy cell formation of the macrophages (Peyron P et al., 2008) but this might not hold true under hypoxic conditions (Daniel J et al., 2011). Peyron P et al., 2008 have shown that these lipid droplets serve as nutritional source to the pathogen and help in its non-replicative life cycle and persistence. One recent report also suggested that mycobacterium prevents lipolysis by interfering with the host lipid metabolic pathways, which leads to lipid accumulation inside the macrophage (Singh V et al., 2012). These lipids serve as a source of nutrition and help the pathogen in its dormant lifestyle. The specific presence of foamy macrophages in the necrotic regions has been suggested that they play crucial role in necrosis and hence in spreading of the bacterium (Peyron P et al., 2008). Although macrophages are the frontline innate immune cells, it is clear that their foamy phenotype helps the pathogen in establishing persistent infection and the host innate and adaptive immune response is no more able to eliminate the pathogen once it happens. Thus the ideal way to target the pathogen is before the establishment of the foamy phenotype of the macrophages harbouring the M Tb.

8. Role of autophagy

In addition to the above discussed mechanisms, hosts also try to clear the pathogen by inducing autophagy-an innate defence against M tb (Kumar D et al., 2010; Jo EK, 2013). Nutrient starvation, stress and activation of the specific cytosolic receptors induce autophagy (Ottenhoff TH, 2012). By this process protein aggregates, damaged organelles and cytosolic pathogens are sequestered inside the autophagosomes. The subsequent fusion of the auophagosome with lysosomes leads to degradation of the trapped entities and this process is prominently involved in the clearance of intracellular pathogens including mycobacteria (Gutierrez MG et al., 2004; Alonso S, 2007; Levine B et al. 2011; Cadwell K and Philips JA, 2013). This process is carried out by the product of autophagy related gene (Atg), Beclin 1 in combination with kinase genes PIP3-VPS34 and the GTPase-IGRM (Deretic V. 2010). The role of autophagy is also suggested in inflammation and related phenomenon (Castillo EF, 2012; Deretic V, 2012).

Autophagy regulates innate and adaptive immune pathways viz. antigen presentation to T cells by macrophages and dendritic cells (Jagannath C, 2009; Ottenhoff TH, 2012) and inflammatory responses (Levine B et al. 2011). Thus autophagy plays an effector function during M tb pathogenesis, however this process itself is regulated by vitamin D. Vitamin D up regulates autophagy and plays bridging role between innate and adaptive immune arms (Deretic V, 2005; Yuk JM et al., 2009).

9. Conclusions and future perspectives

M tb, besides evading host immune response against it also delays the onset of the adaptive immunity (Urdahl KB et al., 2011). M tb engulfed by macrophages tries not only to prevent apoptosis of harbouring macrophage but also promotes its necrosis which helps in spread of the bacterium to the neighbouring cells before establishment of the adaptive immune response (Urdahl KB et al., 2011). Type I interferons regulate the levels of interferon-γ and production of the IL-1β which are critical determinants of immunity to tuberculosis (Novikov A et al., 2011). Eicosanoids play decisive roles in the fate of the infected macrophages (apoptosis versus necrosis) by regulating the level of tumor necrosis factor. Thus, several of the host molecular pathways converge to dictate the delicate balance between host immune response and mycobacterial pathogenesis. We need to further understand their inter-relation and cross regulation in greater details to tackle the mycobacterial infection appropriately. There are intensive research and development activities in progress around the globe to tackle the epidemic of tuberculosis. Bedaquiline-the new drug approved for treatment of the MDR tuberculosis-was released finally in December 2012. According to WHO report on tuberculosis 2013, there are around ten drugs in various phases of clinical trials and many in the preclinical stages (Table 1). Also there are many new TB vaccines in the various phases of clinical development. Whether they are pre-or post-exposure vaccines and other details viz. their immune-therapeutic potential, killed whole cell or extract etc. are nicely elaborated in the WHO report on tuberculosis, 2013.

Lead compounds	Cyclopeptides, Diarylquinoline, DprE Inhibitors, InhA inhibitor, LeuRS inhibitor, Macrolides, Mycobacterial Gyrase inhibitors, Pyrazinamide analogs, Riminophenazines, Ruthenium (II) complexes, Spectinamides, Translocase-1 inhibitors
Preclinical development	CPZEN-45, DC-159a, Q203, SQ609, SQ641, TBI-166
Laboratory toxicity testing	PBTZ-169, TBA-354
Phase II	AZD5847, Bedaquiline (TMC-207), Linezolid, *PA-824, Rifapentine, SQ-109, Sutezolid (PNU-100480)*
Phase III	Delamanid (OPC-67689), Gatifloxacin, Moxiflloxacin, Rifapentine
Note: Four of the drugs in phase II trials (italicized) are novel and part of the combination regimens.	

Table 1. Development Pipeline for new TB drugs (WHO, 2013)

The current research is also helping us to better understand the life cycle and survival strategies of the pathogen. Recently, work by Das B et al., 2013, suggested that M tb persists inside the CD271$^+$/CD45$^-$ mesenchymal stem cells in the bone marrow of tuberculosis patients. They showed that the pathogen remains alive even after the full regimen treatment of the patients with anti-TB drugs. The CD271$^+$/CD45$^-$ mesenchymal stem cells express drug efflux pumps, produce low levels of reactive oxygen species, are quiescent in nature and have self renewal capability. This makes them an ideal place for M tb to survive for a long time. The immune-privileged nature of the bone marrow also supports the dormant life of the pathogen and M tb is able to live a non replicating life inside the bone marrow mesenchymal stem cells (Das B. et al., 2013). The part of the extracellular life of M tb in the form of pellicle or biofilms inside the liquefied granuloma and alternate hiding places has yet to be clearly elucidated. The

http://dx.doi.org/10.5772/58319

growing knowledge about M tb pathogenesis should help us in targeting tuberculosis more precisely in future.

R C Rai is financially supported by the project grant from Department of Biotechnology, Government of India funded to Dr. KVS Rao at ICGEB, New Delhi. Author wish to thank Guiliana Soraya Victoria and editor of the book for critically reading the chapter and their useful suggestions.

Author details

Ramesh Chandra Rai

Immunology Group, International Centre for Genetic Engineering and Biotechnology, Aruna Asaf Ali Marg, New Delhi, India

References

[1] Alonso S, Pethe K, Russell DG, Purdy GE. Lysosomal killing of Mycobacterium mediated by ubiquitin-derived peptides is enhanced by autophagy. Proc Natl Acad Sci U S A. 2007 Apr 3;104(14):6031-6.

[2] Anandaiah A, Sinha S, Bole M, Sharma SK, Kumar N, Luthra K, Li X, Zhou X, Nelson B, Han X, Tachado SD, Patel NR, Koziel H. Vitamin D rescues impaired Mycobacterium tuberculosis-mediated tumor necrosis factor release in macrophages of HIV-seropositive individuals through an enhanced Toll-like receptor signaling pathway in vitro. Infect Immun. 2013 Jan;81(1):2-10.

[3] Berry MP, Graham CM, McNab FW, Xu Z, Bloch SA, Oni T, Wilkinson KA, Banchereau R, Skinner J, Wilkinson RJ, Quinn C, Blankenship D, Dhawan R, Cush JJ, Mejias A, Ramilo O, Kon OM, Pascual V, Banchereau J, Chaussabel D, O'Garra A. An interferon-inducible neutrophil-driven blood transcriptional signature in human tuberculosis. Nature. 2010 Aug 19; 466 (7309): 973-7.

[4] Bloom BR, Small PM. The evolving relation between humans and Mycobacterium tuberculosis. N Engl J Med. 1998 Mar 5;338(10):677-8.

[5] Briken V, Ahlbrand SE, Shah S. Mycobacterium tuberculosis and the host cell inflammasome: a complex relationship. Front Cell Infect Microbiol. 2013 Oct 9;3:62.

[6] Cadwell K, Philips JA. Autophagy meets phagocytosis. Immunity. 2013 Sep 19;39(3): 425-7.

[7] Castillo EF, Dekonenko A, Arko-Mensah J, Mandell MA, Dupont N, Jiang S, Delgado-Vargas M, Timmins GS, Bhattacharya D, Yang H, Hutt J, Lyons CR, Dobos KM,

Deretic V. Autophagy protects against active tuberculosis by suppressing bacterial burden and inflammation. Proc Natl Acad Sci U S A. 2012 Nov 13;109(46):E3168-76.

[8] Daniel J, Maamar H, Deb C, Sirakova TD, Kolattukudy PE. Mycobacterium tuberculosis uses host triacylglycerol to accumulate lipid droplets and acquires a dormancy-like phenotype in lipid-loaded macrophages. PLoS Pathog. 2011 Jun;7(6):e1002093.

[9] Dannenberg, A. M., Jr., and J. A. Rook. 1994. Pathogenesis of pulmonary tuberculosis: an interplay of tissue-damaging and macrophage-activating immune responses. Dual mechanisms that control bacillary multiplication, p. 459–483. *In* B. R. Bloom (ed.), Tuberculosis: pathogenesis, protection, and control. American Society for Microbiology, Washington, D.C.

[10] Das B, Kashino SS, Pulu I, Kalita D, Swami V, Yeger H, Felsher DW, Campos-Neto A. CD271(+) bone marrow mesenchymal stem cells may provide a niche for dormant Mycobacterium tuberculosis. Sci Transl Med. 2013 Jan 30;5(170)

[11] Deretic V. Autophagy in innate and adaptive immunity. Trends Immunol. 2005 Oct; 26(10):523-8.

[12] Deretic, V. (2010) Autophagy in infection. Curr. Opin. Cell Biol. 22, 252–262

[13] Deretic V. Autophagy as an innate immunity paradigm: expanding the scope and repertoire of pattern recognition receptors. Curr Opin Immunol. 2012 Feb;24(1):21-31.

[14] Divangahi M, Behar SM, Remold H. Dying to live: how the death modality of the infected macrophage affects immunity to tuberculosis. Adv Exp Med Biol. 2013;783:103-20.

[15] Divangahi M, Desjardins D, Nunes-Alves C, Remold HG, Behar SM. Eicosanoid pathways regulate adaptive immunity to Mycobacterium tuberculosis. Nat Immunol. 2010 Aug;11(8):751-8. doi: 10.1038/ni.1904. Epub 2010 Jul 11.

[16] Doherty TM, Andersen P. Vaccines for tuberculosis: novel concepts and recent progress. Clin Microbiol Rev. 2005 Oct;18(4):687-702.

[17] Ernst JD. Macrophage receptors for Mycobacterium tuberculosis. Infect Immun. 1998 Apr;66(4):1277-81.

[18] Fernandes-Alnemri T, Yu JW, Juliana C, Solorzano L, Kang S, Wu J, Datta P, McCormick M, Huang L, McDermott E, Eisenlohr L, Landel CP, Alnemri ES. The AIM2 inflammasome is critical for innate immunity to Francisella tularensis. Nat Immunol. 2010 May;11(5):385-93.

[19] Flynn JL, Chan J, Triebold KJ, Dalton DK, Stewart TA, Bloom BR. An essential role for interferon gamma in resistance to Mycobacterium tuberculosisinfection. J Exp Med. 1993 Dec 1;178(6):2249-54.

[20] Galkina E, Ley K. Immune and inflammatory mechanisms of atherosclerosis. Annu Rev Immunol. 2009;27:165-97.

[21] Golden MP, Vikram HR. Extrapulmonary tuberculosis: an overview. Am Fam Physician. 2005 Nov 1;72(9):1761-8.

[22] Green AM, Difazio R, Flynn JL. IFN-γ from CD4 T cells is essential for host survival and enhances CD8 T cell function duringMycobacterium tuberculosis infection. J Immunol. 2013 Jan 1;190(1):270-7.

[23] Gutierrez MC, Brisse S, Brosch R, Fabre M, Omaïs B, Marmiesse M, Supply P, Vincent V. Ancient origin and gene mosaicism of the progenitor of Mycobacterium tuberculosis. PLoS Pathog. 2005 Sep;1(1):e5. Epub 2005 Aug 19.

[24] Gutierrez MG, Master SS, Singh SB, Taylor GA, Colombo MI, Deretic V. Autophagy is a defense mechanism inhibiting BCG and Mycobacterium tuberculosis survival in infected macrophages. Cell. 2004 Dec 17;119(6):753-66.

[25] Harada N. (2006). Characteristics of a diagnostic method for tuberculosis infection based on whole blood interferon-gamma assay. Kekkaku, 81(11): 681-6.

[26] Harari A, Rozot V, Enders FB, Perreau M, Stalder JM, Nicod LP, Cavassini M, Calandra T, Blanchet CL, Jaton K, Faouzi M, Day CL, Hanekom WA, Bart PA,Pantaleo G. Dominant TNF-α+Mycobacterium tuberculosis-specific CD4+T cell responses discriminate between latentinfection and active disease. Nat Med. 2011 Mar;17(3):372-6.

[27] Jagannath C, Lindsey DR, Dhandayuthapani S, Xu Y, Hunter RL Jr, Eissa NT. Autophagy enhances the efficacy of BCG vaccine by increasing peptide presentation in mouse dendritic cells. Nat Med. 2009 Mar;15(3):267-76.

[28] Jayaraman P, Sada-Ovalle I, Nishimura T, Anderson AC, Kuchroo VK, Remold HG, Behar SM. IL-1β promotes antimicrobial immunity in macrophages by regulating TNFR signaling and caspase-3 activation. J Immunol. 2013 Apr 15;190(8):4196-204.

[29] Jo EK. Autophagy as an innate defense against mycobacteria. Pathog Dis. 2013 Mar; 67(2):108-18.

[30] Kang PB, Azad AK, Torrelles JB, Kaufman TM, Beharka A, Tibesar E, DesJardin LE, Schlesinger LS. The human macrophage mannose receptor directs Mycobacterium tuberculosis lipoarabinomannan-mediated phagosome biogenesis. J Exp Med. 2005 Oct 3;202(7):987-99.

[31] Kerrigan AM, Brown GD. C-type lectins and phagocytosis. Immunobiology. 2009 Jul; 214(7):562-75

[32] Kleinnijenhuis J, Joosten LA, van de Veerdonk FL, Savage N, van Crevel R, Kullberg BJ, van der Ven A, Ottenhoff TH, Dinarello CA, van der Meer JW, Netea MG. Transcriptional and inflammasome-mediated pathways for the induction of IL-1beta production byMycobacterium tuberculosis. Eur J Immunol. 2009 Jul;39(7):1914-22.

[33] Kumar D, Nath L, Kamal MA, Varshney A, Jain A, Singh S, Rao KV. Genome-wide analysis of the host intracellular network that regulates survival of Mycobacterium tuberculosis. Cell, 2010 Mar 5;140(5):731-43.

[34] Lazarevic V, Martinon F. Linking inflammasome activation and phagosome maturation. Cell Host Microbe. 2008 Apr 17;3(4):199-200.

[35] Levine B, Mizushima N, Virgin HW. Autophagy in immunity and inflammation. Nature. 2011 Jan 20;469(7330):323-35.

[36] Liu PT, Schenk M, Walker VP, Dempsey PW, Kanchanapoomi M, Wheelwright M, Vazirnia A, Zhang X, Steinmeyer A, Zügel U, Hollis BW, Cheng G, Modlin RL. Convergence of IL-1beta and VDR activation pathways in human TLR2/1-induced antimicrobial responses. PLoS One. 2009 Jun 5;4(6)

[37] Liu PT, Stenger S, Li H, Wenzel L, Tan BH, Krutzik SR, Ochoa MT, Schauber J, Wu K, Meinken C, Kamen DL, Wagner M, Bals R, Steinmeyer A, Zügel U, Gallo RL, Eisenberg D, Hewison M, Hollis BW, Adams JS, Bloom BR, Modlin RL. Toll-like receptor triggering of a vitamin D-mediated human antimicrobial response. Science. 2006 Mar 24;311(5768):1770-3.

[38] Manca C, Tsenova L, Bergtold A, Freeman S, Tovey M, Musser JM, Barry CE 3rd, Freedman VH,Kaplan G. Virulence of a Mycobacterium tuberculosis clinical isolate in mice is determined by failure to induce Th1 type immunity and is associated with induction of IFN-alpha /beta. Proc Natl Acad Sci U S A. 2001 May 8;98(10):5752-7.

[39] Master SS, Rampini SK, Davis AS, Keller C, Ehlers S, Springer B, Timmins GS, Sander P, Deretic V. Mycobacterium tuberculosis prevents inflammasome activation. Cell Host Microbe. 2008 Apr 17;3(4):224-32.

[40] Mayer-Barber KD, Barber DL, Shenderov K, White SD, Wilson MS, Cheever A, Kugler D, Hieny S, Caspar P, Núñez G, Schlueter D, Flavell RA, Sutterwala FS,Sher A. Caspase-1 independent IL-1beta production is critical for host resistance to mycobacterium tuberculosis and does not require TLR signaling in vivo. J Immunol. 2010 Apr 1;184(7):3326-30.

[41] Mishra BB, Rathinam VA, Martens GW, Martinot AJ, Kornfeld H, Fitzgerald KA, Sassetti CM. Nitric oxide controls the immunopathology of tuberculosis by inhibiting NLRP3 inflammasome-dependent processing of IL-1β. Nat Immunol. 2013 Jan;14(1):52-60.

[42] Nnoaham KE, Clarke A. Low serum vitamin D levels and tuberculosis: a systematic review and meta-analysis. Int J Epidemiol. 2008 Feb;37(1):113-9. doi: 10.1093/ije/dym247.

[43] Novikov A, Cardone M, Thompson R, Shenderov K, Kirschman KD, Mayer-Barber KD, Myers TG, Rabin RL, Trinchieri G, Sher A, Feng CG. Mycobacterium tuberculo-

sis triggers host type I IFN signaling to regulate IL-1β production in human macrophages. J Immunol. 2011 Sep 1;187(5):2540-7.

[44] O'Garra A, Redford PS, McNab FW, Bloom CI, Wilkinson RJ, Berry MP. The immune response in tuberculosis. Annu Rev Immunol. 2013;31:475-527.

[45] Ojha AK, Baughn AD, Sambandan D, Hsu T, Trivelli X, Guerardel Y, Alahari A, Kremer L, Jacobs WR Jr, Hatfull GF. Growth of Mycobacterium tuberculosis biofilms containing free mycolic acids and harbouring drug-tolerant bacteria. Mol Microbiol. 2008 Jul;69(1):164-74.

[46] Orme IM. A new unifying theory of the pathogenesis of tuberculosis. Tuberculosis (Edinb). 2013 Aug 4. doi:pii: S1472-9792(13)00142-X. 10.1016/j.tube.2013.07.004.

[47] Ottenhoff TH. New pathways of protective and pathological host defense to mycobacteria. Trends Microbiol. 2012 Sep;20(9):419-28.

[48] Peyron P, Vaubourgeix J, Poquet Y, Levillain F, Botanch C, Bardou F, Daffé M, Emile JF, Marchou B, Cardona PJ, de Chastellier C, Altare F. Foamy macrophages from tuberculous patients' granulomas constitute a nutrient-rich reservoir for M. tuberculosis persistence. PLoS Pathog. 2008 Nov;4(11):e1000204. doi: 10.1371/journal.ppat.1000204.

[49] Portugal LR, Fernandes LR, Pietra Pedroso VS, Santiago HC, Gazzinelli RT, Alvarez-Leite JI. Influence of low-density lipoprotein (LDL) receptor on lipid composition, inflammation and parasitism during Toxoplasma gondii infection. Microbes Infect. 2008 Mar;10(3):276-84.

[50] Rathinam VA, Vanaja SK, Waggoner L, Sokolovska A, Becker C, Stuart LM, Leong JM, Fitzgerald KA. TRIF licenses caspase-11-dependent NLRP3 inflammasome activation by gram-negative bacteria. Cell. 2012 Aug 3;150(3):606-19.

[51] Remoli ME, Giacomini E, Lutfalla G, Dondi E, Orefici G, Battistini A, Uzé G, Pellegrini S, Coccia EM. Selective expression of type I IFN genes in human dendritic cells infected with Mycobacterium tuberculosis. J Immunol. 2002 Jul 1;169(1):366-74.

[52] Russell DG, Cardona PJ, Kim MJ, Allain S, Altare F. Foamy macrophages and the progression of the human tuberculosis granuloma. Nat Immunol. 2009 Sep;10(9): 943-8.

[53] Saiga H, Kitada S, Shimada Y, Kamiyama N, Okuyama M, Makino M, Yamamoto M, Takeda K. Critical role of AIM2 in Mycobacterium tuberculosis infection. Int Immunol. 2012 Oct;24(10):637-44. Epub 2012 Jun 13.

[54] Shah S, Bohsali A, Ahlbrand SE, Srinivasan L, Rathinam VA, Vogel SN, Fitzgerald KA, Sutterwala FS, Briken V. Cutting edge: Mycobacterium tuberculosis but not non-virulent mycobacteria inhibits IFN-β and AIM2 inflammasome-dependent IL-1β production via its ESX-1 secretion system. J Immunol. 2013 Oct 1;191(7):3514-8

[55] Singh SB, Biswas D, Rawat J, Sindhwani G, Patras A, Devrani S, Sarkar P, Mitra S, Gupta SK. Ethnicity-tailored novel set of ESAT-6 peptides for differentiating active and latent tuberculosis. Tuberculosis (Edinb). 2013 Nov;93(6):618-24.

[56] Singh V, Jamwal S, Jain R, Verma P, Gokhale R, Rao KV. Mycobacterium tuberculosis-driven targeted recalibration of macrophage lipid homeostasis promotes the foamy phenotype. Cell Host Microbe. 2012 Nov 15;12(5):669-81.

[57] Smith I. Mycobacterium tuberculosis pathogenesis and molecular determinants of virulence. Clin Microbiol Rev. 2003 Jul;16(3):463-96.

[58] Teles RM, Graeber TG, Krutzik SR, Montoya D, Schenk M, Lee DJ, Komisopoulou E, Kelly-Scumpia K, Chun R, Iyer SS, Sarno EN, Rea TH, Hewison M, Adams JS, Popper SJ, Relman DA, Stenger S, Bloom BR, Cheng G, Modlin RL. Type I interferon suppresses type II interferon-triggered human anti-mycobacterial responses. Science. 2013 Mar 22;339(6126):1448-53.

[59] Tobin DM, Vary JC Jr, Ray JP, Walsh GS, Dunstan SJ, Bang ND, Hagge DA, Khadge S, King MC, Hawn TR, Moens CB, Ramakrishnan L. The lta4h locus modulates susceptibility to mycobacterial infection in zebrafish and humans. Cell. 2010 Mar 5;140(5):717-30. doi: 10.1016/j.cell.2010.02.013.

[60] Trinchieri, G. Type I interferon: friend or foe? J. Exp. Med. 2010, 207: 2053–2063.

[61] Urdahl KB, Shafiani S, Ernst JD. Initiation and regulation of T-cell responses in tuberculosis. Mucosal Immunol. 2011 May;4(3):288-93.

[62] Verway M, Bouttier M, Wang TT, Carrier M, Calderon M, An BS, Devemy E, McIntosh F, Divangahi M, Behr MA, White JH. Vitamin D induces interleukin-1β expression: paracrine macrophage epithelial signaling controls M. tuberculosis infection. PLoS Pathog. 2013 Jun;9(6):e1003407.

[63] Yang Y, Zhou X, Kouadir M, Shi F, Ding T, Liu C, Liu J, Wang M, Yang L, Yin X, Zhao D. The AIM2 inflammasome is involved in macrophage activation during infection with virulentMycobacterium bovis strain. J Infect Dis. 2013 Dec 1;208(11): 1849-58.

[64] Yuk JM, Shin DM, Lee HM, Yang CS, Jin HS, Kim KK, Lee ZW, Lee SH, Kim JM, Jo EK. Vitamin D3 induces autophagy in human monocytes/macrophages via cathelicidin. Cell Host Microbe. 2009 Sep 17;6(3):231-43

[65] World Health Organization, Global tuberculosis report 2013.

[66] Zink AR, Sola C, Reischl U, Grabner W, Rastogi N, Wolf H, Nerlich AG. Characterization of Mycobacterium tuberculosis complex DNAs from Egyptian mummies by spoligotyping.

Section 3

Molecular Diagnostics and Stewardship for Infectious Diseases

Chapter 5

Molecular Diagnostics as an Indispensable Tool for the Diagnosis of Infectious Diseases of Viral Origin and Global Impact

Nora Rosas-Murrieta, Irma Herrera-Camacho, Lourdes Millán-Pérez-Peña, Francisca Sosa-Jurado, Gerardo Santos-López, Verónica Vallejo-Ruíz and Julio Reyes-Leyva

Additional information is available at the end of the chapter

http://dx.doi.org/10.5772/57581

1. Introduction

Infectious diseases are responsible for a considerable number of deaths in infectious in entire world. Infectious diseases are human diseases caused by viruses, bacteria, parasites, fungi and other microorganisms. Most of them have been controlled by vaccines or antimicrobials. However, some of them still represent global public health problems and are being monitored by the WHO and Center for Disease Control and Prevention. This chapter provides an overview of the applications of molecular methods for infectious diseases caused by viruses (intracellular obligate parasites) of global impact such as Dengue virus, Hepatitis B virus or influenza A virus. The infectious diseases not only represent a potential danger to the life of all human beings but also a significant investment in its detection, treatment and control of their spread. The increase in opportunities of infection by globalization, high rates of mobility among most countries around the world, the patient susceptibility to diseases due to genetic variation in populations [1], the ability of the microorganisms to evade the host immune response has forced the World Health Organization (WHO) to establish better methods of detection, prevention and control of infectious diseases caused by viruses as influenza A virus, coronaviruses, dengue virus, among others [2]. On the other hand, some types of cancer are the result of chronic viral infections caused by human papillomavirus, hepatitis B and C virus. Other infectious diseases are related to the development of neurological disorders caused by the measles virus, or human immunodeficiency virus [3]. In the determination of the etiology of such diseases has made extensive use of clinical procedures internationally validated as methods based on viral cultures and serological assays. However, it is increasing the use of nucleic acid tests in the diagnosis of infectious disease of viral etiology, considering that a critical step to proper treatment and control of any virus infection is a correct diagnosis. Diagnostic tests based on nucleic acid (NAT, nucleic acid tests) more used are the nucleic acid sequence-based amplification (NASBA), polymerase chain reaction (PCR) or real-time PCR for virus detection, genotyping and quantification. In addition, the automation of these techniques decrease in test time, low contamination risk, ease of performance, speed and have lower detection limits [4] show the relevance of their use. The detection of the infectious agent can be done by detection of the genomic DNA, genomic ARN and the viral messenger RNA (mRNA) using the follow techniques: Nucleic acids hybridization (Solid-phase, Liquid-phase or *in situ* hybridization), amplification of the signal of nucleic acids (branched-DNA assays and Hybrid capture assays), nucleic acid amplification (PCR, Real-Time PCR, Nested PCR, Multiplex PCR, Transcriptional-based amplification methods coupled to qPCR or NASBA, Strand displacement amplification), Microarrays (DNA microarrays and Multiplexed microsphere-base array) [5]. Currently there are some variants of the above techniques aimed to screening for detection or simultaneous discrimination of various etiological agents using multiplex PCR techniques [6], MassTag PCR, a PCR platform coupled to a mass spectrometer which allows simultaneous detection of >20 different pathogens [7] or microarrays pathogen detection (Virochip) [8]. The routine use of molecular techniques for the fast differential diagnosis of viral infections is vital for a high quality care of the patient with an infectious disease, directs the best therapeutic scheme, thus reducing the likelihood of complications, the proper choice of antiviral drug or the best strategy for control of viral replication, reduces resistance to antivirals and prevent the worsening of the clinical picture, the spread of the disease and the death of the patient [9]. This chapter will present molecular techniques applied to the diagnosis of infectious disease of viral etiology and incidence worldwide. A critical first step to proper treatment and control of any virus infection is a correct diagnosis. Conventional diagnostic tests for viruses it based on amplification of conserved portions of the viral genome, detection of antibodies against to viral proteins, or replication of the virus in cell cultures.

2. Dengue virus

Dengue virus (DENV) infection is the most common arthropodborne viral disease of humans; Aedes mosquitoes, principally *Aedes aegypti*, transmit this disease. According World Health Organization DENV is an emerging infectious agent that infects with an estimated 50–100 million clinical infections occurring annually worldwide [10]. DENV belongs to the family Flaviviridae, genus Flavivirus. DENV is a small are spherical and enveloped virus that contain a positive strand RNA genome of approximately 10,600 nucleotides coding for three structural proteins (capsid C, membrane, M, and the envelope, E) and seven non-structural proteins (NS1, xlinkA, xlinkB, NS3, NS4A, NS4B, NS5) [11], (Figure 1). The envelope protein (E) plays a key role in several important processes including receptor binding, blood cell hemagglutination, and induction of a protective immune response, membrane fusion and virion assembly. Two types of virions are recognized: mature extracellular virions contain M protein, while immature intracellular virions contain prM, which is processed proteolytically during maturation to yield M protein. The envelope of the virus contains the viral surface proteins E and M [12,13].

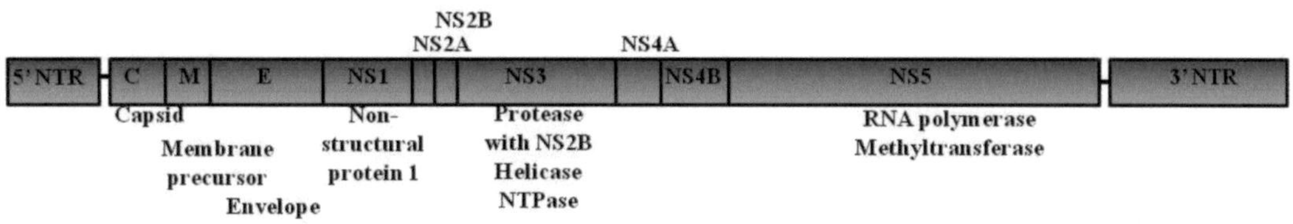

Figure 1. Schematic diagram of dengue virus genome. The DENV genome of positive-sense RNA and single-stranded, comprises approximately 10,600 nucleotides. Any region of genome can be used for genome detection by molecular techniques.

There are 4 antigenically and genetically distinct serotypes (DENV-1,-2,-3 and-4), being the "Asian" genotypes of DEN-2 and DEN-3 the most frequently associated with severe disease accompanying secondary dengue infections [14]. In human, the virus can cause a spectrum of illness, 75% of DENV infections are asymptomatic. But in persons with symptomatic DENV infection (dengue), the illness occurs in three phases. Acute phase, with 2–7 days of fever or self-limiting influenza-like illness (dengue fever or DF), accompanied by headache, retro-orbital eye pain, joint pain, muscle and/or bone pain, rash, mild bleeding manifestations and low white cell count. The critical phase of dengue which marks a 24 to 48 hours, period in which can occur the named severe dengue associated with vascular leakage, hemorrhage (dengue hemorrhagic fever or DHF), potentially leading to vascular shock (dengue shock syndrome or DSS), without appropriate treatment, patients with severe dengue are at risk of death. The convalescent phase of dengue lasts for 4-7 days [15-18]. During the past five decades, the incidence of dengue has increased 30-fold. In 2012, dengue was the most important mosquito-borne viral disease in the world. The emergence and spread of all four dengue viruses ("serotypes") from Asia to the Americas, Africa and the Eastern Mediterranean regions represent a global pandemic threat. Because epidemics of dengue result in human suffering, strained health services and massive economic losses, an international effort to reduce morbidity and mortality is long overdue coordinated by WHO named Global Strategy for Dengue Prevention and Control 2012-2020 [19]. The goal of the global strategy is to reduce the burden of dengue by to reduce mortality and morbidity from dengue by 2020 by at least 50% and 25% respectively. The laboratory diagnosis of dengue can detect severe cases, case confirmation and differential diagnosis with other infectious diseases. Diagnosis of dengue is made by detecting the infective virus, virus genome, dengue antigen or by analyzing, the serological responses (IgM or IgG) present after infection. Serology is currently the most widely applied in routine diagnosis [20] (Table 1). After the mosquito bites occurs an incubation period of 4–10 days, resulting in an asymptomatic or symptomatic dengue infection. In this period, the virus replicates and an antibody response is developed (Figure 2). The development of IgM antibody is coincident with the disappearance of fever and viraemia. In a primary infection (when an individual is infected for the first time with a flavivirus), viraemia develops from 1–2 days before the onset of fever until 4–5 days after and anti-dengue IgM specific antibodies can be detected 3–6 days after fever onset. Low levels of IgM are still detectable around one to three months after fever. In addition, the primary infection is characterized by slowly increasing but low levels of dengue-specific IgG, becoming elevated at days 9–10. Low IgG levels persist for decades, an indication of a past dengue infection. In a secondary infection, there is a rapid and higher increase of anti-dengue specific IgG antibodies. High IgG levels remain for 30–40 days [21]. The serological tests have been used for the diagnosis of dengue infection: hemagglutination-inhibition (HI), complement fixation (CF), neutralization test (NT), immunoglobulin M (IgM) capture enzyme linked immunosorbent assay (MAC-ELISA) and indirect immunoglobulin G ELISA. High cross-reactivity was observed with these tests. MAC-ELISA and rapid tests are the most frequent methods for IgM detection and in the detection of IgG are used HIA or ELISA [22-25]. Dengue non-structural protein 1 (NS1) is secreted from infected cells and produces a very strong humoral response. NS1 is a useful early serum marker for primary and secondary dengue infections, and is typically present between days 1–9 after onset of clinical signs [23]. In febrile patients, the early diagnosis of dengue virus infection on based on NS1 viral antigen [26-27]. At the end of the acute phase of infection, serology is the method of choice for diagnosis by detection anti-DENV IgM and IgG antibodies using MAC-ELISA. High sensitivity for NS1 antigen detection was observed by the association of MAC-ELISA with a commercial anti-DENV IgM/IgG rapid test (PanbioH Dengue Early Rapid test) [28]. A DENV NS1 capture assay using a test NS1 Ag Strip (BioRad Laboratories) is a valuable tool to postmortem dengue confirmation [29]. There are several commercial kits to dengue diagnostic such as the SD Bioline Dengue Duo device (Standard Diagnostic Inc., Korea) this test is composed of 2 tests to detect DENV NS1 antigen (first test) and anti-DENV IgM/IgG (second test) in serum, plasma or whole blood. With this test, still after the onset of illness, the virus can detected in serum, plasma, circulating blood cells and other tissues for 4-5 days.

	SAMPLE	DIAGNOSTIC METHOD	METHODOLOGY
Serological response	Paired sera (acute serum from 1-5 days and second serum 15-21 days after)	IgM or IgG seroconversion	ELISA
			HIA
			Neutralization test
	Serum after day 5 of fever	IgM detection (recent infection)	ELISA
			Rapid tests
		IgG detection	IgG ELISA
			HIA
Virus detection and its components	Acute serum (1-5 days of fever) and necropsy tissues	Viral isolation	Mosquito cell culture inoculation
		Nucleic acid detection	RT-PCR and real time RT-PCR
		Antigen detection	NS1 Ag rapid tests
			NS1 Ag ELISA
			Immuno-histochemistry

ELISA (Enzyme-linked immunosorbent assay). HIA (Haemagglutination inhibition assay). IgG (Immunoglubulin G). IgM (Immunoglobulin M). NS1 Ag (Non-structural protein 1). RT-PCR (Reverse transcriptase polymerase chain reaction). Information based on Chapter 4. Laboratory Diagnosis and Diagnostic Tests. Dengue Guidelines for Diagnosis, Treatment, Prevention and Control. Geneva. TDR/World Health Organization. 2012 [21].

Table 1. Dengue diagnostic methods.

Dengue diagnosis also relies on viral cell culture methods [30,31]. Specimens for virus isolation should be collected early in the course of the infection, during the period of viraemia (usually before day 5). Virus may be recovery from serum, plasma and peripheral blood mononuclear cells. Dengue virus is heat-labile; specimens awaiting transport to the laboratory should be kept in a refrigerator or packed in wet ice. Cell culture is the most widely used method for dengue virus isolation usually takes several days. Four methods of viral isolation have been routinely used for dengue viruses: intracerebral inoculation of newborn mice, inoculation on mammalian cell cultures, intrathoracic inoculation of adult mosquitoes, and inoculation on mosquito cell cultures [32]. The mosquito cell line C6/36 (cloned from *Ae. albopictus*) or AP61 (cell line from *Ae. pseudoscutellaris*) are the host cells of choice for isolation of virus. Indirect fluorescent antibody staining of the infected cell culture is often regarded as the "gold standard" in dengue diagnostics. However, it is tedious, time-consuming, and requires cell culture. All these studies have shown that this can be a valuable approach, especially in the early phase of infection; however, in some cases, they do not identify the viral serotype and these assays may not be as sensitive as the detection of viral RNA by nucleic acid amplification tests (NAAT) using reverse transcriptase-polymerase chain reaction (RT-PCR) and real-time RT-PCR may assume a very important role in dengue diagnosis at confirms an acute dengue infection [33, 20, 21]. Molecular diagnosis methods are usually rapid, sensitive, and simple when correctly standardized and can be used for serotype identification and quantification of genome copies in human clinical samples, biopsies, autopsy tissues, or mosquitoes. NAAT assays may identify viral RNA within 24–48 hours. Although, also be able to detect dengue viruses up to the 10th day after the onset of the symptoms. RNA extraction from clinical samples can be performed with the QIAamp Viral RNA kit [34], VERSANT Molecular System SP (Siemens) or HighPureViral Nucleic Acid Kit (Roche). Several RT-PCR procedures to detect and identify dengue serotypes in clinical specimens have been reported such as one-step, two-step, nested RT–PCR or real time RT–PCR [35]. These PCR assays vary in the amplified gene regions of the genome, in the detection method of RT-PCR products, and the virus typing methods. Real-time RT-PCR assays "singleplex" or "multiplex" can identify all four serotypes from a single sample, in a single reaction and is useful to determine viral titer in a clinical sample. Real-Time-PCR detection and typing of DENV usually addresses to the partially conserved 3′-UTR region of the genome. Due to the typical RNA-viral sequence variations it is difficult to identify one particular probe to be strictly related to one type or which could be used for a melting curve based analysis [36].

Many laboratories utilize a nested RT-PCR assay, using universal dengue primers targeting the C/prM region of the genome for an initial reverse transcription and amplification step, followed by a nested PCR amplification that is serotype-specific. The analysis of the amplification efficiencies of an in-house quantitative real time-PCR (qPCR) assay of DENV, between the region protein-5 (NS5) versus the capsid/pre-membrane region (C-prM) and the 3'-noncoding region (3'NC) showed that the non-structural conserved genomic region the NS5 genomic region provides the best genomic region for optimal detection and typification of DENV in clinical samples [37]. A fragment located at the 5′-UTR region of the virus genome was successfully used to identify and quantify distinct dengue virus strains and serotypes in clinical samples, in sera from patients infected with dengue virus, and in the mosquito *Aedes*

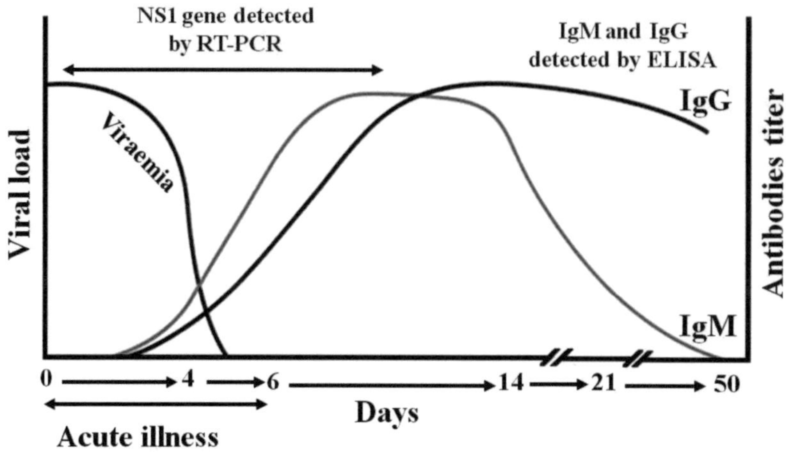

Figure 2. Immune response to virus dengue. In the infection course of dengue virus, the host's B cells produce IgM and IgG antibodies, which are released for recognize and neutralize the dengue virus and molecules such as the dengue NS1 protein with the purpose of eliminates the virus. The figure shows the viremia can detect by the amplification of the NS1 gene by RT-PCR and the antibodies titers by ELISA. Information based on Guzman MG, et al., 2010 [25] and WHO, Geneva, 2009 [10].

aegypti, as well as to study virus replication in different cell lines using TaqMan probes [38]. A real time RT-PCR (qRT-PCR) for DENV using TaqMan Minor Groove Binding (MGB) probe approach was development for detection and quantitation of all four serotypes using a single probe primer set targeted against the 3'UTR of DENV. In this assay, the limit of detection was DENV-1 (0.98 UFP/ml), DENV-2 (0.99 UFP/ml), DENV-3 (0.99 UFP/ml) and DENV-4 (0.99 UFP/ml) [39]. Other option to diagnosis to provide serotype specificity is a multiplex rRT-PCR assay targeting the 5′ untranslated region and capsid gene of the DENV genome using molecular beacons. This assay was linear from 7.0 to 1.0 $\log_{10}$ cDNA equivalents/mL for each serotype. The limit of detection was calculated to be 0.3 cDNA equivalents/mL for DENV-1, 13.8 for DENV-2, 0.8 for DENV-3, and 12.4 for DENV-4 [40]. A technique for the multiplex detection and typing of all DENV serotypes from clinical samples is PCR-ligase detection reaction (LDR). In this technique, a serotype-specific PCR amplifies the regions of genes C and E simultaneously. Then, two amplicons are targeted in a multiplex LDR, and the resultant fluorescently labeled ligation products are detected on a universal array. The sensitivity of the assay was 98.7%, and its specificity was 98.4%, relative to the results of real-time PCR. The detection threshold was 0.017 PFU for DENV-1, 0.004 PFU for DENV-2, 0.8 PFU for DENV-3, and 0.7 PFU for DENV-4. The assay is specific; it does not cross-react with the other flaviviruses tested (West Nile virus, St. Louis encephalitis virus, Japanese encephalitis virus, Kunjin virus, Murray Valley virus, Powassan virus, and yellow fever virus). The detection limit of the assay ranged from 0.004 to 0.7 equivalent PFU/reaction. The assay was 100 times more sensitive for DENV-2 and DENV-1 (LOD, 0.004 and 0.017 equivalent PFU, respectively) than for the others serotypes [41]. Detection of DENV in urine is other diagnostic method, a study by real-time RT-PCR, reported the detection of viral genome in urine between days 6 to 16[42]. Recently, CDC development a CDC DENV-1-4 Real-Time RT-PCR Assay, the first molecular test approved by the US Food and Drug Administration (FDA) for the identification of dengue virus serotypes 1, 2, 3 or 4 from viral RNA in serum or plasma (sodium citrate) collected during the acute phase. The limit of detection (LoD) of assay was determined to be between 1×10^4 and 1×10^3 GCE/mL for all serotypes in both formats in serum and plasma [43]. In all reactions by real-time RT-PCR, a positive PCR result is a definite proof of current infection and it usually confirms the infecting serotype. However, a negative result is interpreted as "indeterminate". Patients receiving negative results before 5 days of illness are usually asked to submit a second serum sample for serological confirmation after the 5th day of illness. Also, it was used other options to diagnostics dengue infection. The first is Virochip is a pan-viral microarray platform; this assay can detect to virus of Herpesviridae, Flaviviridae, Circoviridae, Anelloviridae, Asfarviridae, and Parvoviridae families. In other hand, for viral detection exists the option Deep sequencing and shotgun sequencing of human clinical samples by pyrosequencing using the Illumina GAII platform [44].

3. Influenza virus

Influenza is a highly contagious respiratory disease of humans, with propensity for seasonal epidemics and occasional pandemics. This disease constitutes a global health issue, leading to morbidity, mortality, and economic losses. During influenza season, influenza viruses circulate ubiquitously in the population. Global influenza surveillance forms the primary line of defense against the occurrence of influenza pandemics by identifying emerging influenza virus strains that pose a potential threat [45]. Influenza affects all age groups that result from its pulmonary complications. The virus initially infects the upper airways but can directly extend to the lower airways in severe cases, resulting in a viral pneumonia with significant morbidity and mortality [46, 47]. Influenza viruses belong to the Orthomyxoviridae family and are organize into types A, B and C. Influenza types A and B are responsible for epidemics of respiratory illness in humans and animals. The etiologic agent of influenza is the influenza virus with negative-strand, segmented RNA genome. Influenza type A and B viruses have 8 genes that code for 10 proteins. The virion has two surface glycoproteins (hemagglutinin (HA) and neuraminidase (NA) and the M2 protein protrude through envelop (Figure 3). Influenza virus binds to its sialic (neuraminic) acid receptor on respiratory epithelial cells by means of the HA protein [48]. The influenza type A viruses are sub classified into different subtypes according to HA and NA proteins, there are 16 HA subtypes and 9 NA subtypes, all of them have been identified and isolated from birds, humans and can affect a range of mammal species. The influenza A subtypes that circulated extensively in humans are A(H1N1); A(H1N2); A(H2N2); and seasonal influenza A (H3N2) [49]. Influenza A viruses (IAV) are the cause of pandemics, which are generated by the rearrangement (reassortment) of viral RNA segments in cells infected with two different viral strains [50].

Pandemic viruses of influenza A virus including "Spanish influenza" (H1N1 in 1918) and A/H1N1 or A(H1N1)pdm09 (H1N1 in 2009) [51] or rarely, a novel influenza A virus infection. For the diagnosis, the influenza tests that provide accurate and timely results are the most recommended. The appropriate respiratory samples for influenza testing are upper respiratory

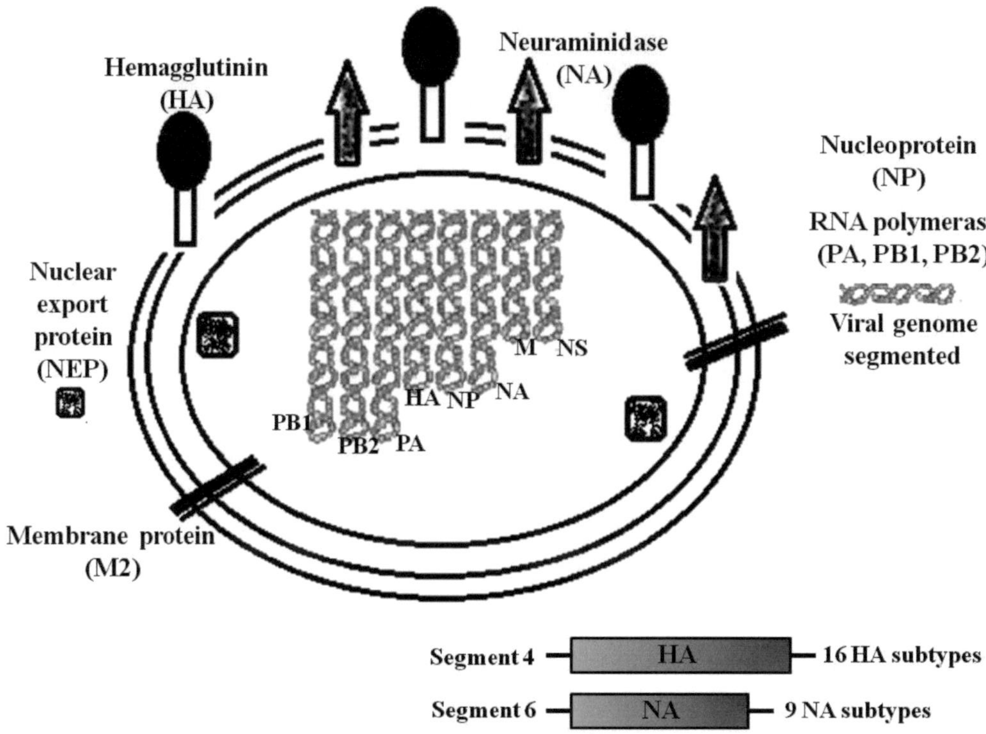

Figure 3. Schematic representation of influenza virus A (not drawn to scale). On the envelope viral are anchored: HA, M2 (ion channel protein) and NA protein. Inside the virion the negative-RNA single-stranded and segmented viral genome with ARN polymerase formed for PB1, P2 and PA. Also, there is a NEP protein.

tract specimen such as deep nostrils (nasal swab), throat (throat swab) and nasopharynx (nasopharyngeal swab). Nasopharyngeal aspirate and bronchial aspirate are also useful. Samples should be collected within the first 4 days of illness [52,53]. According to WHO the diagnosis of influenza is based in enzyme-linked immunosorbent assay (ELISA), haemagglutination inhibition (HI) and neuraminidase inhibition (NI) tests, egg and cell culture inoculation, and conventional reverse transcriptase PCR (RT-PCR) and Real-Time PCR (Table 2). The reference standards for laboratory confirmation of influenza virus infection are reverse transcription-polymerase chain reaction (RT-PCR) or viral culture [54]. Serologic testing is usually not recommended to detect evidence of human influenza virus infection for management of acute illness. However, a variety of serological tests, including the hemagglutination inhibition (HAI) test, complement fixation and EIA are used for testing paired acute and convalescent phase sera to detect antibody titers. The Rapid Influenza Diagnostic Tests (RIDTs) can identify the presence of influenza A and B viral nucleoprotein antigens, the result only is positive or negative. The RIDTs are immunoassays than provide results in 10–30 min but exhibit decreased sensitivity (70%–90% in children and 40% to 60% in adults), compared with RT-PCR and with viral culture. There is a potential for false negative results. Negative results of RIDTs do not exclude influenza virus infection in patients with signs and symptoms suggestive of influenza, follow-up testing with RT-PCR and/or viral culture should be considered to confirm negative test results [55]. Besides, of its low sensitivity RIDTs may be used to help with diagnostic and treatment decisions for patients in clinical settings, such as whether to prescribe antiviral medications [45]. These tools are continuously improved, a double-sandwich ELISA (pH1N1 ELISA), based on two monoclonal antibodies against haemagglutinin (HA) of the pH1N1 virus has a sensitivity of 92.3% (84/91, 95% CI 84.8–96.9%), being significantly higher than that of the BD Directigen EZ Flu A+B test (70.3%, $p < 0.01$). In addition, this assay can directly differentiate pandemic (H1N1) 2009 (pH1N1) virus from other respiratory pathogens, including seasonal influenza virus [56]. A hemagglutination inhibition assay is an extremely reliable tool for typing, subtyping and analyze the antigenic characteristics of influenza viral isolates if the reference antisera used contain antibodies to currently circulating viruses [53]. An HAI test showed that the patients with influenza A H1N1 have effective immune response [57]. The Directigen EZ Flu A+B test is a rapid chromatographic immunoassay for the qualitative detection of influenza A and B viral antigens, it has an accuracy of 95.5% and 96.8%, respectively. This kit has the ability to detect H5N1 isolates and of the A/California/07/2004 strain [BD Diagnostics, Becton Dickinson and Company, 2005]. Viral culture is considering one "gold standard" for detection of infection with human influenza viruses. Although, viral isolation is not a screening routine test in outbreaks, during periods of low influenza activity, could performed on respiratory specimens collected from persons with suspected influenza. Viral culture does not provide timely results (1-14 days) [58, 59]. In the influenza seasonal and in outbreaks, the viral culture is essential as a source of virologic data about strain characteristics, such as antigenic comparison to influenza vaccine strains and antiviral susceptibility that are important for clinicians and public health. Shell vial centrifugation cultures have been used to shorten the time to results to 1 to 5 days, to detect viral antigens [60]. Immunofluorescence using direct fluorescent antibody or indirect fluorescent antibody staining for influenza antigen detection are used as screening tests. This test exhibits slightly lower sensitivity and specificity than viral isolation in cell culture, but results are obtained within hours [45]. An example is the Respiratory Screen direct immunofluorescence antibody (DFA) (direct fluorescent antibody) staining of cells collected using nasopharyngeal (NP) swabs or NP aspirates can detects not only influenza, but RSV, parainfluenza types 1,2,3, and adenovirus. DFA is reported within 2-3 hrs [61]. However, for detection of respiratory viruses in clinical specimens, the nucleic acid tests (NATs) are fast, accurate and sensitive test. Several nucleic acid based amplification approaches have been applied for the detection of individual respiratory viruses including PCR, nucleic acid sequence-based amplification (NASBA), loop mediated isothermal amplification (LAMP), and multiplex ligation-dependent probe amplification (MLPA) [62-65]. For NATs, the nucleic acid is extracted from the samples by using commercial kits, like QIAamp viral RNA extraction kit (Qiagen, Hilden, Germany) using silica gel membrane technology. KingFisher mL (ThermoFisher Scientific Inc., Worcester, MA, USA) and easyMAG (bioMérieux, Marcy l'Etoile, France) kits using magnetic beads-based technology [66, 67]. TruTip (Akonni Biosystems, Inc., Frederick, MD, USA) use a porous nucleic acid binding matrix embedded within a pipette tip [68]. Reverse transcriptase-PCR (RT-PCR) or Real-time RT-PCR can be considered the other "gold standard" for detection of influenza viruses due to its high sensitivity and specificity for detection of influenza A and B viruses. The results are available within 4–6 h after specimen submission. These molecular tools are used as a confirmatory test. Several different gene targets have been used for amplification such as the matrix (*m*) to detect all influenza A subtypes, *ha* to distinguish between influenza A, B and C or between influenza A subtypes and non-structural protein genes (*nsp*) [69-71]. In all eight segments of influenza A virus, the first 12 nucleotides of the 3′ terminus (Uni12) and the first 13 nucleotides of 5' terminus (Uni13) are conservative and are the target to designed a primers pair. Detection of influenza A virus in human nasal swabs can performed by RT-PCR with Uni12 and Uni13 primers. The coupling of RT-PCR with sequencing analysis provides information about viral genotype [72]. Multiplex RT-PCR assays have been widely used for detection and differentiation of a panel of respiratory viral pathogens. FluPlex is a multiplex RT-PCR enzyme hybridization assay, capable of typing influenza viruses and subtyping HA (H1, H2, H3, H5, H7, and H9) and NA (human N1, animal N1, N2, and N7) with high sensitivity (10–100 copies/reaction) [73]. As the Qiagen ResPlex II multiplex RT-PCR kit, an test with high specificity for detection of 17 viral pathogens in nasopharyngeal swab samples such as influenza A virus (FluA), FluB, FluA 2009 pandemic A(H1N1)pdm09 and others pathogens as parainfluenza virus 1 (PIV1), PIV2, PIV3, PIV4, respiratory syncytial virus (RSV), human metapneumovirus (hMPV), rhinoviruses (RhV), adenoviruses (AdV), four coronaviruses (229E, OC43, NL63 and HKU1) [74]. The TrueScience RespiFinder Identification Panels (Applied Biosystems) is other multiplex PCR test to detect and differentiate 15 respiratory pathogens, using the multiplex ligation-dependent probe amplification (MLPA) technology, which starts by a preamplification step, which ensures the detection of both RNA and DNA viruses.

Follow is performed a reverse transcription, a PCR reaction, the hybridization probes to their target regions to the PCR product. A ligation probes and the final PCR exponentially amplifies the ligated probes with only two primers. The targets are detected through capillary electrophoresis. The pathogens potentially identified are Influenza A, Influenza B, Influenza A H5N1, Parainfluenza 1, Parainfluenza 2, Parainfluenza 3, Parainfluenza 4, RSV-A, RSV-B, Corona 229E, Corona NL63, Corona OC43, Adenovirus, Rhinovirus, Bordetella pertussis, Chlamydophila pneumoniae, Legionella pneumophila and Mycoplasma pneumoniae. MPLA shows specificities and sensitivities of 98.2% and 100%, respectively, for influenza A virus [75]. A successful test to detect a H5N1 virus was based on Loop-Mediated Isothermal Amplification (LAMP) method. For other side, detection, quantification and subtyping of influenza viruses can be performed by real-time RT-PCR (qRT-PCR). There are many papers of this technique applied to influenza A diagnosis such as TaqMan qRT-PCR method, which detects HA and NA genes of HPAI H5N1 virus [76]. A new generation qRT-PCR approach designated as Super high-speed qRT-PCR (SHRT-PCR) is a version of qRT-PCR with an extremely short reaction time (less than 20 min per run for 40 cycles) capable to detects viral RNA segments of influenza A [77]. RealTime ready Influenza A/H1N1 Detection Set (Roche) is an assay to detect the M2 gene (M2 PCR) of a generic influenza virus A and a specific PCR targeting the HA of A/H1N1-pdm09 (HA PCR, 2009 H1N1), to detect and quantify the 2009 H1N1 virus in clinical samples [78]. CDC developed the CDC Human Influenza Virus Real-Time RT-PCR Diagnostic Panel-Influenza A/H7 (Eurasian Lineage) assay for patients with signs and symptoms of respiratory infection. The kit contains a dual-labeled hydrolysis probe (TaqMan). The limit of detection of

METHOD	TYPE INFLUENZA VIRUS	TYPE SPECIMENS
Cell culture (Madin-Darby canine kidney (MDCK), mink lung epithelial cell line (Mv1Lu), rhesus monkey kidney (LLC MK2), and buffalo green monkey kidney (BGMK)	A and B	NP swab, throat swab, NP or bronchial wash, nasal or endotracheal aspirate, sputum
Rapid cell culture (commercial shell vials, single or mixed cell lines)	A and B	NP swab, throat swab, NP or bronchial wash, nasal or endotracheal aspirate, sputum
Immunofluorescence microscopy by direct fluorescent antibody (DFA) test or an immunofluorescent antibody (IFA) test, using commercial monoclonal antibody for influenza A and B viruses; or non commercial monoclonal antibody specific for H1, H3 H5, H7 and H9	A and B Identification of subtypes of A	NP swab, thrat swab, NP or bronchial wash, NP or endotracheal aspirate, sputum
Immunospecific assay for viral antigen detection Rapid influenza diagnostic test (RIDT's)	A and B	NP swab, nasal wash, NP aspirate, throat swab
Viral antibody detection Virus neutralization test Haemmaglutination inhibition ELISA using commercially anti-human antibody conjugates Complement fixation	A and B	Serum
Nucleic acid testing (Conventional RT-PCR singleplex and multiplex, Multiplex PCR, Degenerate PCR, Probe-based real-time PCR (TaqMan), SBRY Green I-based real-time PCR, Microarrays, NABA, LAMP, Pyrosequencing	A and B Identification of subtypes of A	NP swab, throat swab, NP or bronchial wash, NP or endotracheal aspirate, sputum

Information based on Centers for Disease Control and Prevention, National Center for Immunization and Respiratory Diseases (NCIRD). Guidance for Clinicians on the Use of Rapid Influenza Diagnostic.2011. Petric M, et al. 2006 [64]; Wang&Taubenberger, 2010 [65].

Table 2. Methods of diagnosis of influenza virus.

this kit was $10^{3.4}$ [79]. On April 1, 2013, an outbreak of human infections with a new avian influenza A (H7N9) virus was first reported in China by the World Health Organization. The diagnostics of this virus used the real time RT-PCR by TaqMan assay. Other molecular technique to diagnosis is DNA microarray such as FluChip-55 [Sakurai & Shibasaki, 2012] used in influenza diagnosis and others viruses such as parainfluenza, respiratory syncytial virus, human metapneumovirus, adenovirus, rhrinoviruses, coronaviruses causes pneumonia, which can be analyzed by multiplex PCR that assist in the discrimination of the etiologic agent [Pavia, 2011; Mahony, 2008]. The NGEN respiratory virus analyte-specific assay (Nanogen, San Diego, CA) detects influenza A, influenza B and others pathogens such as PIV type 1 (PIV-1), PIV-2, PIV-3, and RSV on a NanoChip 400 electronic microarray. The FilmArray Respiratory Panel (RP) is a PCR array test (Idaho Technology, Inc., Salt Lake City, UT) that can detect up to 21 viral and bacterial respiratory pathogens within about an hour as Adenovirus, Bocavirus, Coronavirus 229E, Coronavirus HKU1, Coronavirus NL63, Coronavirus OC43, Human Metapneumovirus, Parainfluenza virus 1, Parainfluenza virus 2, Parainfluenza virus 3, Parainfluenza virus 4, Rhinovirus/Enterovirus, Respiratory Syncytial Virus, Bordetella pertussis, Chlamydophila pneumoniae, and Mycoplasma pneumonia and Influenza A, Influenza A subtype H1, Influenza A subtype H3, Influenza A subtype H1 2009, Influenza B. This assay is a feasible alternative to viral culture in an acute clinical setting [80]. Recently, it was reported the method for the detection of genetic markers associated with high pathogenicity of influenza virus [81].

4. Human papillomavirus

Human papillomavirus (HPV) is a pathogen associated to development of cervical cancer, which is the second more common cancer in women worldwide. These viruses typically infect the skin and mucosal surfaces of humans. HPV is a non-enveloped virus with a circular and supercoiled double-stranded DNA genome of approximately 8,000 bp long within an icosahedral coat or capsid comprised by 72 pentameric capsomers. The open reading frames (ORFs) in the viral genome are organized in three regions: the early expression region (E), the late region (L) and the long control region (LCR) that bears the origin of viral replication and transcription. The E region codes for proteins related to replication (E1) and to activation or repression of the viral DNA (E2), and the oncogenes E6, E7, E5 [82]. The L1 and L2 genes encode the mayor and minor capsid proteins. Late genes L6 and L7 code for structural capsid proteins which encapsidate the viral genome (Figure 4) [83]. The L1 gene is the region most conserved between individual types and used to analyze phylogenetic relationship.

Those HPVs with L1 sequence divergence of 2–10% are known as subtypes and less than 2%, variants. The term "genus" is used for the higher order clusters, named using the Greek alphabet, and within genus, small clusters are referred to as species and given a number [84-86]. There are more than 200 different types, of which approximately 100 are fully sequenced and classified according to their biological niche, phylogenetic position and oncogenic potential [87]. About 40 can infect the anogenital mucosa of humans (mucosotrophic HPVs) [88-89]. According to their association with cervical cancer, there are low-risk HPV, which can cause benign or low-grade cervical cell changes, genital warts, and recurrent respiratory papillomatosis. High-risk HPV types act as carcinogens in the development of cervical cancer and other anogenital cancers [90]. Cervical cancer is a commonly-encountered malignant tumor in women. The surveys demonstrated that the increase of women with cervical cancer

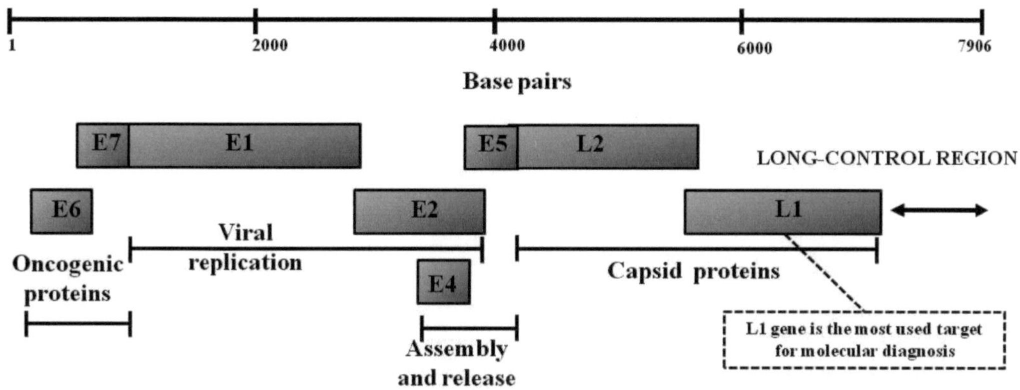

Figure 4. Linear representation of Human Papillomavirus (HPV) genome. The circular HPV genome has approximately 7900 base pairs, in the schematic with eight overlapping reading frames. L1 is signaled as the most used genomic target for detection of HPV.

less than 35 years old is particularly significant. The possible causes that result in cervical cancer to tend to occur in young include remarkable increase of HPV infection rate, especially the high-risk HPV 16 and 18 infection closely related to cervical cancer [91]. The primary screening and diagnostic methods have been cytology and histology. Papanicolaou (Pap) staining is the gold standard for detecting abnormal cervical epithelial cells, using microscopic analyses of conventional cervical smears or cell suspensions from liquid cytology medium. The limitation of Pap smear are low specificity, is need repeat the screening at short intervals [92]. Morphological findings from a cytology analysis determine the level of risk for developing cervical malignancies. Cervical epithelial cells atypical or abnormal are known as "atypical squamous cells of undetermined significance" (ASCUS). Some ASCUS signals the presence of low-grade squamous intraepithelial lesions (LSIL). However, some ASCUS are associated with underlying high-grade disease, including cervical intraepithelial neoplasia (CIN) [93-95]. HPV serology is not used diagnostically. Detection of the humoral antibody response is type-specific and first detected 6–18 months after infection. The response is weak and only between 50–60% of patients positive to HPV DNA-positive mount a measurable antibody response [96]. Although, the role played by the humoral immune response during the HPV infection is not very well understood; it was observed that this response is generated all throughout the malignant process; 54%-69% of women with incident HPV 16, 6, or 18 infections had antibodies. Serum antibodies against many different viral products of HPV have been detected by ELISA. The best characterized and most type-specific antibodies are those directed against conformational epitopes of the L1 capsid protein assembled as VLPs (virus-like particles) such as HPV-16 L1 VLP (virus-like particle)-based ELISA [97]. There is some high-throughput single-serum-dilution enzyme-linked immunoassay (ELISA) system for determining anti-HPV antibody titers following vaccination against HPV [98].

At present there is no "gold standard" for HPV detection. Guidelines for the management of women with cervical neoplasia or abnormal cervical cancer screening tests indicates the immediate colposcopy (cervical exam), cytologic follow-up, and triage by HPV DNA testing

[99]. HPV serves as paradigm for the use of NAATs due to how difficult it is to obtain the virus via cell cultures or to develop indirect diagnosis techniques [100]. There are several molecular techniques for HPV DNA detection (Table 3). They include DNA hybridization, PCR-RFLP, reverse-line hybridization and hybrid capture assay. The method most commonly used is the polymerase chain reaction (PCR). All target amplification techniques such as PCR for HPV virus detection currently use consensus or type-specific primers group-or type-specific conventional PCR, to amplify a broad-spectrum of HPV genotypes by targeting a conserved region within the HPV genome [101, 102]. L1 and E1 regions are the most conserved parts of the genome [103]. Many assays use primers targeted to the viral capsid L1 gene, which can detect numerous HPV types [104]. There are several PCR primer sets as GP5+/6+that amplify a 140 bp region in the L1 gene allowing the identification of 30 HPV genotypes. This method is useful in predicting high-grade cervical intraepithelial neoplasia. The MY09/11 system identifies high-risk HPV genotypes by amplifying a 450 bp sequence in the conserved L1 region. The MY09/11 primer set uses degenerate bases to reduce variability due to different genotypes. The SPF10 system primers amplify a 65 bp sequence from a highly conserved region of the viral L1 gene for the identification of 16 different genotypes of the human papillomavirus (HPV) [105]. Commonly used L1 consensus primer sets include PGMY09/11, GP5+/6+, and SPF10, having the ability to identify a large range of HPV types with 1 amplification [106, 107]. Hybridization on PCR products (Cervista HPV HR Test, INNO-LiPa HPV Genotyping, Linear Array HPV Genotyping Test, Digene HPV Genotyping RH Test) [Estrade et al., 2011; Jeney et a., 2007; Chan et a., 2012]. Linear Array HPV Genotyping Test (Roche Diagnostics, Indianapolis, IN) is able to identify 37 types of HPV, 14 are high-risk genotypes. Linear Array also includes PGMY primers and is a commonly used method for genotyping HPV using Probes for multiple HPV types are fixed on a membrane strip, and the PCR product is hybridized to the strip, followed by visual detection [108]. Other assay so used is INNO-LiPA HPV Genotyping Extra (Innogenetics, Ghent, Belgium). This kit amplifies HPV DNA with SPF10 primers at the L1 region. The probes are fixed to membrane strips in sequence-specific lines and visualized as purple/brown bands. The test can detect and distinguish 24 low-and high-risk HPV types. [INNO-LiPA HPV Genotyping Extra. Ghent, Belgium: Innogenetics; 2007. A HPV viral target to detect is the L1 gene to amplify a broad spectrum of HPV types with a single set of degenerated primers or a cocktail of primers (Amplicor HPV Test) [Sepehr et al., 2012] and HPV mRNA amplification against HPV E6/E7 mRNA (APTIMA HPV Assay, NucliSENS EasyQ HPV, PreTect HPV-Proofer). Another test is the Multiplex Genotyping Kit (Multimetrix, Heidelberg, Germany). The test is a PCR-based fluorescent bead array that can detect 24 low-and high-risk HPV types [109]. The quadruplex quantitative PCR method (AllGlo fluorescent probes) was established to simultaneously detect and differentiate HPV 6, 11, 16 and 18 [110]. Between the signal amplification methods are liquid-phase or in situ hybridization as Hybrid Capture 2 HPV DNA Test for to detect 13 high-risk types (HPV 16, 18, 31, 33, 35, 39, 45, 51, 52, 56, 58, 59 and 68) and five low-risk types [111, 112]. Microarray on PCR products is other molecular technique to detect influenza virus such as Infiniti HPV-HR QUAD Assay, PapilloCheck or HybriMax for HPV genotyping [113]. PapilloCheck (Greiner Bio-One, Monroe, NC) for HPV genotyping PapilloCheck identifies 24 types of low-and high-risk HPV with a high specificity and sensitivity [114]. Genotyping with this method is based

on PCR amplification of the E1 gene by a group of new E1-specific primers, followed by hybridization to a DNA chip with immobilized HPV oligoprobes. A novel assay for molecular diagnostics and typing application known as Sequencing Bead Array (SBA) is an alternative method to HPV diagnosis. SBA is a digital suspension array using Next-Generation Sequencing (NGS) that in the case of HPV could distinguish ten Human Papillomavirus (HPV) genotypes associated with cervical cancer progression. This is a robust system capable to identify genetic signatures or single nucleotide polymorphisms (SNPs). SBA has the potential to change the probe-based diagnostics, and allow for a transition towards the technology by genomic sequencing [115]. Some groups are studying other molecular factors as possible markers of infection by HPV as a complementary diagnostics. The overexpression of the HPV E6 and E7 genes is indicated in HPV-induced carcinogenesis, making these genes a potential measure of virulence. Monitoring the expression levels of these genes may allow for screening and monitoring of cancer progression [116].

MOLECULAR DIAGNOSIS METHOD	NAME TEST	GENOTYPES AND TARGET DETECTED
Real time	Real Time High risk HPV test (Abbott Molecular)	14 high risk HPV genotypes: 16, 18, 31, 33, 35, 39, 45, 51, 52, 56, 58, 59, 66, 68 and to partially genotype 16, 18 from other 12 high risk genotypes using L1 gene.
	Cobas 4800 HPV Test Amplification/Detection kit (Roche Molecular Diagnostics)	HPV 16 and HPV 18 and concurrently detecting the rest of the high risk types (31, 33, 35, 39, 45, 51, 52, 56, 58, 59, 66 and 68), using L1 gene
Hybrid capture	Hybrid Capture 2 High-Risk HPV DNA Test	High-risk HPV types 16, 18, 31, 33, 35, 39, 45, 51, 52, 56, 58, 59 and 68 using all genome.
PCR and hybridization	AMPLICOR Human Papillomavirus Test (Roche Molecular Diagnostics)	HPV types: 16, 18, 31, 33, 35, 39, 45, 51, 52, 56, 58, 59 and 68 using L1 gene.
TMA	APTIMA HPV assay (Hologic)	Qualitative detection of E6/E7 viral messenger RNA (mRNA) from 14 high-risk types of HPV: 16, 18, 31, 33, 35, 39, 45, 51, 52, 56, 58, 59, 66 and 68.
Reverse hybridization	Digene HPV Genotyping RH Test (Qiagen)	Detection of HPV subtypes 16, 18, 26, 31, 33, 35, 39, 45, 51, 52, 53, 56, 58, 59, 66, 68, 73 and 82 using L1 gene.
	INNO-LiPA HPV Genotyping Extra (Innogenetics)	Detection of at least 54 HPV types using L1 gene.
	Linear Array HPV Genotyping test (Roche Molecular Diagnostics)	Linear Array detects thirty seven anogenital HPV DNA genotypes 6, 11, 16, 18, 26, 31, 33, 35, 39, 40, 42, 45, 51, 52, 53, 54, 55, 56, 58, 59, 61, 62, 64, 66,

MOLECULAR DIAGNOSIS METHOD	NAME TEST	GENOTYPES AND TARGET DETECTED
		67, 68, 69, 70, 71, 72, 73 (MM9), 81, 82, 83, 84, IS39 and CP6108.
Invader chemistry	Cervista HPV HR Test (Hologic)	Detection of 14-type High Risk HPV genotypes: 16, 18, 31, 33, 35, 39, 45, 51, 52, 56, 58, 59, 66, 68 using L1 gene.
PCR-microarray	PapilloCheck HPV-Screening Test (Greiner Bio-One)	Type-specific identification of 18 high-risk(16,18, 31,33, 35, 39, 45, 51, 52, 53, 56, 58, 59, 66, 68, 70, 73, 82) and 6 low-risk types of HPV (6, 11, 40, 42, 43, 44) using E1 gene.
	Clart HPV 2 (Genomics)	Identification of HPV 6, 11, 16, 18, 26, 31, 33, 35, 39, 40, 42, 43, 44, 45, 51, 52, 53, 54, 56, 58, 59, 61, 62, 66, 68, 70, 71, 72, 73, 81, 82, 83, 84, 85 and 89 genotypes using L1 gene.
	Infiniti HPV Genotyping assay (AutoGenomics)	Genotyping of HPV 6, 11, 16, 18, 26, 30, 31, 33, 34, 35, 39, 45, 51, 52, 53, 56, 58, 59, 66, 67, 68, 69, 70, 73, 82 and 85 using E1 gene.
NASBA amplification and real-time detection using molecular beacon probes	NucliSENS EasyQ HPV (BioMérieux)	Discriminates the E6/E7 mRNA between genotypes 16, 18, 31, 33 and 45.
Next-Generation assay	NextGen HPV Screening Assay and Platform (Qiagen)	15 high risk subtypes (+ types 66 and 82)

Information based on Kroupis C, et al., 2011 [90]; Arney A, et al., 2010 [100].

Table 3. Principal methods of molecular diagnosis of HPV.

Analysis of the host factor p16INK4a (p16), a cyclin-dependent kinase inhibitor could be a molecular marker to HPV infection. The increase of p16 indicates removal of the negative feedback control supplied by the retinoblastoma gene, pRB. When oncogenic HPV E7 proteins bind to pRB, p16 is overexpressed and elevated, representing active expression of HPV oncogenes [117]. The sialylation modification observed during oncogenic transformation, tumor metastases and invasion, has been associated with enhanced sialyltransferases (STs) transcription such as ST3Gal III, ST3Gal IV and ST6Gal I in CIN [118].

5. Viral hepatitis

Viral hepatitis is a necroinflammatory liver disease of variable severity. Persistent infection by HBV is often associated with chronic liver disease that can lead to the development of cirrosis and hepatocellular carcinoma being a global public health as chronic diseases, cause of infectious disease mortality globally, each year causing approximately 1.4 million deaths. In addition, viral hepatitis are cause of liver cancer and the most common reason for liver transplantation [119]. The viruses more common are Hepatitis A, Hepatitis B, and Hepatitis C. Approximately 400 million persons living with chronic hepatitis B virus (HBV) or hepatitis C virus infection who die from cirrhosis or liver cancer, years and decades after of their infection [120]. Hepatitis B is caused by infection with HBV, which may lead to acute or chronic hepatitis. HBV is the 9th leading cause of death worldwide. It causes cirrhosis, liver failure and hepatocellular carcinoma. HBV is a small nonenveloped DNA virus that is a member of the Hepadnaviridae family, HBV contains a 3.2-kb partially double-stranded DNA genome with 4 open reading frames encoding 7 proteins (P/viral polymerase, S/Surface antigen proteins/HBsAg, C/core protein, HBeAg y X/HBx protein) [121]. Eight genotypes of HBV (designated-H) have been identified by sequence divergence of >8% over the entire genome of HBV DNA [122]. HBV is efficiently transmitted by percutaneous or mucous membrane exposure to infectious blood or body fluids that contain blood. Acute HBV infection can be either asymptomatic or symptomatic. Symptoms in acute HBV infection are clinically indistinguishable from those in other acute viral hepatitis infections [123]. Diagnosis of hepatic viral infection is carried out by studying biochemical as liver function tests, serologic assays and histological parameters. Serological HBV diagnosis identifies virally-encoded antigens and their corresponding antibodies in serum. Three clinical useful antigen-antibody systems have been identified for hepatitis B: hepatitis B surface antigen (HBsAg) and antibody to HBsAg (anti-HBs), antibody (anti-HBc IgM and anti-HBc IgG) to hepatitis B core antigen (HBcAg), hepatitis B e antigen (HBeAg) and antibody to HBeAg (anti-HBe) [124]. B surface antigen (HBsAg) is the first serological marker to appear during the course of HBV infection, is present in both acute and chronic infection. The immunoassays to detect HBsAg are highly specific and show a sensitivity, allowing the detection of <0.15 ng/ml of HbsAg [125]. Detection of HBsAg allowed for the first time screening of inapparently infected blood donors for a dangerous pathogen. The simultaneous detection of antibodies against HBsAg (anti-HBs) and HBcAg (anti-HBc) can be useful to know the evolution of disease. The presence of IgM antibody to hepatitis B core antigen (IgM anti-HBc) is diagnostic of acute or recently acquired HBV infection. Antibody to HBsAg (anti-HBs) is produced after a resolved infection and is the only HBV antibody marker present after immunization. The presence of HBsAg and total anti-HBc, with a negative test for IgM anti-HBc, indicates chronic HBV infection. The presence of anti-HBc alone might indicate a false-positive result or acute, resolved, or chronic infection [126, 127]. Chronic HBV infection is defined by the persistence of serum HBsAg for more than 6 months [128]. Serologic assays for HBV are the mainstay diagnostic tools for HBV infection. The clinically silent HBV infections are a strong driving force in the development of modern virus diagnostics to analyze the HBV replication profile, HBV DNA levels and the viral protein expression [129]. When serological testing could be inconclusive for the diagnosis of a HBV infection (due to the presence of genetic variants of HBV), the molecular detection of HBV DNA may help to resolve the uncertainties. The NAT assays in plasma or serum can detect to 10 copies/mL [130]. The viral genomes can be detected and quantified by polymerase chain reaction (PCR), transcription-mediated amplification (TMA), and with signal amplification methods such as hybrid-capture and the branched DNA assay. Quantification of genome of HBV can be used for diagnosing HBV infection and monitoring the effect of antiviral therapy. HBV DNA is the earliest detectable marker in acute HBV infection and the gold standard for the diagnosis of occult HBV infection. HBV DNA testing is particularly useful in the detection of the early phase of acute HBV infection prior to the appearance of serum HBsAg as well as in occult HBV infection [131, 132]. Several commercial molecular assays have been developed for quantitation of HBV DNA. Such as COBAS Amplicor HBV Monitor, which is based on the amplification of DNA targets by PCR with HBV-specific primers. Between the hybridizations methods are Hybrid capture Ultrasensitive hybrid capture II and Branched DNA VERSANT hepatitis B virus DNA 3.0. Recently developed real-time target amplification methods have improved viral genome detection and quantification for clinical and research purposes. Real time PCR for HBV DNA has reached an excellent level of performance with a detection limit close to the theoretical minimum of 1 DNA molecule per reaction mix and a huge dynamic range up to 10^7 or more. In 1991 the WHO introduced International Standard preparations and an arbitrary International Unit (IU) of HBV DNA. The number of molecules per IU depends on the assay; but typically 5 molecules correspond to one IU HBV DNA [133]. Real-Time PCR (Real Time Abbott PCR, Smart HBVTM, Real Art HBV, COBAS AmPliprep, Cobas TaqMan HBV, Aptima HBV Quantitative assay) [134-136]. Fosun real-time PCR HBV kit is a comercial assay for quantitation of serum HBV DNA based on TaqMan PCR technology, which is useful for monitoring HBV DNA levels in patients with chronic hepatitis B. The limit of the duplex real-time PCR assay was 29.5 IU/ml, whereas the specificity was 100% for the detection of HBV DNA [137]. A trial has been tested, a TaqMan locked nucleic acid (LNA) real-time polymerase chain reaction (PCR) probe for the accurate quantification and detection of hepatitis B virus (HBV) DNA in serum (plasma) [138]. The genotyping analysis of HBV can performed by real-time PCR using (GQ-PCR) method or the direct sequencing and reverse hybridization with INNO-LiPA HBV genotyping assay [139]. Other option to diagnostics of hepatotrophic viruses is Real-time PCR array, useful in the rapid detection of multiple viral pathogens, between them hepatitis B virus (HBV), hepatitis C virus (HCV) using the SYBR Green chemistry. The array detected: 10 genome equivalents (geq)/ml of HCV, 50 geq of HBV (genotype A) [140]. Micro-RNAs (miRNAs) are noncoding RNAs that regulate gene expression primarily at the post-transcriptional level by binding to mRNAs. The circulating miRNA in serum or plasma might be a very useful biomarker for the diagnosis and prognosis of HBV-related diseases, indicating a promising future in the treatment of HBV-related diseases [141]. Hepatitis C virus (HCV) is a major public health problem and a leading cause of chronic liver disease. An estimated 180 million people are infected worldwide, several of these patients go on to develop chronic HCV infection, often developing into liver cirrhosis, hepatic failure and hepatocellular carcinoma [142]. Hepatitis C virus is a single stranded RNA, enveloped virus, belongs to the Flaviviridae family and is the only member of the Hepacivirus genus [143]. The commercially-available diagnostic tests are based on enzyme immunosorbent assays (EIA) for the detection of HCV-specific antibodies and recombinant immunoblot assays (RIBA). Although, in the diagnosis of influenza is applied the algorithm showed in figure 5 [144-146]. Testing for circulating HCV by genomic sequence amplification (PCR and branched DNA assay) has been successfully utilized for confirmation of serological results and the effectiveness of antiviral therapy [134,

147]. An alternative to HCV diagnosis is Loop-mediated isothermal amplification (LAMP) assay for rapid detection of HCV genomic RNA [148]. The molecular HCV assays includes to RT-PCR (AmpliScreen 2.0, Amplicor HCV 2.0, Cobas Amplicor Monitor HCV 2.0, Versant HCV RNA, Procleix HIV/HCV assay, Procleix Ultrio assay). The methods for accurate quantification of HCV RNA levels are key tools in the clinical management of patients. The HCV RNA Assay by RT-PCR includes to Amplicor HCV Monitor 2.0, Cobas Amplicor Monitor HCV 2.0, Cobas AmliPrep/Cobas TaqMan HCV, Versant HCV RNA 3.0 Quantitative assay, LCx HCV RNA Quantitative assay, SuperQuant, Abbott RealTime [135]. To evaluate the response to antiviral therapies is possible analyze the absence or alteration of genetic material in clinical specimens from successfully treated patients. In situ hybridization (ISH) enables visualization of specific nucleic acid in morphologically preserved cells and tissue sections. The anti-sense probe detected HCV RNA, with a sensitivity and specificity of 95% and 100%, respectively. HCV genomic RNA can be variably distributed in tissue sections and was located primarily in the perinuclear regions in hepatocytes [149]. Viral hepatitis is one of the major health problems worldwide. Hepatitis delta virus (HDV) is also not uncommon world-wide. Hepatitis D virus (HDV) or delta virus is a defective virus. It requires the help of another virus that is hepatitis B virus for its multiplication. It always occur with HBV either in the form of co-infection or super-infection [150]. HCV, HBV, and HDV share parallel routes of transmission due to which dual or triple viral infection can occur in a proportion of patients at the same time. HBV and HCV are important factors in the development of liver cirrhosis (LC) and hepatocellular carcinoma [151]. In the diagnosis of co-infections, individually each infection (HBV, HCV and HDV) is confirmed by the presence of the serum surface antigen, hepatitis B, C and D envelope antigen and specific antibodies to the hepatitis B, C and D core [152]. By Deep Sequencing were readily detected at high coverage in plasma of patients with chronic viral hepatitis B and C. Although, this protocol also is adapted to other samples such as urine, bile, saliva and other body fluids by viral metagenomic survey [153]. For other side, other molecular technique as the protein micro-array gives a way to diagnosis multiple viral infections; using two viral antigens (HBsAg, HBeAg) and seven viral antibodies (HBsAb, HBcAb, HBeAb, HCVAb, HDVAb, HEVAb, HGVAb) of human hepatitis viruses [154]. Finally, the successful simultaneous detection of HAV, HBV and HCV was performed with the Magicplex HepaTrio Real-time Detection test, whose sensitivity and specificity of the HepaTrio test were 93.8% and 98.2%, respectively, for detecting HBV infection, and 99.1% and 100.0%, respectively, for HCV infection [155].

6. Mumps virus

Mumps is an acute viral infection caused by a member of the *Rubulavirus* genus in the *Paramyxoviridae* family. Mumps virus (MuV) is pleomorphic, enveloped, comprising a nucleocapsid core with helical structure composed of the 15384 nucleotide. Nonsegmented negative-sense RNA genome has the organization: 3′-NP-P-M-F-SH-HN-L-5′ [156]. The molecular epidemiology of MuV is characterized by the co-existence of 10 (or more) distinct genotypes named A-J based on the nucleotide sequence of the SH gene. MuV genotypes (C,

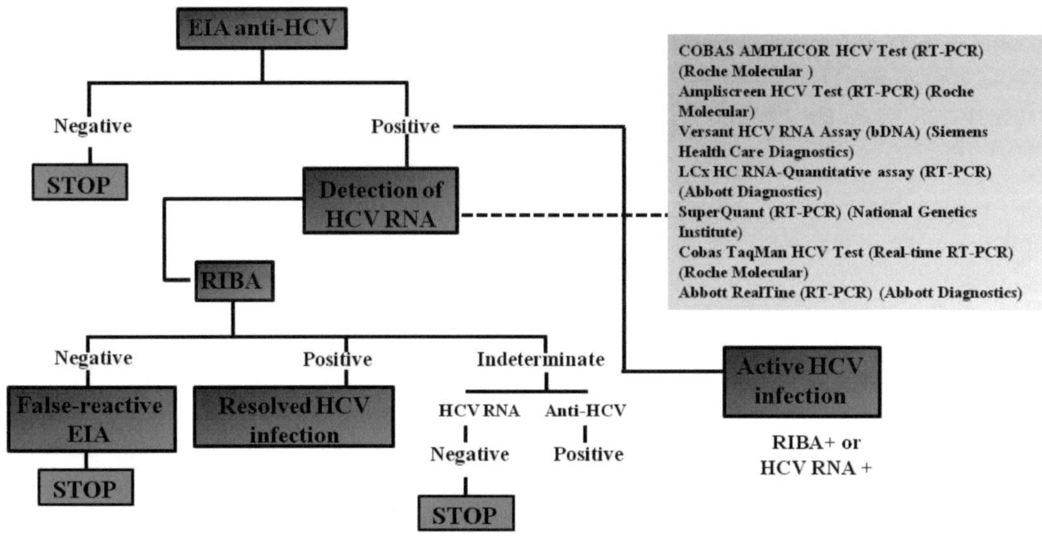

Figure 5. HCV Testing Algorithm and molecular assays.

D, H, J) and vaccine strains (Urabe Am9) have been associated with enhanced neurovirulence [157]. MuV is known to affect the salivary glands causing parotid swelling lasting at least two days, but may persist longer than ten days [158]. The mumps incubation period ranges from 12–25 days, but parotitis typically develops 16 to 18 days after exposure to mumps virus. The MuV also produce an acute systemic infection involving glandular, lymphoid and nervous tissues, leading to some important complications, the main central nervous system (CNS) complication of mumps virus infection is aseptic meningitis (in up to 15% of cases) [159, 160, 161]. Mumps epidemics are usually caused by airborne transmission of mumps virus (MuV) and have high morbidity in non-immunized children. Massive vaccination programs have decreased the incidence of MuV infection worldwide. The annual incidence of mumps in the absence of immunization was in the range of 100–1000 cases/100 000 people, outbreaks have not been completely eliminated even in populations with high vaccination coverage [162]. Laboratory confirmation of mumps infection can be made by the detection of immunoglobulin M (IgM) antibodies specific to mumps virus in acute-phase serum samples (gold standard for mumps diagnosis). Mumps virus can be detected from fluid collected from the parotid duct, other affected salivary gland ducts, the throat, from urine, and from cerebrospinal fluid (CSF). Parotid duct swabs yield the best viral sample. With previous contact with mumps virus either through vaccination or natural infection, serum mumps IgM test results may be negative; IgG test results may be positive at the initial blood draw. The serologic tests available for laboratory confirmation of mumps acute infection and confirmation of previous exposure to mumps vary among laboratories. Tests for IgM antibody includes Enzyme Immunoassay (EIA): a highly specific test for diagnosing acute mumps infection and Immunofluorescence assay (IFA) a test that is relatively inexpensive and simple, but the test is particularly susceptible to interference by high levels of mumps-specific IgG. A significant rise in IgG antibody titer, in acute-and convalescent-phase serum specimens is a positive result of infection. The presence of mumps-

http://dx.doi.org/10.5772/57581

specific IgG, detected using a serologic assay (EIA or IFA), is considered evidence of mumps immunity but does not predict the presence of neutralizing antibodies or protection from mumps disease [163]. A near patient test (NPT) for the detection of mumps-specific IgM in oral fluid specimens was developed and evaluated using 196 oral fluid specimens from suspected cases of mumps and measles. Compared to EIA, the sensitivity, specificity, positive and negative predictive value of the mumps IgM NPT were 79.5%, 100%, 100%, and 72.6%, respectively. Mumps IgM NPT is rapid and simple to perform for confirmation of a clinical diagnosis. The NPT strip is also a suitable matrix for preserving nucleic acid, enabling virus-specific RT-PCR to be performed [164]. Standard diagnostics that detect virus or virus-specific antibody are dependable for confirming primary mumps infection in immunologically naïve persons, but these methods perform inconsistently for individuals with prior immune exposure. Detection of activated mumps-specific antibody-secreting B cells (ASCs) by an enzyme-linked immunospot (ELISPOT) assay has the potential for use as an alternative method of diagnosis when suspect cases cannot be confirmed by detection of IgM or virus. The mumps-specific memory B cells are detected at a much lower frequency than measles-or rubella-specific cells, suggesting that mumps infection may not generate robust B-cell memory [165]. Successful virus isolation by cell culture should always be confirmed by immunofluorescence with a mumps-specific monoclonal antibody or by molecular techniques such as RT-PCR, nested-PCR or real-time RT-PCR [166-168]. In patients vaccinated, pre-existing vaccine-induced antibodies. Moreover, acute infection has to be demonstrated by direct detection of the virus by viral isolation or genomic amplification. RT-PCR allows a diagnosis and also forms the basis for genotype characterization by sequencing the SH gene, useful tool for mumps surveillance, management and control, according to WHO recommendations. Virus genotyping allows the building of a sequence database that will help to know transmission pathways of mumps strains circulating in the world and to distinguish wild-type mumps virus from vaccine virus [169]. Standard RT-PCR to detect the SH gene of mumps virus can be used to detect mumps RNA in clinical samples or in infected cell culture [170]. The sequence of the PCR product containing the coding region of the SH gene can be used to determine the viral genotype [171]. A multiplex real-time RT-PCR test for the detection of RNA from mumps virus in patient specimens, using primers and probes that target the mumps SH gene [172]. Several test of real-time RT-PCR are performed with TaqMan Assay [173]. A multiplex real-time RT-PCR assay, for rapid mumps diagnosis in a clinical setting. The assay used oligonucleotide primers and a TaqMan probe targeting the mumps SH gene. This test showed 100% correlation with results from viral culture. [172]. Other qRT-PCR assay is directed to the mumps virus F gene [174]. Recently, by RT-PCR it was detect a case of corneal endothelitis following the mumps parotitis [175].

7. Measles virus

Measles produces a highly contagious respiratory infection and may cause extensive epidemics. Measles is one of the most important causes of child morbidity and mortality. [176]. A safe and efficacious live attenuated virus vaccine is available toward global measles control [177,

178]. Measles vaccination is highly effective, safe and relatively cost-effective and has interrupted measles transmission in most parts of the world [179]. Despite tremendous achievements towards global measles mortality reduction and measles elimination goals, globally, in 2010, there were 327305 measles cases reported and an estimated 139300 measles deaths) [180, 181]. Mortality is highest in children and most acute measles deaths are due to secondary infections that result from a poorly understood measles-induced suppression of immune responses [182]. In addition to the risks of acute infection, children under the age of 2 years are also vulnerable to development of subacute sclerosing panencephalitis (SSPE), a progressive, uniformly fatal neurologic disease associated with persistent measles virus infection of the nervous system, have documented high levels of antibody to measles virus [183]. Other diseases related to measles are systemic lupus erythematosus [184] and multiple sclerosis [185]. The measles virus is a member of the Morbillivirus genus of the family Paramyxoviridae. The virions are pleomorphic and range in size from 100 to 300 nm. The measles virus is antigenically stable and genetic differences are few among vaccine strains. Wild-type viruses are more variable. Several different genotypes of wild measles virus are currently circulating worldwide and this genetic variation provides the basis for the application of molecular epidemiological techniques to study the transmission of measles virus [186]. Laboratory confirmation of clinically diagnosed measles was traditionally based on methods such as immunofluorescence antibody for detection of viral antigen and haemagglutination inhibition (HI), haemolysin inhibition, complement fixation, and plaque-reduction neutralization (PRN) for detection of measles antibody in serum (Table 4) [187]. Currently, detection of measles-specific IgM antibody and measles RNA by real-time RT-PCR are the most common methods for confirmation of measles infection [168]. Initially laboratory confirmation of cases of measles infection is performed by detection of measles-specific immunoglobulin M (IgM) antibodies, the test of choice for rapid diagnosis of measles cases in a single serum specimen collected within the first few days of rash onset, usually become detectable in serum after four days post onset of rash (90-100% sensitivity) and decline rapidly after one month. The virus can be detected in serum samples, blood spots, throat swab (or nasopharyngeal swab), urine and or collection of both respiratory and urine samples that can increase the likelihood of detecting virus. [188]. Oral fluids can also be used to detect viral ribonucleic acid (RNA) [189]. The enzyme immunoassay is the most commonly used method for detecting measles-specific IgM or IgG antibodies. Both capture and indirect formats for IgM detection are available commercially. Some tests available are LIAISON IgM measles (DiaSorin, Saluggia, Italy) a new automated chemiluminescence immunoassay and the enzyme immunoassay (EIA) Enzygnost (Siemens, Marburg, Germany), which have a a sensitivity of 93.7% and 98.8%, whereas the specificity was 96.8% and 97.9%, respectively [190]. DiaSorin Liaison (Saluggia, Italy) is other option for measles diagnosis, with a sensitivity and specificity for measles IgM of 92% and 100% respectively [191]. Commercially, there are some test directs to simultaneous detection of measles and rubella as Enzygnost (Siemens) and Platelia (Bio-Rad), useful for detecting IgM against measles and rubella [192].

In acute, uncomplicated measles, there is a significant rise in measles-specific IgG antibodies between acute-and convalescent-phase serum specimens. A positive test result for specific IgG antibodies in a serum indicates past infection with measles virus or measles vaccination, but does not ensure protection from infection or re-infection. Screening the young adult population about to enter college or the military, pregnant women, and other individuals at risk, for seropositivity, is a valuable tool for determining their immune status.

LABORATORY TEST
Serological assays Using serum sample Detection of IgM antibody by indirect IgM ELISA, IgM-capture ELISA or EIA for IgM Detection of IgG antibody by IgG ELISA Virus neutralization test HI
Cell culture and immunofluorescence microscopy Using urine, nasopharyngeal swabs or blood lymphocytes and detect to virus using specific measles antibody
NAT analysis measles RNA can be detected from nasopharyngeal swab, urine or peripheral blood lymphocytes (oral fluid/ throat swabs) up to 5 days post disease manifestation. RT-PCR, RT-nested PCR, Real-Time RT-PCR and sequencing

Table 4. Laboratory diagnosis for measles in clinical materials.

Enzyme-linked immunosorbent assay (ELISA) is normally used to quantify the amount of serum IgG antibodies against measles (measles in addition to mumps, rubella, and varicella-zoster virus, MMRV). However, a multiplex immunoassay for the simultaneous detection of antibodies against MMRV showed be a good alternative to conventional ELISAs and suitable for use in serosurveillance and vaccine studies [193]. An enzyme linked Immunosorbent commercial assay is Captia Measles IgG based (Trinity, Biotech, USA). In countries where disease prevalence is low, intensified surveillance typically implemented during and after an importation will result in some false positive IgM results since no assay is 100% specific. So, it is necessary to introduce other techniques of diagnosis related to ARN genome. In the Fifth Hands-on Training on the Laboratory Diagnosis of Measles and Rubella focusing on Molecular Detection and Sequence Analysis, in Hong Kong, China. It was exposed the need of introduce the molecular detection of measles and rubella viruses using new real-time polymerase chain reaction (PCR) as well as conventional PCR, quantitative real-time PCR and others molecular techniques such as sequencing. Dr Paul Rota (Chief, Measles Virus Section, Centers for Disease Control and Prevention USA), presented on the use of real-time and conventional RT-PCR for case classification and molecular surveillance of measles virus. These tests can detect 10-100 copies of RNA/sample in a high throughput format and produce results within two hours. It can help to confirm a case when serologic results are inconclusive but negative results do not rule out a case. These molecular tests are more sensitive than conventional (endpoint) RT-PCR. Sequence information from the conventional PCR is required for genotype assignment and confirmation of vaccine reactions [194].

Measles RNA can be detected (oral fluid/ throat swabs) up to 5 days post disease manifestation. Molecular assays to measles virus includes measles H (haemagglutinin) gene real-time PCR and hybridization [195] and nucleic acid sequence analysis of the nested N-gene PCR amplicons (nucleocapsid) [196, 197]. A nested reverse transcriptase PCR (RT-PCR) that detected measles virus (MV) from dried filter papers was set up using MV infected cells diluted in sterile phosphate-buffered saline. Although, the nested RT-PCR results of low titer viruses dried onto filter papers are not reproducible and reliable [198, 199]. Detection of RNA in PBMC by RT-PCR is the most effective method for diagnosis of measles. A study performed in 2010, analyzed sixty-three throat swabs, 84 peripheral blood mononuclear cell (PBMC) samples, and 85 plasma samples were collected from 85 cases of suspected measles. The percentage of positive results from PBMC by RT-PCR and virus isolation was 100 and 91.7%, respectively. The percentage of positive results from throat swabs by RT-PCR and virus isolation was 91.2 and 52.8%, respectively [200]. Measles can produce congenital infections with a risk of neurological complications in the newborn. Mother-to-child transmission of the measles virus, it has been widely documented in the newborns either by RT-PCR in saliva or by IgM detection in blood. An early viral RT-PCR detection allows successful immunoglobulin prophylaxis in one newborn avoiding the development classical or neurological clinical signs of measles infection [201]. Molecular detection of measles virus has been optimized by amplification of nucleocapsid (N) and human RNase P mRNA for a one-step quantitative reverse transcription (qRT)-PCR [202]. The qRT-PCR for measles diagnosis can use SYBR Green or TaqMan (ABI) in real-time reverse transcription-polymerase chain reaction (RT-PCR) assays. For the real-time RT-PCR, primer sets are design from a region of the MV H gene of the Edmonston strain (genotype A) and a TaqMan probe specific for the H gene of genotype D MV [203]. Currently, is possible estimate the titer of measles, mumps and rubella (MMR) viruses by a TaqMan-based real-time reverse transcription-polymerase chain reaction (qPCR-RT) assay optimized in infected cell culture supernatants [204]. For genetic typing of measles virus in clinical samples is xMAP technology that employs specific oligonucleotide probes of genotypes D4, D6 and D7 of virus [205]. Other alternative employed for the genotype analysis of measles virus is sequencing of the 450 nucleotide of nucleoprotein gene (N450) that contributes to the genetic characterization of wild-type measles viruses and offers data in the study of viral transmission pathways. N450 is amplifying with the primer pair, MeV216/MeV214. It is clear that the molecular tools improvement the molecular characterization of circulating measles viruses globally and provides enhanced quality control measures [206]. Demonstration of the usefulness of molecular tests in the diagnosis of measles during outbreaks or epidemic peaks was reported in an outbreak in Paris (France) in 2011. 171 oral fluid samples and 235 serum samples collected from 270 patients were tested using a novel one-step real-time RT-PCR assay. This study showed that the detection rate of MV-RNA by RT-PCR was 98% (100/102) for oral fluid and 95% (97/102) for serum samples. The detection rate of MV-IgM was 85% (87/102). In addition, it was found than during the early stage of infection, the MV-RNA viral load in serum was lower in patient's positive than in those negative for MV-IgG [207]. The detection and identification of the virus in cell culture may take several weeks. The samples should undergo virus isolation on sensitive cell lines, such as B95a cells. Measles virus can be isolated from clinical specimens, including; throat swab, conjunctival swabs, nasopharyngeal aspirates or urine [208].

8. HIV

Acquired Immunodeficiency Syndrome (AIDS) is one of the most critically acclaimed endemic diseases, caused by two lentiviruses HIV-1 and 2. Human immunodeficiency virus (HIV) is the pathogen causing the acquired immunodeficiency syndrome (AIDS) [209, 210]. HIV is an enveloped virus with tropism for CD4+lymphocytes and monocytes. HIV is classified in the family *Retroviridae*, subfamily *Lentivirinae*, and genus *Lentivirus*. HIV comprising a single stranded, positive-sense ribonucleic acid (RNA) genome of about 9.7 kilobases. From the 5' end of genome are located the three genes that characterize retroviruses: *gag-pol-env*. The *gag* gene codes for the internal structural proteins, the *pol* gene for the three viral enzymes, and the *env* gene for the envelope glycoproteins. LTR (Long Terminal Repeat) sequences are found at each extremity of the genome, containing the signals for the regulation of expression of the viral genes. The genome also has six additional genes called "accessory" genes: *vif, nef, vpr, tat, rev* and *vpu* (HIV-1) or *vpx* (HIV-2) [211]. There are two strands of HIV RNA and each strand has a copy with nine genes, which encode 15 proteins. The RNA is surrounding by a cone - shaped capsid which consists of approximately 2000 copies of the p24 viral protein. Surrounding the capsid is the viral envelope. Each envelope subunit consists of two non-covalently linked membrane proteins: glycoprotein (gp) 120, the outer envelope protein, and gp41, the transmembrane protein that anchors the glycoprotein complex to the surface of the virion. The envelope protein is the most variable component of HIV, although gp120 itself is structurally divided into highly variable (V) and more constant (C) regions. The variability of the HIV envelope also confers a uniquely complex antigenic diversity. The virion contains three enzymes necessary for multiplication: reverse transcriptase (enables the viral RNA to be transcribed into DNA), and endonuclease (enables the DNA to be integrated into the host cell, the viral genome then becomes proviral DNA) and the protease (enables the virus to mature at a late stage in the cycle of intracellular multiplication). The presence of two copies of the retroviral genome in each particle promotes genetic recombination between the RNAs. This and the high error rate of the viral reverse transcriptase leads to considerable genetic variation in the viral progeny. AIDS is characterized by the selective targeting of the CD4+/CD8+T cells by HIV which fatally impairs the immune system. The window period for this retrovirus is from several weeks to few months altogether before detection of earliest antibodies in blood serum raised against HIV [210]. HIV infection is one of the major threats to human health due to the lack of relevant vaccine and drugs to cure AIDS. Its early diagnosis is thus important in controlling HIV transmission. With acute HIV infection, high levels of infectious virus are detectable in serum and genital secretions. The rate of transmission during acute HIV infection is higher than the established HIV infection, for this reason, new HIV testing strategies need to focus on sensitivity, especially for this highly contagious phase immediately after infection. There are two types of virus, HIV-1 and HIV-2, which are further divided into groups and/or subtypes. The pandemic is caused by HIV-1 group M. HIV-1 and HIV-2 have differences as clinical progression of the disease is slower and mother-to-child transmission is less likely with HIV-2 than with HIV-1 (maternal-fetal transmission < 2% in the absence of treatment). Recombinant HIV strains are known as CRF (Circulating Recombinant Forms). Although HIV-2 is also associated with AIDS, it is not transmitted as readily and, generally speaking, progression toward immunodeficiency is much slower in individuals with an HIV-2 infection. HIV-1 is responsible for a chronic infection that gradually develops and causes the destruction of the body's CD4+T lymphocytes. HIV-1 is responsible for a chronic infection that gradually causes the destruction of $CD4^{+}T$ lymphocytes [212]. To detect a HIV infection several tests are used to analyze the HIV infection status of a patient, evaluate the progression of disease, and monitor the effectiveness of antiretroviral therapy (ART). HIV infection can be diagnosed by direct visualization of virions or electron microscopy; cultivation by lymphocyte culture; measurement of HIV-specific serologic responses; detection of viral antigens; and detection of viral nucleic acids [213]. For many years, laboratory diagnosis of HIV is based on the identification of HIV antibodies using immuno-enzymatic (ELISA) tests or other immunological techniques of equivalent sensitivity. Still considering the limitation of this approach in the known 'window period' between the time of infection and the initial instance of detectable antibody, this may last for several weeks. Primary infection is asymptomatic in more than 50% of cases. In the remaining cases, symptoms appear two to three weeks after infection and clinical signs usually resemble those of flu-like or mononucleosis syndromes. Plasma viraemia levels are generally high ($\geq 10^6$ copies of viral genome/ml) during primary infection.

An assay useful in Multispot HIV-1/HIV-2 Rapid Test (BIO-RAD) directed to a rapid test for detection and differentiation of HIV-1 and HIV-2 antibodies in human serum and plasma. This test have a time of results of 10 minute and shows HIV-1 sensitivity: 100%, HIV-2 sensitivity: 100% and specificity: 99.9% [214]. BIO-RAD also has an assay know as HIV-1/HIV-2 PLUS O, an ELISA-immuno assay utilizing recombinant proteins and synthetic peptides for the detection of antibodies to HIV-1 (groups M and O) and/or HIV-2.

New HIV screening tests approved by the US FDA in 2010-2011 include immunoassays capable of detecting p24 antigen and HIV antibody simultaneously. The fourth generation combo assays could reduction the window period due to their ability to detect viral protein s in addition to IgG and IgM class antibodies against both HIV-1 and HIV-2 [215], but the monitoring of HIV disease progression is mostly accomplished by the quantitation of CD4 T cells and viral RNA [216]. The use of combined ELISA tests called "4th generation" tests, enables for more effective early detection of infections which are very often asymptomatic. Also, these assays can detect acute and chronic infections. An example is the ARCHITECT HIV Ag/Ab Combo assay (Abbott Diagnostics), which uses anti-HIV-1 p24 antibodies as reagents to detect HIV-1 p24 antigen, thereby decreasing the window period and improving early detection of HIV infection. The assay is useful to determine the presence of HIV-1 p24 antigen, antibodies to HIV-1 (group M and group O), and antibodies to HIV-2 in human serum or plasma using chemiluminescent microparticle immunoassay A technology. The test has an analytical sensitivity of <50 pg/mL for HIV-1 p24 antigen [217]. There are others fourth-generation human immunodeficiency virus-1 (HIV-1) screening assays as the AxSYM HIV Ag/Ab Combo (Abbott

http://dx.doi.org/10.5772/57581

diagnostics, Delkenheim, Germany), Elecsys 2010 HIV Combi (Roche Diagnostics GmbH, Mannheim, Germany) and Vidas HIV Duo Quick (Biomerieux, France). All of the assays had sensitivities of 100% on clinical samples. The specificities of the AxSYM, ARCHITECT, Elecsys 2010 HIV Combi, and Elecsys HIV Combi PT were 99.6, 99.6, 99.0, and 99.5%, respectively [218]. Genscreen Ultra HIV Ag-Ab is other new version of the HIV p24 antigen and antibody combination assays [218]. The commercial ELISAs such as Vironostika HIV Ag/Ab, Enzygnost Anti-HIV 1/2 Plus Genscreen HIV-1/2 Version 2 and INNO-LIA HIV I/II are suitable tools for making HIV test performance accessible to people [219]. The accurate diagnosis of HIV infection demands that to consider a positive result, at least three assays with different antigenic base should be used, one of them, Western-Blot being mandatory for confirmation. Confirmatory techniques which are used most frequently they are the Western Blot (WB) and the recombinant immunoblot or immunoassay online (LIA) who have at least the same sensitivity than ELISA and a higher specificity. Both techniques they can incorporate antigens of HIV-2. It detects antibodies against the glycoprotein gp160 envelope, gp120 and gp41, p55, p24 and p17 encoded-gag and p66, p51 and p311. The interpretation of the results is crucial; a negative test is the total absence of reactivity. To assess, the positivity numerous criteria applied, according to the Center for Disease Control (CDC) a positive result occurs with at least 2 bands of p24, gp41, and gp160gp120 are detected. WHO recognizes a positive test with 2 bands. The ARC (American Red Cross) indicates three bands, one of each structural gene, and the Consortium for Retrovirus Serology Standardization indicates at least one of gp120 or gp160 and one of p24 or p31 [220, 221]. It is interpreted as an undetermined result, any reactivity that does not meet the minimum criteria of positivity. Since, the causes of WB indeterminate are diverse and they may correspond to early phases or advanced stages of infection associated to severe immune impairment, or to the presence of immune complexes than can reduce the antibodies circulating, between other causes. Detection of some band of envelope with or without bands of gag gene, may be due to HIV infection. In these cases, is necessary performed others confirmatory tests as LIA and sometimes complement them with the determination of proviral DNA or viral load or p24 antigen to assess a possible primoinfeccion. In any case on an indeterminate WB is required a new sample [222-224]. The comparison between the Ag/Ab combo assay and RNA viral load showed that in an acute HIV infection in human gave a similar result. HIV Combo detected 97% of infections acute. The ARCHITECT HIV Combo assay can detect p24 Ag when RNA is above approximately 58,000 copies/mL [225]. However, the comparison between the results of HIV RNA nucleic acid test (NAT) and 4th-generation Ag/Ab assay (ARCHITEC HIV Ag/Ab Combo [HIV Combo] assay, Abbott Diagnostics) in 2744 HIV antibody-negative samples were identified fourteen people with acute HIV infection (HIV antibody negative/NAT positive). The HIV Combo assay detected nine of these individuals [226 delete these rows, from the stage word to the HIV Word [226In the 2012 HIV Diagnostics Conference: the molecular diagnostics perspective, gives in Atlanta, GA, USA, 12–14 December 2012. The forum was foccusing in the evaluation of molecular diagnostics and their role in HIV diagnosis. Many scientific presentations exposed the role played by RNA testing and new developments in molecular diagnostics, including detection of total and integrated HIV-1 DNA, detection and quantification of HIV-2 RNA, and rapid formats for detection of HIV-1 RNA [227]. HIV infection monitoring is based on counting the number of $CD4^{+}$lymphocytes and quantification of plasma viral RNA. These tests are performed every 6 months if the CD4 count is > 500/mm^3 and every 3 to 4 months if the CD4 count is between 200 and 500/mm^3. Plasma viral load is measured using quantitative tests based on molecular tools: gene amplification (PCR-polymerase chain reaction, LCR-ligase chain reaction, TMA-transcription mediated amplification, NASBA-nucleic acid sequence based amplification) or hybridization followed by signal amplification (bDNA-branched DNA). Most tests have sensitivity of the order of 50-100 copies/ml. Although the new HIV diagnostic algorithm relies on RNA assays as a supplemental test, it is not clear how accessible these assays will be for clinical laboratories. Currently, only one HIV RNA test is approved by the US FDA for HIV diagnosis (Hologic Gen-Probe APTIMA HIV-1 RNA Qualitative Assay) and some clinical laboratories may need to send specimens out for RNA testing. Currently, molecular diagnosis of HIV infection is only used as a complementary diagnosis although viral load test is used to monitor disease progression and responsiveness to antiviral therapy. Recently, it was proposed to the first-line HIV molecular techniques performed on a routine basis routed to the use of HIV molecular tools for the screening of blood products, organs and tissue from human origin. Directed to medically assisted procreation and in neonates from HIV-infected mothers [228]. In 2012 HIV Diagnostics Conference was presented the design of a new HIV-1 proviral DNA assay capable of detecting two copies of HIV-1 DNA in a qualitative format and quantitatively of three to 30,000 copies per ml. Since the lack a nucleic acid test for HIV-2, in this meeting was described a novel HIV-2 RNA viral load assay based on the 5′ long terminal repeat of HIV-2, with a lower quantification limit of 29 infectious units per ml. In addition, an assay capable of detecting HIV-2 proviral DNA, which combines three separate amplification reactions from three regions of the proviral genome, detected both A and B HIV-2 subtypes at between five and ten copies of the HIV-2 proviral genome [228]. For other side, HIV-1 detection in plasma samples with a molecular beacon-based multiplex NASBA assay of a region in the HIV-1 pol gene showed a limit of quantification of the assay was <1000 copies/ml for HIV-1 with 98% sensitivity and 100% specificity [229]. Also, it was reported the detection and quantification of HIV-1 group O RNA in plasma by an RT-qPCR assay [230]. In addition, there are several HIV molecular assays showed in the table 5 [231].

Routine follow-up of HIV-infected individuals includes measurement of CD4$^+$T cell count to evaluate the immune status, of viral load to assess virus replication directed to events of therapeutic failure (therapeutic escape), and of changes in the viral genome to characterize resistance to drugs and tropism. Genotype resistance testing can detect a potential viral escape due to poor compliance with the treatment regimen, metabolic problems or the selection of resistant mutants. In summary, the diagnosis of HIV infection is established by one of the following methods: detecting antibodies to the virus; detecting the viral p24 antigen; detecting viral nucleic acid; or culturing HIV.

The most widely used test is the detection of antibodies to HIV [232]. Rapid serological tests take only 15 minutes with acceptable specificity and sensibility. But, there is the possibility of have a negative false result with them. NATs are assays more sensitive in HIV diagnosis, but more expensive. The expanded use of point-of-care (POC) tests to HIV testing plays an important role in HIV prevention, both in developed and in developing countries [233]. The

http://dx.doi.org/10.5772/57581

METHOD AND NAME TEST
DNA/RNA qualitative assays used to diagnosis HIV
APTIMA HIV-1 RNA Qualitative assay or Procleix HIV-1/HCV Assay (Gen Probe)
RNAviral load testing used for clinical diagnosis and/or monitoring of HIV-1
COBAS AmpliPrep/TaqMan HIV-1 (Roche Molecular)
Versant HIV-1RNA (Siemens)
NucliSens HIV RNA QT (bioMérieux)
RealTime m2000 HIV-1 (Abbott Molecular)
Genotyping drug used to Antiretroviral drug resistance
TruGene HIV-1 genotyping (Siemens)
ViroSeq HIV-1 genotyping (Abbott Molecular)
HIV PRT GeneChip assay (Affymetrix)
HIV RT Line Probe assay (Innogenetics)
Phenotyping drug used to Antiretroviral drug resistance
AntiVirogram assay (Virco Lab)
Trofile (MonoGram BioSciences)
SensiTrop II HIV (Pathway Diagnostics)
Information based on Tang YW, et al. 2012 [231].

Table 5. Main molecular diagnostics methods for HIV-1.

access to immediate HIV test results could improve the application of prophylactic regimens to reduce vertical transmission when used intrapartum or postpartum [234].

The analysis of the cost-effectiveness of initial diagnosis with a rapid HIV test, to screen out HIV-uninfected infants shows that in the comparison of DNA-PCR and rapid HIV test approaches, the first assay identified 94.3% (91.8–94.7%) of HIV-infected infants, as compared with 87.8% (79.4–90.5%) for the latter. Moreover, the total cost of the POC testing program was about 40% less than that of DNA-PCR ($59 vs. $38 per infant aged 6–9 months). Assessing the cost-effectiveness of several HIV testing as well as establishing a specific threshold of positivity for routine testing of HIV dignosis will be critical in AIDS control [235, 236]. Despite the global effort to control the AIDS pandemic, human immunodeficiency virus (HIV) infection continues to spread relatively unabated in many parts of the world. As the AIDS epidemic continues is necessary establish new strategies of prevention, treatment and molecular diagnostics assays to discriminate "window phase" infections from those that are serologically positive. There is opportunity to implement and evaluate the incremental diagnostic usefulness of new test modalities that are based on sophisticated molecular diagnostic technologies and that can be performed in settings where laboratory infrastructure is minimal [237]. Human immunodeficiency virus type 1 (HIV-1) is a highly diverse virus, a global scale, and within individual HIV-1 infected subjects [238]. The genetic variants constituting the viral population are called haplotypes, and these haplotypes form a viral quasispecies [239]. This viral diversity is highly relevant on pathogenesis, drug resistance, and vaccine development. Currently, virus populations can be studied much faster using next-generation sequencing (NGS) platforms. NGS is a valuable tool for the detection and quantification of HIV-1 variants *in vivo* [240, 241]. As Venet exhibited in 2004, a major evolution in the near future will be the generalization of NAT for the diagnosis of viral etiology in patients, mostly with respiratory, CNS or hepatic diseases. Major technical improvements have been made to avoid obstacles that still limit this generalization, related to genetic variability of viruses, multiplex detection or contamination risk [242]. Real-time amplification has allowed the development of new NAT platforms and the introduction of others techniques as NGS than contributes with data that support to global diagnostic [243].

In this chapter was presented the some methods applied to diagnosis and monitoring of an infectious disease of viral etiology with global incidence, such as hepatitis, mumps or influenza that have been authorized by WHO and CDC. In addition, new applications of molecular techniques that facilitate fast identification of the etiology of an infectious disease were presented.

Author details

Nora Rosas-Murrieta[1], Irma Herrera-Camacho[1], Lourdes Millán-Pérez-Peña[1], Francisca Sosa-Jurado[2], Gerardo Santos-López[2], Verónica Vallejo-Ruíz[2] and Julio Reyes-Leyva[2]

*Address all correspondence to: nora.rosas@correo.buap.mx

1 Laboratorio de Bioquímica y Biología Molecular. Centro de Química, Instituto de Ciencias, Benemérita Universidad Autónoma de Puebla, México

2 Laboratorio de Biología Molecular y Virología, Centro de Investigación Biomédica de Oriente, Instituto Mexicano del Seguro Social, Metepec, Puebla, México

References

[1] Baker C, Antonovics J. Evolutionary Determinants of Genetic Variation in Susceptibility to Infectious Diseases in Humans. *PLoS ONE* 2012; 7(1): e29089.

[2] Wilson ME. The traveller and emerging infections: Sentinel, courier, transmitter. *J Appl Microbiol.* 2003; 94(Suppl): 1S–11S.

[3] Speers DJ. Clinical applications of molecular biology for infectious diseases. *Clin Biochem Rev.* 2006; 27(1): 39-51.

[4] Cobo F. Application of molecular diagnostic techniques for viral testing. *The Open Virology Journal*. 2012; 6, (Suppl 1: M7) 104-114.

[5] Muldrew KL. Molecular diagnostics of infectious diseases. *Current Opinion in Pediatrics*. 2009, 21: 102–111.

[6] Liao Y, Wang X, Sha C, Xia Z, Huang Q, Li Q. Combination of fluorescence color and melting temperature as a two-dimensional label for homogeneous multiplex PCR detection. *Nucleic Acids Res*. 2013; 41(7):e76.

[7] Briese T, Palacios G, Kokoris M, Jabado O, Liu Z, Renwick N, Kapoor V, Casas I, Pozo F, Limberger R, Perez-Brena P, Ju J, Lipkin WI. Diagnostic system for rapid and sensitive differential detection of pathogens. Emerg Infect Dis. 2005; 11(2):310-3.

[8] Chen EC, Miller SA, DeRisi JL, Chiu CY.Using a pan-viral microarray assay (Virochip) to screen clinical samples for viral pathogens. *J Vis Exp*. 2011; (50). pii: 2536.

[9] Mosammaparast N, McAdam AJ. Molecular testing for infectious diseases should be done in the clinical microbiology laboratory. *Journal of Clinical Microbiology*. 2012; 50(6): 1836–1840.

[10] Dengue. Guidelines for diagnosis, treatment prevention and control. Geneva, TDR/WHO, 2009. WHO/HTM/NTD/DEN/2009.

[11] Rodenhuis-Zybert IA, Wilschut J, Smit JM. Dengue virus life cycle: viral and host factors modulating infectivity. *Cell. Mol. Life Sci.* 2010; 67 (16): 2773–2786.

[12] Chambers TJ, Hahn CS, Galler R, Rice CM. Flavivirus genome organization, expression and replication. *Annu Rev Microbiol.* 1990; 44: 649—688.

[13] Guzman MG, Rosario D, Kouri G. In: Kalitzky M and Borowski P, eds. Diagnosis of dengue virus infection. Molecular Biology of the flaviviruses. Horizon Bioscience, UK, 2009.

[14] Halstead SB. Dengue: the syndromic basis to pathogenesis research. Inutility of the 2009 WHO case definition. *Am J Trop Med Hyg*. 2013; 88(2): 212-215.

[15] WHO. Dengue and dengue haemorrhagic fever. Factsheet No 117, revised May 2008. Geneva, World Health Organization, 2008.

[16] Rigau-Pérez JG, Clark GG, Gubler DJ, Reiter P, Sanders EJ, Vorndam AV. Dengue and dengue haemorrhagic fever. *Lancet.* 1998; 352(9132): 971-977.

[17] Deen JL, Harris E, Wills B, Balmaseda A, Hammond SN, Rocha C, Dung NM, Hung NT, Hien TT, Farrar JJ. The WHO dengue classification and case definitions: time for a reassessment. *Lancet.* 2006; 368(9530): 170-173.

[18] Oishi K, Saito M, Mapua CA, Natividad FF. Dengue illness: clinical features and pathogenesis. *J Infect Chemother*. 2007; 13(3): 125-133.

[19] WHO. Global strategy for dengue prevention and control 2012-2020. Geneva. TDR/World Health Organization, 2009.

[20] De Paula SO, Fonseca BA. Dengue: a review of the laboratory tests a clinician must know to achieve a correct diagnosis. *Braz J Infect Dis.* 2004; 8(6): 390-398.

[21] Handbook for clinical management of dengue. Geneva. TDR/World Health Organization. 2012. Chapter 4. Laboratory Diagnosis and Diagnostic Tests. Dengue Guidelines for Diagnosis, Treatment, Prevention and Control. Geneva. TDR/World Health Organization. 2012.

[22] Nunes MR, Nunes Neto JP, Casseb SM, Nunes KN, Martins LC, Rodrigues SG, Matheus S, Dussart P, Casseb LM, Vasconcelos PF. Evaluation of an immunoglobulin M-specific capture enzyme-linked immunosorbent assay for rapid diagnosis of dengue infection. *J Virol Methods.* 2011; 171(1): 13-20.

[23] Ho TS, Wang SM, Lin YS, Liu CC. Clinical and laboratory predictive markers for acute dengue infection. *J Biomed Sci.* 2013; 20(1): 75.

[24] Guzman MG, Kouri G. Dengue diagnosis, advances and challenges. *Int J Infect Dis.* 2004; 8: 69-80.

[25] Guzman MG, Halstead SB, Artsob H, Buchy P, Farrar J, Gubler DJ, Hunsperger E, Kroeger A, Margolis HS, Martínez E, Nathan MB, Pelegrino JL, Simmons C, Yoksan S, Peeling RW. Dengue: a continuing global threat. *Nat Rev Microbiol.* 2010; 8(12 Suppl): S7-S16.

[26] Chaiyaratana W, Chuansumrit A, Pongthanapisith V, Tangnararatchakit K, Lertwongrath S, Yoksan S. Evaluation of dengue nonstructural protein 1 antigen strip for the rapid diagnosis of patients with dengue infection. *Diagn Microbiol Infect Dis.* 2009, 64(1): 83–84.

[27] Lima MR, Nogueira RM, Schatzmayr HG, dos Santos FB. Comparison of three commercially available dengue NS1 antigen capture assays for acute diagnosis of dengue in Brazil. *PLoS Negl Trop Dis.* 2010; 4: e738.

[28] Fry SR, Meyer M, Semple MG, Simmons CP, Sekaran SD, Huang JX, McElnea C, Huang CY, Valks A, Young PR, Cooper MA.The diagnostic sensitivity of dengue rapid test assays is significantly enhanced by using a combined antigen and antibody testing approach. *PLoS Negl Trop Dis.* 2011; 5(6): e1199.

[29] Lima Mda R, Nogueira RM, Schatzmayr HG, de Filippis AM, Limonta D, dos Santos FB. A new approach to dengue fatal cases diagnosis: NS1 antigen capture in tissues. *PLoS Negl Trop Dis.* 2011; 5(5): e1147.

[30] Kyle JL, Harris E. Global spread and persistence of dengue. *Annu Rev Microbiol.* 2008; 62: 71-92.

[31] Peeling RW, Artsob H, Pelegrino JL, Buchy P, Cardosa MJ, Devi S, Enria DA, Farrar J, Gubler DJ, Guzman MG, Halstead SB, Hunsperger E, Kliks S, Margolis HS, Nathan-

son CM, Nguyen VC, Rizzo N, Vázquez S, Yoksan S. Evaluation of diagnostic tests: dengue. *Nat Rev Microbiol.* 2010; 8(12 Suppl): S30-S38.

[32] De Paula SO, Fonseca BA. Dengue: a review of the laboratory tests a clinician must know to achieve a correct diagnosis. *Braz J Infect Dis.* 2004; 8(6): 390-398.

[33] Bhatnagar J, Blau DM, Shieh WJ, Paddock CD, Drew C, Liu L, Jones T, Patel M, Zaki SR. Molecular detection and typing of dengue viruses from archived tissues of fatal cases by rt-PCR and sequencing: diagnostic and epidemiologic implications. *Am J Trop Med Hyg.* 2012; 86(2): 335-340.

[34] De Paula SO, Nunes C, Matos R, de Oliveira ZM, Lima DM, da Fonseca BA. Comparison of techniques for extracting viral RNA from isolation-negative serum for dengue diagnosis by the polymerase chain reaction. *J Virol Methods.* 2001; 98(2): 119-125.

[35] De Paula SO, Pires Neto RJ, Corrêa JA, Assumpção SR, Costa ML, Lima DM, Fonseca BA. The use of reverse transcription-polymerase chain reaction (RT-PCR) for the rapid detection and identification of dengue virus in an endemic region: a validation study. *Trans R Soc Trop Med Hyg.* 2002; 96(3): 266-269.

[36] Houng HS, Chung-Ming Chen R, Vaughn DW, Kanesa-thasan N. Development of a fluorogenic RT-PCR system for quantitative identification of dengue virus serotypes 1-4 using conserved and serotype-specific 3' noncoding sequences. *J Virol. Methods.* 2001; 95: 19-32.

[37] Odreman-Macchioli M, Vielma S, Atchley D, Comach G, Ramirez A, Pérez S, Téllez L, Quintero B, Hernández E, Muñoz M, Mendoza J. Analysis of real time PCR amplification efficiencies from three genomic region of dengue virus. *Invest Clin.* 2013; 54(1): 5-19.

[38] Thaís M. Conceic¸ ão, Andrea T. Da Poian, Marcos H.F. Sorgine. A real-time PCR procedure for detection of dengue virus serotypes 1, 2, and 3, and their quantitation in clinical and laboratory samples. Journal of Virological Methods. 2010; 163: 1–9.

[39] KR Gurukumar, D Priyadarshini, JA Patil, A Bhagat, A Singh, PS Shah and D Cecilia. Development of real time PCR for detection and quantitation of Dengue Viruses. *Virology J.* 2009; 6: 10-18.

[40] Jesse J. Waggoner, Janaki Abeynayake, Malaya K. Sahoo, Lionel Gresh, Yolanda Tellez, Karla Gonzalez, Gabriela Ballesteros, Anna M. Pierro, Paolo Gaibani, Frances P. Guo, Vittorio Sambri, Angel Balmaseda, Kumudu Karunaratne, Eva Harris, Benjamin A. Pinsky. Single-Reaction, Multiplex, Real-Time RT-PCR for the Detection, Quantitation, and Serotyping of Dengue Viruses. *PLoS Negl Trop Dis.* 2013; 7(4): e2116.

[41] Das S, Pingle MR, Muñoz-Jordán J, Rundell MS, Rondini S, Granger K, Chang GJ, Kelly E, Spier EG, Larone D, Spitzer E, Barany F, Golightly LM. Detection and sero-

typing of dengue virus in serum samples by multiplex reverse transcriptase PCR-ligase detection reaction assay. *J Clin Microbiol.* 2008; 46(10): 3276-84.

[42] Takanori Hirayama, Yasutaka Mizuno, Nozomi Takeshita, Akira Kotaki, Shigeru Tajima, Tsutomu Omatsu, Kouichi Sano, Ichiro Kurane, Tomohiko Takasaki. Detection of Dengue Virus Genome in Urine by Real-Time Reverse Transcriptase PCR: a Laboratory Diagnostic Method Useful after Disappearance of the Genome in Serum. *J Clin Microbiol.* 2012; 50(6): 2047–2052.

[43] Santiago GA, Vergne E, Quiles Y, Cosme J, Vazquez J, Medina JF, Medina F, Colón C, Margolis H, Muñoz-Jordán JL. Analytical and clinical performance of the CDC real time RT-PCR assay for detection and typing of dengue virus. P*LoS Negl Trop Dis.* 2013; 7(7): e2311.

[44] Yozwiak NL, Skewes-Cox P, Stenglein MD, Balmaseda A, Harris E, DeRisi JL. Virus identification in unknown tropical febrile illness cases using deep sequencing. *PLoS Negl Trop Dis.* 2012; 6(2): e1485.

[45] Harper SA, Bradley JS, Englund JA, File TM, Gravenstein S, Hayden FG, McGeer AJ, Neuzil KM, Pavia AT, Tapper ML, Uyeki TM, Zimmerman RK; Expert Panel of the Infectious Diseases Society of America. Seasonal influenza in adults and children--diagnosis, treatment, chemoprophylaxis, and institutional outbreak management: clinical practice guidelines of the Infectious Diseases Society of America. *Clin Infect Dis.* 2009; 48(8):1003-1032.

[46] Kuiken T, Taubenberger JK. Pathology of human influenza revisited. *Vaccine* 2008; 26(Suppl 4): D59-D66.

[47] Bogoch II, Andrews JR, Zachary KC, Hohmann EL.Diagnosis of influenza from lower respiratory tract sampling after negative upper respiratory tract sampling. *Virulence.* 2013; 4(1): 82-84.

[48] Wright, F.; Neumann, G.; Kawaoka, Y. Orthomyxoviruses. In Fields Virology; Wolters Kluwer, Lippincott Willams & Wilkins: Philadelphia, 2007; pp. 1691-1740.

[49] A revision of the system of nomenclature for influenza viruses: a WHO memorandum. Bull. World Health Organ. 1980, 58, 585-591.

[50] Webster RG. Influenza virus: transmission between species and relevance to emergence of the next human pandemic. *Arch. Virol.*1997; ; 13: 105-113.

[51] Peiris JS, Poon LL, Guan Y. Emergence of a novel swine-origin influenza A virus (S-OIV) H1N1 virus in humans. *J. Clin. Virol.* 2009; 45(3): 169–173.

[52] Irving SA, Vandermause MF, Shay DK, Belongia EA. Comparison of nasal and nasopharyngeal swabs for influenza detection in adults. *Clin Med Res.* 2012; 10(4): 215-218.

[53] WHO global influenza surveillance network: Manual for the laboratory diagnosis and virological surveillance of influenza. World Health Organization. 2011.

[54] Akira Sakurai and Futoshi Shibasaki. Updated values for molecular diagnosis for highly pathogenic Avian Influenza Virus. *Viruses 2012*; 4: 1235-1257.

[55] Centers for Disease Control and Prevention (CDC). Evaluation of rapid influenza diagnostic tests for detection of novel influenza A (H1N1) Virus-United States, 2009. *MMWR Morb Mortal Wkly Rep*. 2009; 58(30): 826-829.

[56] Yuan Q, Cheng XD, Yang BC, Zheng QB, Chen YX, Chen QR, Zeng F, Zhang R, Ge SX, Hao XK, Chen H, Zhang J, Xia NS. Differential diagnosis of pandemic (H1N1) 2009 infection by detection of haemagglutinin with an enzyme-linked immunoassay. *Clin Microbiol Infect*. 2011; 17(10): 1574-80.

[57] Shen HH, Hou J, Zhao M, Xu J, Bai BK, Zhao J, Hu Y, Mao PY, Li BA, Mao YL. Analysis of hemagglutination inhibition antibody level in patients with influenza A H1N1]. Zhonghua Shi Yan He Lin Chuang Bing Du Xue Za Zhi. 2012; 26(4):270-2.

[58] Landry M L. Rapid viral diagnosis. In: Rose N R, Conway de Macario E, Folds J D, Lane H C, Nakamura R M, editors. Manual of clinical laboratory immunology. 5th ed. Washington, D.C.: ASM Press; 1997. pp. 608–617.

[59] Matthey S, Nicholson D, Ruhs S, Alden B, Knock M, Schultz K, Schmuecker A. Rapid detection of respiratory viruses by shell vial culture and direct staining by using pooled and individual monoclonal antibodies. J Clin Microbiol. 1992; 30: 540–544.

[60] Landry ML, Ferguson D. SimulFluor Respiratory Screen for rapid detection of multiple respiratory viruses in clinical specimens by immunofluorescence staining. *J Clin Microbiol*. 2000; 38: 708-711.

[61] Landry, ML, Ferguson D. Suboptimal detection of influenza in adults by Directigen Flu A+B and correlation with number of antigen-positive cells detected by cytospin immunofluorescence. *J Clin Microbiol*. 2003; 41: 3407-3409.

[62] Mahony JB. Detection of respiratory viruses by molecular methods. *Clin Microbiol Rev*. 2008; 21: 716–747.

[63] Mahony JB. Nucleic acid amplification-based diagnosis of respiratory virus infections. *Expert Rev Anti Infect Ther*. 2010; 8: 1273–1292.

[64] Petric M, Comanor L, Petti CA. Role of the laboratory in diagnosis of influenza during seasonal epidemics and potential pandemics. *J Infect Dis*. 2006; 194(Suppl 2): S98-110.

[65] Wang R, Taubenberger JK. Methods for molecular surveillance of influenza. *Expert Rev Anti Infect Ther*. 2010; 8(5): 517-27.

[66] Loens K, Bergs K, Ursi D, Goossens H, Ieven M. Evaluation of NucliSens easyMAG for automated nucleic acid extraction from various clinical specimens. *J Clin Microbiol*. 2007; 45(2): 421-425.

[67] Yang G, Erdman DE, Kodani M, Kools J, Bowen MD, Fields BS. Comparison of commercial systems for extraction of nucleic acids from DNA/RNA respiratory pathogens. *J Virol Methods*. 2011; 171(1): 195-199.

[68] Chandler DP, Griesemer SB, Cooney CG, Holmberg R, Thakore N, Mokhiber B, Belgrader P, Knickerbocker C, Schied J, St George K. Rapid, simple influenza RNA extraction from nasopharyngeal samples. *J Virol Methods*. 2012; 183(1): 8-13.

[69] Ellis JS, Fleming DM, Zambon MC. Multiplex reverse transcription-PCR for surveillance of influenza A and B viruses in England and Wales in 1995 and 1996. *J Clin Microbiol*. 1997; 35: 2076–2082.

[70] Beck ET, Henrickson KJ. Molecular diagnosis of respiratory viruses. *Future Microbio.l* 2010; 5: 901–916.

[71] Mahony JB, Petrich A, Smieja M. Molecular diagnosis of respiratory virus infections. *Crit Rev Clin Lab Sci*. 2011; 48(5-6): 217-49.

[72] Hoffmann E, Stech J, Guan Y, Webster RG, Perez DR. Universal primer set for the full-length amplification of all influenza A viruses. *Arch Virol*. 2001;146(12): 2275-89.

[73] He J, Bose ME, Beck ET, Fan J, Tiwari S, Metallo J, Jurgens LA, Kehl SC, Ledeboer N, Kumar S, Weisburg W, Henrickson KJ. Rapid multiplex reverse transcription-PCR typing of influenza A and B virus, and subtyping of influenza A virus into H1, 2, 3, 5, 7, 9, N1 (human), N1 (animal), N2, and N7, including typing of novel swine origin influenza A (H1N1) virus, during the 2009 outbreak in Milwaukee, Wisconsin. *J Clin Microbiol*. 2009; 47(9): 2772-2778.

[74] Deng J, Ma Z, Huang W, Li C, Wang H, Zheng Y, Zhou R, Tang YW. Respiratory virus multiplex RT-PCR assay sensitivities and influence factors in hospitalized children with lower respiratory tract infections. *Virol Sin*. 2013; 28(2): 97-102.

[75] Reijans M, Dingemans G, Klaassen CH, Meis JF, Keijdener J, Mulders B, Eadie K, van Leeuwen W, van Belkum A, Horrevorts AM, Simons G. RespiFinder: a new multiparameter test to differentially identify fifteen respiratory viruses. *J Clin Microbiol*. 2008; 46(4): 1232-1240.

[76] Ellis JS, Smith JW, Braham S, Lock M, Barlow K, Zambon MC. Design and validation of an H5 TaqMan real-time one-step reverse transcription-PCR and confirmatory assays for diagnosis and verification of influenza A virus H5 infections in humans. *J Clin Microbiol*. 2007; 45(5): 1535-1543.

[77] Sakurai A, Nomura N, Nanba R, Sinkai T, Iwaki T, Obayashi T, Hashimoto K, Hasegawa M, Sakoda Y, Naito A, Morizane Y, Hosaka M, Tsuboi K, Kida H, Kai A, Shibasaki F. Rapid typing of influenza viruses using super high-speed quantitative real-time PCR. *J Virol Methods*. 2011; 178(1-2): 75-81.

[78] Tham Nt, Hang Vt, Khanh TH, Viet do C, Hien TT, Farrar J, Chau Nv, van Doorn HR. Comparison of the Roche RealTime ready Influenza A/H1N1 Detection Set with

CDC A/H1N1pdm09 RT-PCR on samples from three hospitals in Ho Chi Minh City, Vietnam. *Diagn Microbiol Infect Dis*. 2012; 74(2): 131-6.

[79] CDC Human Influenza Virus Real-Time RT-PCR Diagnostic Panel – Influenza A/H7 (Eurasian Lineage) Assay. For Emergency Use Only. To Be Used in Conjunction With CDC Human Influenza Virus Real-Time RT-PCR Diagnostic Panel. Catalog # FluEUA-01. Centers for Disease Control and Prevention Influenza Division, 2013.

[80] Layman CP, Gordon SM, Elegino-Steffens DU, Agee W, Barnhill J, Hsue G. Rapid multiplex PCR assay to identify respiratory viral pathogens: moving forward diagnosing the common cold. *Hawaii J Med Public Health*. 2013; 72: 24-26.

[81] Negri P, Dluhy RA. Detection of genetic markers related to high pathogenicity in influenza by SERS. *Analyst*. 2013; 138(17): 4877-884.

[82] de Villiers EM, Fauquet C, Broker TR, Bernard HU, zur Hausen H. Classification of Papillomaviruses. *Virol*. 2004; 324: 17-27.

[83] Doorbar J. Molecular biology of human papillomavirus infection and cervical cancer. *Clin Sci (Lond)*. 2006; 110(5): 525-541.

[84] Muñoz N, Bosch FX, de Sanjosé S, Herrero R, Castellsagué X, Shah KV, Snijders PJ, Meijer CJ; International Agency for Research on Cancer Multicenter Cervical Cancer Study Group. Epidemiologic classification of human papillomavirus types associated with cervical cancer. *N Engl J Med*. 2003; 348: 518–27.

[85] van Ranst, M., R. Tachezy, and R. D. Burk. 1996. Human papillomaviruses: a never-ending story? p. 1–19. In C. Lacey (ed.), Papillomavirus reviews: current research on papillomaviruses. Leeds University Press, Leeds, United Kingdom.

[86] Burk RD, Harari A, Chen Z. Human papillomavirus genome variants. *Virology*. 2013; 445(1-2): 232-43.

[87] De Villiers EM. Taxonomic classification of papillomaviruses. *Papillomavirus Rep*. 2001; 12: 57-63.

[88] Bernard HU, Burk RD, Chen Z, van Doorslaer K, Hausen Hz, de Villiers EM. Classification of papilllomaviruses (PVs) based on 189 PV types and proposal of taxonomic amendments. *Virology*. 2010; 401(1): 70-79.

[89] Schiffman M, Clifford G, Buonaguro FM. Classification of weakly carcinogenic human papillomavirus types: addressing the limits of epidemiology at the borderline. *Infect Agent Cancer*. 2009; 4: 1-8.

[90] Kroupis C, Vourlidis N. Human papilloma virus (HPV) molecular diagnostics. *Clin Chem Lab Med*. 2011; 49(11): 1783–1799.

[91] Wang JL, Yang YZ, Dong WW, Sun J, Tao HT, Li RX, Hu Y. Application of human papillomavirus in screening for cervical cancer and precancerous lesions. *Asian Pac J Cancer Prev*. 2013; 14(5): 2979-2982.

[92] Molijn A, Kleter B, Quint W, van Doorn LJ. Molecular diagnosis of human papillomavirus (HPV) infections. *J Clin Virol*. 2005; 32(suppl 1): S43–S51.

[93] Solomon D, Davey D, Kurman R, Moriarty A, O'Connor D, Prey M, Raab S, Sherman M, Wilbur D, Wright T Jr, Young N; Forum Group Members; Bethesda 2001 Workshop. The 2001 Bethesda System: terminology for reporting results of cervical cytology. *JAMA*. 2002; 287(16): 2114-2119.

[94] Genital HPV Infection-CDC Fact Sheet. Centers for Disease Control and Prevention. 2010.

[95] Schiffman M, Solomon D. Findings to date from the ASCUS-LSIL Triage Study (ALTS). *Arch Pathol Lab Med*. 2003; 127: 946–949.

[96] Carter JJ, Koutsky LA, Hughes JP, Lee SK, Kuypers J, Kiviat N, Galloway DA. Comparison of human papillomavirus types 16, 18, and 6 capsid antibody responses following incident infection. Journal of Infectious Diseases, 2000; 181(6): 1911–1919.

[97] Kemp TJ, Safaeian M, Hildesheim A, Pan Y, Penrose KJ, Porras C, Schiller JT, Lowy DR, Herrero R, Pinto LA. Kinetic and HPV infection effects on cross-type neutralizing antibody and avidity responses induced by Cervarix. *Vaccine*. 2012; 31(1): 165-70.

[98] Jin Y, Kim HJ, Yim GW, Kim YT, Chang DY, Kim HJ. A single serum dilution enzyme-linked immunosorbent assay for determining anti-human papillomavirus (HPV) antibody titers in humans immunized with prophylactic HPV vaccines. *J Pharm Biomed Anal*. 2012; 66: 352-355.

[99] The Consensus Guidelines for the Management of Women with Abnormal Cervical Cancer Screening Tests. American Society for Colposcopy and Cervical Pathology. 2010.

[100] Arney A, Bennett KM. Molecular Diagnostics of Human Papillomavirus. *LABMEDICINE*. 2010; 41: 523-530.

[101] Ting Y, Manos M. Detection and typing of genital human papillomaviruses. In: Innis M, Gelfand D, Sninsky J, White T, eds. PCR Protocols: A Guide to Methods and Applications. San Diego: Academic Press, 1990: 356–366.

[102] Velázquez-Márquez N, Paredes-Tello MA, Pérez-Terrón H, Santos-López G, Reyes-Leyva J, Vallejo-Ruiz V. Prevalence of human papillomavirus genotypes in women from a rural region of Puebla, Mexico. *Int J Infect Dis*. 2009; 13(6): 690-705.

[103] Tieben LM, ter Schegget J, Minnaar RP, Bouwes Bavinck J, Berkhout RJ, Vermeer BJ. Detection of cutaneous and genital HPV types in clinical samples by PCR using consensus primers. *J Virol. Methods* 1993; 42: 265-279.

[104] Villa LL, Denny, L. Chapter 7: Methods for detection of HPV infection and its clinical utility. *International Journal of Gynecology & Obstetrics*. 2006; 94(suppl 1): S71–S80.

[105] Piana A, Sotgiu G, Castiglia P1, Pischedda S, Dettori M, Cocuzza C, Muresu E, Maida A. Molecular methods for the detection of human papillomavirus infection: new in-

sights into their role in diagnostics and epidemiological surveillance. *Italian Journal of Public Health.* 2009; 6(2): 1644-1671.

[106] Molijn A, Kleter B, Quint W, van Doorn LJ. Molecular diagnosis of human papillomavirus (HPV) infections. *J Clin Virol.* 2005; 32(Suppl 1): S43-51.

[107] Chin-Hong PV, Klausner JD. New diagnostic tests for HPV in the developed and the developing world. *MLO Med Lab Obs.* 2008; 40(11):48, 50, 52-3.

[108] Women's Health Diagnostic Assays (IVDD). 2007. Available at rochediagnostics.ca/lab/molecular/wh.php#wh2. Accessed March 16, 2010.

[109] Multiplex HPV Genotyping Kit for Research in Epidemiology [package insert]. In: Multimetrix, ed. Heidelberg, Germany.

[110] Yu D, Chen Y, Wu S, Wang B, Tang YW, Li L. Simultaneous detection and differentiation of human papillomavirus genotypes 6, 11, 16 and 18 by AllGlo quadruplex quantitative PCR. *PLoS One.* 2012; 7(11): e48972.

[111] Lörincz A. Hybrid capture method for detection of human papillomavirus DNA in clinical specimens: a tool for clinical management of equivocal Pap smears and for population screening. *J Obstet Gynaecol Res.* 1996; 22: 629–36.

[112] Clavel C, Masure M, Putaud I, Thomas K, Bory JP, Gabriel R, Quereux C, Birembaut P. Hybrid capture II, a new sensitive test for human papillomavirus detection. Comparison with hybrid capture I and PCR results in cervical lesions. *J Clin Pathol.* 1998; 51(10): 737-40.

[113] Tao P, Zheng W, Wang Y, Bian ML. Sensitive HPV genotyping based on the flow-through hybridization and gene chip. *J Biomed Biotechnol.* 2012; 2012: 938780.

[114] PapilloCheck HPV-Screening Brochure. Available at: www.greinerbioone.com/UserFiles/File/PailloCheck/Papillo_Laborinfo_074%20046.pdf. Accessed March 16, 2010.

[115] Akhras MS, Pettersson E, Diamond L, Unemo M, Okamoto J, Davis RW, Pourmand N. The Sequencing Bead Array (SBA), a Next-Generation Digital Suspension Array. *PLoS One.* 2013; 8(10): e76696.

[116] Lie AK, Kristensen G. Human papillomavirus E6/E7 mRNA testing as a predictive marker for cervical carcinoma. *Expert Rev Mol Diagn.* 2008; 8: 405–415.

[117] Klaes R, Benner A, Friedrich T, Ridder R, Herrington S, Jenkins D, Kurman RJ, Schmidt D, Stoler M, von Knebel Doeberitz M. p16INK4a immunohistochemistry improves interobserver agreement in the diagnosis of cervical intraepithelial neoplasia. *Am J Surg Pathol.* 2002; 26(11): 1389-1399.

[118] López-Morales D, Velázquez-Márquez N, Valenzuela O, Santos-López G, Reyes-Leyva J, Vallejo-Ruiz V. Enhanced sialyltransferases transcription in cervical intraepithelial neoplasia. Invest Clin. 2009; 50(1): 45-53.

[119] Lozano R, Naghavi M, Foreman K,, Murray CJ, AlMazroa MA, Memish ZA.Global and regional mortality from 235 causes of death for 20 age groups in 1990 and 2010: a systematic analysis for the Global Burden of Disease Study 2010. *Lancet*. 2012; 380: 2095–128.

[120] World Health Organization. Outbreak surveillance and response in humanitarian emergencies: WHO guidelines for EWARN implementation. Geneva, Switzerland: World Health Organization; 2012.

[121] Beck J, Nassal M. Hepatitis B virus replication. World J. Gastroenterol. 2007; 13: 48–64.

[122] Bonino F, Piratvisuth T, Brunetto MR, Liaw YF. Diagnostic markers of chronic hepatitis B infection and disease. *Antivir Ther*. 2010; 15 (Suppl 3): 35-44.

[123] Beasley RP. Hepatitis B virus. The major etiology of hepatocellular carcinoma. Cancer. 1988; 61(10): 1942-1956.

[124] Servoss JC, Friedman LS. Serologic and molecular diagnosis of hepatitis B. *Infect Dis Clin North Am*. 2006; 20(1): 47-61.

[125] Jia JD, Hong M, Wei L, Zhang XX, Mao YL, Wang LL, Gao ZL, Hou JL, Zhang J. Multicentre evaluation of the Elecsys hepatitis B surface antigen II assay for detection of HBsAg in comparison with other commercially available assays. *Med Microbiol Immunol*. 2009; 198(4): 263-269.

[126] Servoss JC, Friedman LS. Serologic and molecular diagnosis of hepatitis B virus. Infect Dis Clin North Am. 2006; 20(1):47-61.

[127] Cacciola I, Pollicino T, Squadrito G, Cerenzia G, Orlando ME, Raimondo G. Occult Hepatitis B Virus Infection in Patients with Chronic Hepatitis C Liver Disease. N Engl J Med. 1999; 341:22-26.

[128] Ganem D, Prince AM. Hepatitis B virus infection-natural history and clinical consequences. N. Engl. J. Med. 2004; 350:1118 –1129.

[129] Wong CH, Chan SK, Chan HL, Tsui SK, Feitelson M. The molecular diagnosis of hepatitis B virus-associated hepatocellular carcinoma. Crit Rev Clin Lab Sci. 2006; 43(1): 69-101.

[130] Servoss JC, Friedman LS. Serologic and molecular diagnosis of hepatitis B virus. *Infect Dis Clin North Am*. 2006; 20(1): 47-61.

[131] Samal J, Kandpal M, Vivekanandan P. Molecular mechanisms underlying occult hepatitis B virus infection. *Clin Microbiol Rev*. 2012; 25(1): 142-63.

[132] Dettori S, Candido A, Kondili LA, Chionne P, Taffon S, Genovese D, Iudicone P, Miceli M, Rapicetta M. Identification of low HBV-DNA levels by nucleic acid amplification test (NAT) in blood donors. *J Infect*. 2009; 59(2): 128-33.

[133] Saldanha J, Gerlich W, Lelie N, Dawson P, Heermann K, Heath A, WHO Collaborative Study Group: An international collaborative study to establish a World Health Organization international standard for hepatitis B virus DNA nucleic acid amplification techniques. *Vox Sang* 2001; 80: 63–71.

[134] Vivekanandan P, Singh OV. Molecular methods in the diagnosis and management of chronic hepatitis B. *Expert Rev Mol Diagn* 2010; 10(7): 921-933.

[135] Cabezas-Fernandez M, Cabeza-Barrera M. Introduction of an automated system for the diagnosis and quantification of hepatitis B and hepatitis C viruses. *Open Virol J.* 2012; 6: 122-134.

[136] Ismail AM, Sivakumar J, Anantharam R, Dayalan S, Samuel P, Fletcher GJ, Gnanamony M, Abraham P. Performance Characteristics and Comparison of Abbott and artus Real-Time Systems for Hepatitis B Virus DNA Quantification. *J Clin Microbiol.* 2011; 49(9): 3215–3221.

[137] Sun S, Meng S, Zhang R, Zhang K, Wang L, Li J. Development of a new duplex real-time polymerase chain reaction assay for hepatitis B viral DNA detection. *Virol J.* 2011; 8: 227.

[138] Wang Q, Wang X, Zhang J, Song G. LNA real-time PCR probe quantification of hepatitis B virus. *Exp Ther Med.* 2012; 3(3): 503–508.

[139] Zhao Y, Zhang XY, Hu Y, Zhang WL, Hu JL, Zeng AZ, Guo JJ, Huang WX, Chen WX, Shan YL, Huang AL. Comparison of a novel real-time PCR assay with sequence analysis, reverse hybridization, and multiplex PCR for hepatitis B virus type B and C genotyping. *J Clin Microbiol.* 2011; 49(9): 3392-3394.

[140] Pripuzova N, Wang R, Tsai S, Li B, Hung GC, Ptak RG, Lo SC. Development of Real-Time PCR Array for Simultaneous Detection of Eight Human Blood-Borne Viral Pathogens. *PLoS ONE.* 2012; 7(8): e43246.

[141] Wei YF, Cui GY, Ye P, Chen JN, Diao HY. MicroRNAs may solve the mystery of chronic hepatitis B virus infection. *World J Gastroenterol.* 2013; 19(30): 4867–4876.

[142] Hugo R, Rosen MD. Chronic hepatitis C infection. N Engl J Med 2011; 364: 2429-2438.

[143] Hoofnagle JH, Doo E, Liang TJ, Fleischer R, Lok AS. Management of hepatitis B: summary of a clinical research workshop. *Hepatology* 2007; 45: 1056-75.

[144] Chevaliez S, Pawlotsky JM. Hepatitis C virus serologic and virologic tests and clinical diagnosis of HCV-related liver disease. *Int J Med Sci.* 2006; 3(2):35-40.

[145] Kamili S, Drobeniuc J, Araujo AC, Hayden TM. Laboratory diagnostics for hepatitis C virus infection. *Clin Infect Dis.* 2012; 55: S43-S48.

[146] CDC. Guidelines for laboratory testing and result reporting of antibody to hepatitis C virus. *MMWR* 2003; 52(No. RR–3).

[147] Ho SK, Chan TM, Cheng IK, Lai KN. Comparison of the second generation digene hybrid capture assay with the branched-DNA assay for measurement of hepatitis B virus DNA in serum. *J Clin Microbiol*. 1999; 37: 2461-2465.

[148] Kargar M, Askari A, Doosti A, Ghorbani-Dalini S. Loop-Mediated Isothermal Amplification Assay for Rapid Detection of Hepatitis C virus. *Indian J Virol*. 2012; 23(1): 18-23.

[149] Li G, Li K, Lea AS, Li NL, Abdulla NE, Eltorky MA, Ferguson MR. In situ hybridization for the detection of hepatitis C virus RNA in human liver tissue. *J Viral Hepat*. 2013; 20(3): 183-92.

[150] Zuberi BF, Salahuddin A, Quraishy MS. Triple hepatitis: frequency and treatment outcome of co/super infection of hepatitis C and D among patient of hepatitis B. *J Coll Physicians Surg Pak*. 2008; 18: 404-407.

[151] Kumar, Vijay and Das, Saumitra and Jameel, Shahid (2010) The biology and pathogenesis of hepatitis viruses. In: Current Science (Bangalore), 98 (3). pp. 312-325.

[152] Riaz M, Idrees M, Kanwal H, Kabir F. An overview of triple infection with Hepatitis B, C and D viruses. *Virology J*. 2011; 8: 368.

[153] Law J, Jovel J, Patterson J, Ford G, O'keefe S, Wang W, Meng B, Song D, Zhang Y, Tian Z, Wasilenko ST, Rahbari M, Mitchell T, Jordan T, Carpenter E, Mason AL, Wong GK. Identification of hepatotropic viruses from plasma using deep sequencing: a next generation diagnostic tool. *PLoS One*. 2013; 8(4): e60595.

[154] Xu R, Gan X, Fang Y, Zheng S, Dong Q. A simple, rapid and sensitive integrated protein microarray for simultaneous detection of multiple antigens and antibodies of five human hepatitis viruses (HBV, HCV, HDV, HEV, and HGV). *Anal Biochem* 2007; 362: 69-75.

[155] Park Y, Kim BS, Choi KH, Shin DH, Lee MJ. A Novel Multiplex Real-Time PCR Assay for the Concurrent detection of Hepatitis A, B and C viruses in patients with acute hepatitis. *PLoS ONE. 2012;* 7(11): e49106.

[156] Elango N, Varsanyi T, Kovamees J, Norrby E. Molecular cloning and characterization of six genes, determination of gene order and intergenic sequences and leader sequence of mumps virus. *J. Gen. Virol*. 1988; 69: 2893–2900.

[157] Mühlemann K. The molecular epidemiology of mumps virus. *Infect Genet Evol*. 2004; 4(3): 215-9.

[158] Plotkin SA and Rubin SA. Mumps vaccine. In: Plotkin S, Orenstein W, and Offit P, editors. Vaccines. Philadelphia, PA: Saunders; 2008. p. 435–65.

[159] Carbone KM & Rubin S. Mumps virus, In: Fields Virology, D.M. Knipe & P.M. Howley Eds., 2007. pp. 1528-1551, Lippincott Williams & Wilkins, ISBN 0781760607.

[160] Hviid A, Rubin S, Muhlemann K. Mumps. *Lancet*, 2008; 371 (9616): 932-944.

[161] WHO (December 2010). Mumps, In: Immunization surveillance, assessment and monitoring, Available from: http://www.who.int/immunization_monitoring/diseases/mumps/en/index.html

[162] Lara-Sampablo A, Rosas-Murrieta N, Herrera-Camacho I, Vallejo-Ruiz V, Santos-López G, Reyes-Leyva J (2012). Chapter 10. Studies on the Association of Meningitis and Mumps Virus Vaccination. Insight and Control of Infectious Disease in Global Scenario. Dr. Roy Priti (Ed.), pp. 179-200 ISBN: 978-953-51-0319-6, InTech, Available from: http://www.intechopen.com/books/insight-and-control-of-infectious-disease-in-global-scenario/studies-on-the-association-of-meningitis-and-mumps-virus-vaccination

[163] Parker-Fiebelkorn A, Barskey A, Hickman C, Bellini W. Chapter 9: Mumps. Manual for the Surveillance of Vaccine-Preventable Diseases. 5th Edition, 2012.

[164] Warrener L, Slibinskas R, Brown D, Sasnauskas K, Samuel D. Development and evaluation of a rapid immunochromatographic test for mumps-specific IgM in oral fluid specimens and use as a matrix for preserving viral nucleic acid for RT-PCR. *J Med Virol.* 2010; 82(3): 485-93.

[165] Latner DR, McGrew M, Williams N, Lowe L, Werman R, Warnock E, Gallagher K, Doyle P, Smole S, Lett S, Cocoros N, DeMaria A, Konomi R, Brown CJ, Rota PA, Bellini WJ, Hickman CJ. Enzyme-linked immunospot assay detection of mumps-specific antibody-secreting B cells as an alternative method of laboratory diagnosis. *Clin Vaccine Immunol.* 2011; 18(1): 35-42.

[166] Poggio GP, Rodriguez C, Cisterna D, Freire MC, Cello J. Nested PCR for rapid detection of mumps virus in cerebrospinal fluid from patients with neurological diseases. *J Clin Microbiol.* 2000; 38(1): 274-278.

[167] Uchida K, Shinohara M, Shimada S, Segawa Y, Doi R, Gotoh A, Hondo R. Rapid and sensitive detection of mumps virus RNA directly from clinical samples by real-time PCR. *J Med Virol.* 2005; 75(3): 470-4.

[168] Tipples G, Hiebert J. Detection of measles, mumps, and rubella viruses. *Methods Mol Biol.* 2011; 665:183-93.

[169] Royuela E, Castellanos A, Sánchez-Herrero C, Sanz JC, De Ory F, Echevarria JE. Mumps virus diagnosis and genotyping using a novel single RT-PCR. *J Clin Virol.* 2011; 52(4): 359-62.

[170] Jin L, Rima B, Brown D, Orvell C, Tecle T, Afzal M, Uchida K, Nakayama T, Song JW, Kang C, Rota PA, Xu W, Featherstone D Proposal for genetic characterisation of wild-type mumps strains: preliminary standardisation of the nomenclature. *Arch Virol.* 2005; 150(9): 1903-1909.

[171] Palacios G, Jabado O, Cisterna D, de Ory F, Renwick N, Echevarria JE, Castellanos A, Mosquera M, Freire MC, Campos RH, Lipkin WI. Molecular identification of mumps

virus genotypes from clinical samples: standardized method of analysis. *J Clin Microbiol.* 2005; 43(4): 1869-1878.

[172] Boddicker JD, Rota PA, Kreman T, Wangeman A, Lowe L, Hummel KB, Thompson R, Bellini WJ, Pentella M, Desjardin LE. Real-time reverse transcription-PCR assay for detection of mumps virus RNA in clinical specimens. *J Clin Microbiol.* 2007; 45(9): 2902-2908.

[173] Ammour Y, Faizuloev E, Borisova T, Nikonova A, Dmitriev G, Lobodanov S, Zverev V. Quantification of measles, mumps and rubella viruses using real-time quantitative TaqMan-based RT-PCR assay. *J Virol Methods.* 2013; 187(1): 57-64.

[174] Leblanc JJ, Pettipas J, Davidson RJ, Tipples GA, Hiebert J, Hatchette TF. Detection of mumps virus RNA by real-time one-step reverse transcriptase PCR using the LightCycler platform. *J Clin Microbiol.* 2008; 46(12): 4049-4051.

[175] Ando K, Ishihara M, Kusumoto Y, Shibuya E, Nakamura S, Mizuki N. A case of corneal endotheliitis with mumps virus RNA in aqueous humor detected by rt-PCR. *Ocul Immunol Inflamm.* 2013; 21(2): 150-152.

[176] Wolfson LJ, Grais RF, Luquero FJ, Birmingham ME, Strebel PM. Estimates of measles case fatality ratios: a comprehensive review of community-based studies. *Int J Epidemiol.* 2009; 38: 192–205.

[177] Bellini WJ, Rota JS, Lowe LE, Katz RS, Dyken PR, Zaki SR, Shieh WJ, Rota PA. Subacute sclerosing panencephalitis: more cases of this fatal disease are prevented by measles immunization than was previously recognized. *J Infect Dis.* 2005; 192: 1686–1693.

[178] Griffin DE, Lin WH, Pan CH. Measles virus, immune control, and persistence. *FEMS Microbiol Rev.* 2012; 36(3): 649-662.

[179] Cairns KL, Perry RT, Ryman TK, Nandy RK, Grais RF. Should outbreak response immunization be recommended for measles outbreaks in middle-and low-income countries? An update. *J Infect Dis.* 2011; 204: S35–S46.

[180] Simons E, Ferrari M, Fricks J, Wannemuehler K, Anand A, Burton A, Strebel P. Assessment of the 2010 global measles mortality reduction goal: results from a model of surveillance data. *Lancet.* 2012; 379(9832): 2173-2178.

[181] World Health Organization. Measles fact sheet No.286 External Web Site Icon. Accessed Feb 2013.

[182] Shanks GD, Lee S-H, Howard A, Brunden KR. Extreme mortality after first introduction of measles virus to the Polynesian Island of Rotuma, 1911. *Am J Epidemiol.* 2011; 173:1211–1222.

[183] Anlar B. Subacute sclerosing panencephalitis and chronic viral encephalitis. *Handb Clin Neurol.* 2013; 112: 1183-1189.

[184] Rima BK, Duprex WP. Morbilliviruses and human disease. J Pathol. 2006; 208(2): 199-214.

[185] Sips GJ, Chesik D, Glazenburg L, Wilschut J, De Keyser J, Wilczak N. Involvement of morbilliviruses in the pathogenesis of demyelinating disease. *Rev Med Virol.* 2007; 17(4): 223-244.

[186] Kutty P, Rota J, Bellini W, Redd SB, Barskey A, Wallace G. Chapter 7: Measles. Manual for the Surveillance of Vaccine-Preventable Diseases. 6th Edition, 2013.

[187] Bellini WJ, Helfand RF. The challenges and strategies for laboratory diagnosis of measles in an international setting. *J Infect Dis*. 2003; 187 Suppl 1: S283-90.

[188] Centers for Disease Control and Prevention. Recommendations from an ad hoc meeting of the WHO measles and Rubella Laboratory Network (LabNet) on use of alternative diagnostic samples for measles and rubella surveillance. *MMWR Morb Mortal Wkly Rep* 2008; 57: 657–660.

[189] Hutse V, Van Hecke K, De Bruyn R, Samu O, Lernout T, Muyembe JJ, Brochier B. Oral fluid for the serological and molecular diagnosis of measles. *Int J Infect Dis*. 2010; 14(11): e991.

[190] Sampedro A, Rodríguez-Granger J, Gómez C, Lara A, Gutierrez J, Otero A. Comparative evaluation of a new chemiluminiscent assay and an ELISA for the detection of IgM against measles. *J Clin Lab Anal*. 2013; 27(6): 477-480.

[191] Haywood B, Patel M, Hurday S, Copping R, Webster D, Irish D, Haque T. Comparison of automated chemiluminescence immunoassays with capture enzyme immunoassays for the detection of measles and mumps IgM antibodies in serum. *J Virol Methods*. 2013; 196C: 15-17.

[192] Sanz JC, Mosquera M, Ramos B, Ramírez R, de Ory F, Echevarria JE. Assessment of RNA amplification by multiplex RT-PCR and IgM detection by indirect and capture ELISAs for the diagnosis of measles and rubella. *APMIS*. 2010; 118(3): 203-209.

[193] Smits GP, van Gageldonk PG, Schouls LM, van der Klis FR, Berbers GA. Development of a bead-based multiplex immunoassay for simultaneous quantitative detection of IgG serum antibodies against measles, mumps, rubella, and varicella-zoster virus. *Clin Vaccine Immunol*. 2012; 19(3): 396-400.

[194] The Fifth Regional Hands-On Training Workshop. On The Laboratory Diagnosis of Measles And Rubella. World Health Organization. Regional Office for The Western Pacific. Hong Kong (China). 29 October to 3 November 2012.

[195] Thomas B, Beard S, Jin L, Brown KE, Brown DWG. Development and evaluation of a real-time PCR assay for rapid identification and semiquantitation of measles virus. *J Med Virol*. 2007; 79: 1587–92.

[196] Kühne M, Brown DW, Jin L. Genetic variability of measles virus in acute and persistent infections. *Infect Genet Evol.* 2006; 6: 269–276.

[197] Lenesha Warrener, Rimantas Slibinskas, Kaw Bing Chua, Wondatir Nigatu, Kevin E Brown, Kestutis Sasnauskas, Dhanraj Samuel, David Brown. A point-of-care test for measles diagnosis: detection of measles-specific IgM antibodies and viral nucleic acid. *Bull World Health Organ.* 2011; 89(9): 675–682.

[198] Sheikhakbari S, Mokhtari-Azad T, Salimi V, Norouzbabaei Z, Abbasi S, Zahraei SM, Shahmahmoodi S. The use of oral fluid samples spotted on filter paper for the detection of measles virus using nested rt-PCR. *J Clin Lab Anal.* 2012; 26(3): 215-222.

[199] Uzicanin A, Lubega I, Nanuynja M, Mercader S, Rota P, Bellini W, Helfand R. Dried blood spots on filter paper as an alternative specimen for measles diagnostics: detection of measles immunoglobulin M antibody by a commercial enzyme immunoassay. *J Infect Dis.* 2011; 204 Suppl 1: S564-S569.

[200] Akiyoshi K, Suga T, Nukuzuma S, Kon-no M, Shibata M, Itoh M, Ito M, Ihara T. Reevaluation of laboratory methods for diagnosis of measles. *Jpn J Infect Dis.* 2010; 63(4): 225-8.

[201] Giusti D, Burette J, Nguyen Y, Lévêque N, Graesslin O, Andreoletti L. Virological diagnosis and management of two cases of congenital measles. *J Med Virol.* 2013; 85(12): 2136-2138.

[202] Ikeno S, Suzuki MO, Muhsen M, Ishige M, Kobayashi-Ishihara M, Ohno S, Takeda M, Nakayama T, Morikawa Y, Terahara K, Okada S, Takeyama H, Tsunetsugu-Yokota Y. Sensitive detection of measles virus infection in the blood and tissues of humanized mouse by one-step quantitative RT-PCR. *Front Microbiol.* 2013; 4: 298.

[203] Ito M, Suga T, Akiyoshi K, Nukuzuma S, Kon-no M, Umegaki Y, Kohdera U, Ihara T. Detection of measles virus RNA on SYBR green real-time reverse transcription-polymerase chain reaction. *Pediatr Int.* 2010; 52(4): 611-615.

[204] Ammour Y, Faizuloev E, Borisova T, Nikonova A, Dmitriev G, Lobodanov S, Zverev V. Quantification of measles, mumps and rubella viruses using real-time quantitative TaqMan-based RT-PCR assay. *J Virol Methods.* 2013; 187(1): 57-64.

[205] Maksimov NL, Agafonov AP, Drozdov IG. The application of xMAP technology in genetic typing of measles virus. *Klin Lab Diagn.* 2011; (8): 46-58.

[206] Bankamp B, Byrd-Leotis LA, Lopareva EN, Woo GK, Liu C, Jee Y, Ahmed H, Lim WW, Ramamurty N, Mulders MN, Featherstone D, Bellini WJ, Rota PA. Improving molecular tools for global surveillance of measles virus. *J Clin Virol.* 2013; 58(1): 176-82.

[207] Michel Y, Saloum K, Tournier C, Quinet B, Lassel L, Pérignon A, Grimprel E, Carbajal R, Vabret A, Freymuth F, Garbarg-Chenon A, Schnuriger A. Rapid molecular di-

agnosis of measles virus infection in an epidemic setting. *J Med Virol*. 2013; 85(4): 723-30.

[208] Measles Lab Manual from the World Health Organization. Manual for the Laboratory Diagnosis of Measles and Rubella Virus Infection, 2nd edition, August 2007 from the World Health Organization (WHO).

[209] Amadi K, Sabo AM, Ogunkeye OO, Oluwole FS. Thyroid hormone: a "prime suspect" in human immunodeficiency virus (HIV/AIDS) patients?. Nigerian Journal of Physiological Sciences: official publication of the Physiological Society of Nigeria. 2008; 23: 61– 66.

[210] McCutchan FE. Global epidemiology of HIV. *J Med Virol*. 2006; 78: S7-S12.

[211] HIV and its transmission. Centers for Disease Control and Prevention HIV/AIDS Fact Sheets Web site. http://www.cdc.gov/hiv/resources/factsheets/transmission.htm. July 1999.

[212] Centers for Disease Control and Prevention. HIV-2 Infection Surveillance-United States, 1987-2009. *MMWR*. 2011; 60(29): 985-988.

[213] Branson BM, Stekler JD. Detection of acute HIV infection: we can't close the window. *J Infect Dis 2012*; 205: 521–524.

[214] O'Conell RJ, Peel SA. Multispot HIV-1/HIV-2 Rapid Test: advantages over other rapid HIV tests. *Expert Rev Mol Diagn*. 2007; 7(5): 499-505.

[215] Bentsen C, McLaughlin L, Mitchell E, Ferrera C, Liska S, Myers R, Peel S, Swenson P, Gadelle S, Shriver MK. Performance evaluation of the Bio-Rad Laboratories GS HIV Combo Ag/Ab EIA, a 4th generation HIV assay for the simultaneous detection of HIV p24 antigen and antibodies to HIV-1 (groups M and O) and HIV-2 in human serum or plasma. *J Clin Virol*. 2011; 52 (Suppl 1): S57-S61.

[216] Branson BM. The future of HIV testing. *J. Acquir. Immune Defic. Syndr*. 2010; 55 (Suppl. 2): S102–S105.

[217] Song EY, Hur M, Roh EY, Park MH, Moon HW, Yun YM. Performances of four fourth-generation human immunodeficiency virus-1 screening assays. *J Med Virol*. 2012; 84(12): 1884-8.

[218] Sano T, Kondo M, Yoshimura Y, Tachikawa N, Sagara H, Itoda I, Yamanaka K, Sudo K, Kato S, Imai M. Evaluation of a new vesion of the human immunodeficiency virus antigen and antibody combination assay with improved sensitivity in HIV-1 p24 antigen detection. *Kansenshogaku Zasshi*. 2013; 87(4): 415-23.

[219] Fransen K, Vermoesen T, Beelaert G, Menten J, Hutse V, Wouters K, Platteau T, Florence E. Using conventional HIV tests on oral fluid. *J Virol Methods*. 2013; 194(1-2): 46-51.

[220] O'Gorman MR, Weber D, Landis SE, Schoenbach VJ, Mittal M, Folds JD. Interpretive criteria of the Western blot assay for serodiagnosis of human immunodeficiency virus type 1 infection. *Arch Pathol Lab Med*. 1991; 115: 26–30.

[221] The Consortium for Retrovirus Serology Standardization Serologial diagnosis of human immunodeficiency virus infection by Western blot testing. *JAMA*. 1988; 260: 674–679.

[222] Tebourski F, Slim A, Elgaaied A. The significance of combining World Health Organization and Center for Disease Control criteria to resolve indeterminate human immunodeficiency virus tipe-1 Western blot results. *Diagn Microbiol Infect Dis*. 2004; 48: 59–61.

[223] García F, Álvarez M, Bernal C, Chueca N, Guillot V. Laboratory diagnosis of HIV infection, viral tropism and resistance to antiretrovirals. *Enferm Infecc Microbiol Clin*. 2011; 29(4): 297-307.

[224] Grossman Z, Kra-Oz Z. HIV testing: the medical laboratory role in HIV diagnosis and monitoring. *Harefuah*. 2013; 152(8): 477-80, 498.

[225] Brennan CA, Yamaguchi J, Vallari A, Swanson P, Hackett JR Jr. ARCHITECT HIV Ag/Ab Combo assay: correlation of HIV-1 p24 antigen sensitivity and RNA viral load using genetically diverse virus isolates. *J Clin Virol*. 2013; 57(2): 169-172.

[226] Karris MY, Anderson CM, Morris SR, Smith DM, Little SJ. Cost savings associated with testing of antibodies, antigens, and nucleic acids for diagnosis of acute HIV infection. *J Clin Microbiol*. 2012; 50(6): 1874-1878.

[227] Branson BM, Mark Pandori M. 2012 HIV Diagnostics Conference: the molecular diagnostics perspective. *Expert Rev. Mol. Diagn*. 2013; 3(3): 243–245.

[228] Bourlet T, Memmi M, Saoudin H, Pozzetto B. Molecular HIV screening. *Expert Rev Mol Diagn*. 2013; 13(7): 693-705.

[229] Mohammadi-Yeganeh S, Paryan M, Mirab Samiee S, Kia V, Rezvan H. Molecular beacon probes-base multiplex NASBA Real-time for detection of HIV-1 and HCV. *Iran J Microbiol*. 2012; 4(2): 47-54.

[230] Gueudin M, Leoz M, Lemée V, De Oliveira F, Vessière A, Kfutwah A, Plantier JC. A new real-time quantitative PCR for diagnosis and monitoring of HIV-1 group O infection. *J Clin Microbiol*. 2012; 50(3):831-6.

[231] Tang YW, Ou CY. Past, present and future molecular diagnosis and characterization of human immunodeficiency virus Infections. *Emerg Microbes Infect*. 2012; 1(8): e19.

[232] Yoshimura Y, Techikawa N. HIV tests. *Rinsho Byori*. 2008; 56(11): 1019-25.

[233] Vickerman P, Watts C, Peeling RW, Mabey D, Alary M. Modelling the cost effectiveness of rapid point of care diagnostic tests for the control of HIV and other sexually

transmitted infections among female sex workers. *Sex Transm Infect.* 2006; 82: 403–412.

[234] De Cock KM, Fowler MG, Mercier E et al. Prevention of mother-to child HIV transmission in resource-poor countries: translating research into policy and practice. *JAMA* 2000; 283: 1175–1182.

[235] Menzies NA, Homsy J, Chang Pitter JY, Pitter C, Mermin J, Downing R, Finkbeiner T, Obonyo J, Kekitiinwa A, Tappero J, Blandford JM. Cost-effectiveness of routine rapid human immunodeficiency virus antibody testing before DNA-PCR testing for early diagnosis of infants in resource-limited settings. *Pediatr Infect Dis J.* 2009; 28: 819–825.

[236] Loubiere S, Moatti JP.Economic evaluation of point-of-care diagnostic technologies for infectious diseases. Clin Microbiol Infect. 2010 Aug;16(8):1070-6.

[237] Schito ML, D'Souza MP, Owen SM, Busch MP. Challenges for rapid molecular HIV diagnostics. *J Infect Dis.* 2010; 201 (Suppl 1): S1-S6.

[238] Korber B, Gaschen B, Yusim K, Thakallapally R, Kesmir C, Detours V. Evolutionary and immunological implications of contemporary HIV-1 variation. *Br Med Bull.* 2001; 58: 19–42.

[239] Lauring AS, Andino R Quasispecies theory and the behavior of RNA viruses. *PLoS Pathog.* 2010; 6: e1001005.

[240] Di Giallonardo F, Zagordi O, Duport Y, Leemann C, Joos B, Künzli-Gontarczyk M, Bruggmann R, Beerenwinkel N, Günthard HF, Metzner KJ. Next-Generation Sequencing of HIV-1 RNA Genomes: Determination of Error Rates and Minimizing Artificial Recombination. *PLoS One.* 2013; 8(9):e74249.

[241] Mild M, Hedskog C, Jernberg J, Albert J. Performance of ultra-deep pyrosequencing in analysis of HIV-1 pol gene variation. PLoS One. 2011; 6: e22741.

[242] Guy Vernet. Molecular diagnostics in virology. Journal of Clinical Virology. 2004; 31-8(4): 239-247.

[243] Gorzer I, Guelly C, Trajanoski S, Puchhammer-Stockl E. The impact of PCR-generated recombination on diversity estimation of mixed viral populations by deep sequencing. J Virol Methods. 2010; 169: 248–252.

Chapter 6

Phenotypic and Molecular Methods for the Detection of Antibiotic Resistance Mechanisms in Gram Negative Nosocomial Pathogens

Meletis Georgios, Tzampaz Egki and
Sianou Effrosyni

Additional information is available at the end of the chapter

http://dx.doi.org/10.5772/57582

1. Introduction

Antibiotic resistance among clinical isolates of *Klebsiella pneumoniae, Pseudomonas aeruginosa, Acinetobacter baumannii, Escherichia coli, Enterobacter* spp and *Proteus* spp is causing worldwide concern [1-5] especially when mediated by transferable genetic elements.

The role of the Clinical Microbiology Department in this regard is crucial for the isolation of non-susceptible bacteria and the detection of the underlying mechanisms leading to their resistant phenotype. Rapid and reliable results are of the utmost importance in order to apply the appropriate treatment and to contain the spread of resistance determinants within hospital settings.

In the present chapter, laboratory procedures for the detection of antibiotic resistance mechanisms will be discussed focusing mainly on those more frequently used for Gram negative clinical isolates around the world.

2. Antibiotic resistance mechanisms among Gram negative nosocomial pathogens

Antibiotic resistance may be intrinsic (the microorganism is by definition resistant against a certain antibiotic) or acquired. Acquired refers to resistance that is a consequence of mutational events or gene acquisition via horizontal gene transfer.

Four general mechanisms leading to acquired antibiotic resistance have been described: (1) decreased entrance of the antibiotic into the bacterial cell; (2) increased extrusion of the antibiotic by bacterial efflux systems; (3) mutational modification of the antibiotic's target and; (4) production of antibiotic-inactivating enzymes. Characteristic examples for each mechanism are presented in Table 1.

Mechanism	Examples
Decreased permeability	Diminished expression or loss of the OprD porin in *Pseudomonas aeruginosa* and OmpK35, OmpK36 porins in *Klebsiella pneumoniae* [6-9]
Efflux	Overexpression of MexAB-OprM and MexXY-OprM in *Pseudomonas aeruginosa* and OqxAB in *Klebsiella pneumoniae* [10-13]
Target modification	Mutations of gyrases and topoisomerases leading to fluoroquinolone resistance [14-16]
Inactivating enzymes	Production of beta-lactamases and aminoglycoside modifying enzymes [17-19]

Table 1. Examples of antibiotic resistance mechanisms.

Among the aforementioned mechanisms, the production of beta-lactamases is considered of major importance because these enzymes are commonly transferable and inactivate multiple beta-lactam antibiotics. Within this large enzymatic family, carbapenemases (class B metallo-beta-lactamases (MBLs) [20] that contain zinc in their active center and class A KPC [21]) hydrolyze in vitro all or almost all beta-lactams, including carbapenems [22]. Class A extended spectrum beta-lactamases (ESBLs) hydrolyze penicillins, monobactams and cephalosporins whereas are inhibited by the beta-lactamase inhibitors [23,24]. Class C cephalosporinases (AmpC) present various spectrums of cephalosporin hydrolysis but are not inhibited by the beta-lactamase inhibitors [25]. Additionaly, AmpC enzymes may be inducible in *Serratia* spp, *Pseudomonas* spp, Indole-positive *Proteus*, *Citrobacter* spp and *Enterobacter* spp (SPICE group of bacteria) complicating the treatment of infections caused by these pathogens. Finally, molecular class D beta-lactamases (OXA) comprise numerous enzymes with variable spectrums of beta-lactam hydrolysis [26].

3. Phenotypic tests

Phenotypic tests may be used in the everyday laboratory practice in order to identify the presence of acquired resistance mechanisms among frequently isolated nosocomial pathogens. In the present chapter, the procedure and the interpretation of seven useful phenotypic tests are described. Special attention has been given to the phenotypic detection of beta-lactamases and especially those hydrolyzing carbapenems together with other beta-lactams (carbapenemases).

http://dx.doi.org/10.5772/57582

3.1. Double Disc Synergy Test (DDST)

The DDST is used for the detection of beta-lactamases that are inhibited by beta-lactamase inhibitors such as clavulanic acid (Ambler class A beta-lactamases and especially ESBLs). For SPICE organisms, cloxacillin should be incorporated in Mueller-Hinton agar during its preparation in order to prevent any AmpC interference [27].

3.1.1. Procedure

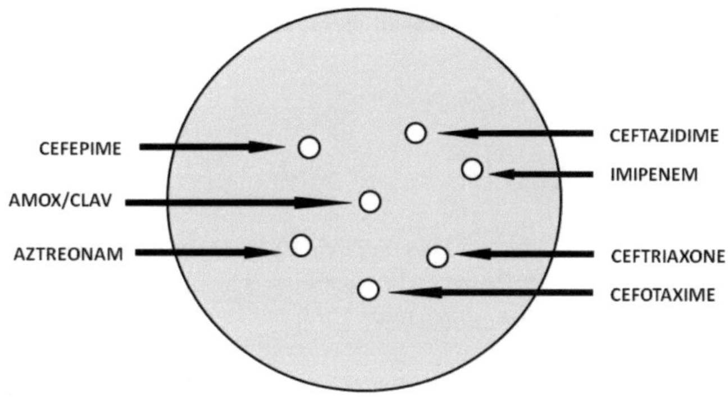

Figure 1. Double Disc Synergy Test preparation.

Step 1: Prepare agar plates containing 200μg/ml cloxacillin (by adding 1ml solution containing 80 mg cloxacillin in 399 ml Mueller-Hinton agar at the liquid phase). Omit this step when testing non-SPICE bacteria.

Step 2: Make a 0.5 McFarland bacterial suspension.

Step 3: Inoculate with a sterile cotton swab and place an amoxicillin/clavulanic acid disc at the center of the plate (20 μg amoxicillin+10 μg clavulanic acid).

Step 4: Place ceftazidime, imipenem, ceftriaxone, cefotaxime, aztreonam and cefepime discs around the central amoxicillin/clavulanic acid disc (Figure 1).

Step 5: Incubate at 37°C for 18-24h.

3.1.2. Interpretation

The DDST is considered positive when the inhibition zone of any of the antibiotics is larger towards the clavulanic acid disc (Figure 2-lower left plate) or a ghost inhibition zone appears between the central disc and any of the other antibiotics (Figure 2-lower right plate). This is happening because of the ESBL's inhibition by the clavulanic acid. In proximity to the central disc the enzyme's activity is blocked. Thus, the growth inhibition zone appears only towards the clavulanic acid disc. If resistance to cephalosporins is not due to ESBL production, the test results negative (Figure 2-upper plates).

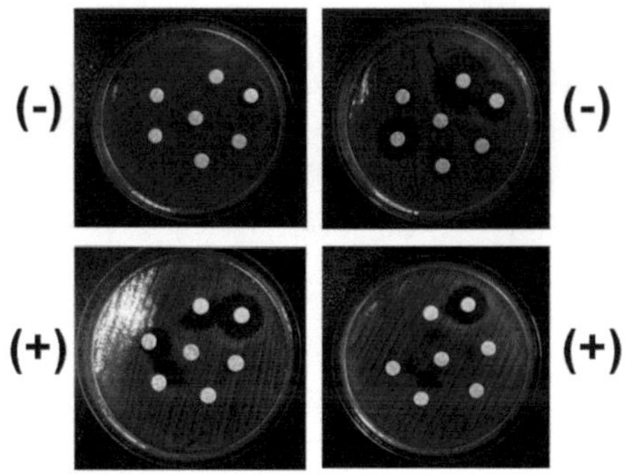

Figure 2. Interpretation of the DDST. (-): Negative; (+): Positive.

3.2. Imipenem-EDTA synergy test

EDTA (ethylene-diamine-tetraacetic acid) is a polyamino carboxylic acid that binds metal ions like zinc and can inactivate the metallo-beta-lactamases. Therefore, it is used for the phenotypic detection of MBL production in clinical isolates [28].

3.2.1. Procedure

Step 1: Soak paper discs within a 0.1 M EDTA solution.

Step 2: Make a 0.5 McFarland bacterial suspension.

Step 3: Inoculate with a sterile cotton swab and place an imipenem and a ceftazidime disc at the center of the plate.

Step 4: Place the EDTA discs at both sides in respect to the antibiotics as shown in Figure 3.

Step 5: Incubate at 37°C for 18-24h.

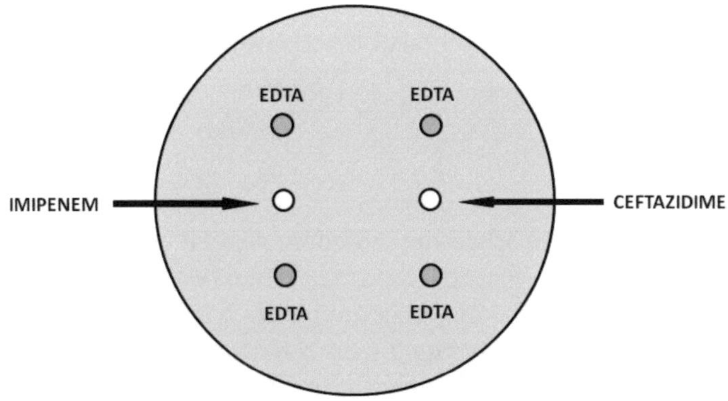

Figure 3. Preparation of the imipenem-EDTA synergy test.

3.2.2. Interpretation

The imipenem-EDTA synergy test is positive when the inhibition zone takes a characteristic keyhole shape because of the MBL inactivation by the EDTA (Figure 4). In proximity to the EDTA discs, the hydrolytic activity of MBLs is blocked. Consequently, imipenem and ceftazidime inhibition zones may appear larger towards the EDTA discs.

3.3. Boronic acid test

Phenylboronic acid acts as an inhibitor for KPC carbapenemases and class A and C beta-lactamases. The boronic acid test has been proposed for the phenotypic detection of KPC-producers because it is easier to perform than the DDST and also presents less false positive results because of the presence of ESBLs or AmpC beta-lactamases [29-31].

3.3.1. Procedure

Step 1: Make a 0.5 McFarland bacterial suspension.

Step 2: Inoculate with a sterile cotton swab and place two meropenem discs (Figure 5).

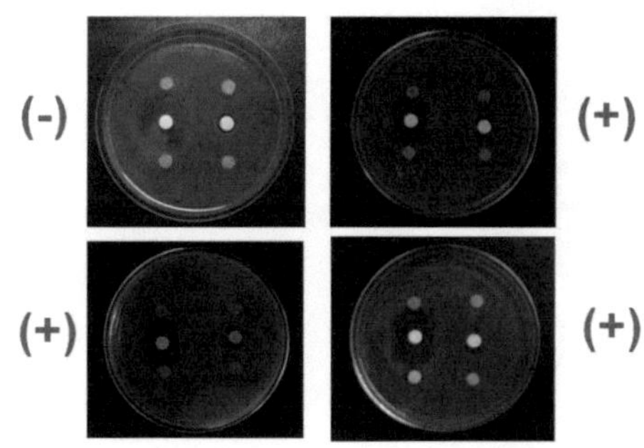

Figure 4. Interpretation of the imipenem-EDTA synergy test. (-): Negative; (+): Positive. Note that the upper left isolate is negative for MBL production but shows positive D-test between imipenem and ceftazidime indicating for the presence of inducible AmpC beta-lactamases (The D-test is described in paragraph 3.6).

Step 3: Add 20 μl of phenylboronic acid 20 g/L on one of the two meropenem discs.

Step 4: Incubate at 37°C for 18-24h.

3.3.2. Interpretation

In case of KPC production, the phenylboronic acid that has been added to the second meropenem disc will block the hydrolytic activity of the enzyme. As a consequence, the second disc will have a larger inhibition halo. The test is considered positive when the inhibition zone of the meropenem+phenylboronic acid is ≥ 5mm larger than the inhibition zone of meropenem alone (Figure 6).

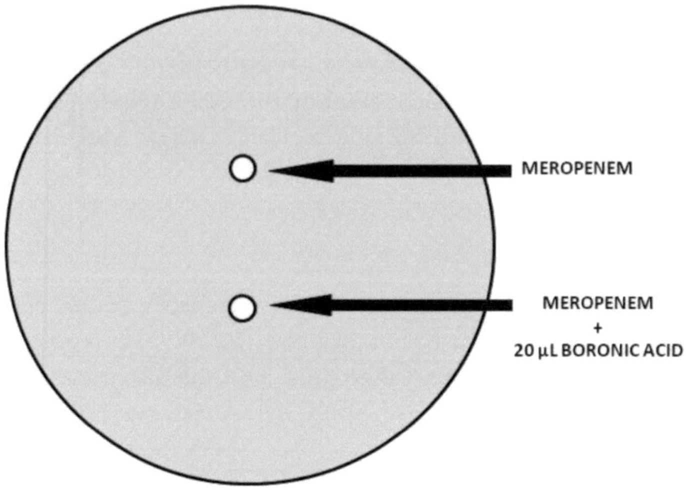

Figure 5. Preparation of the boronic acid test.

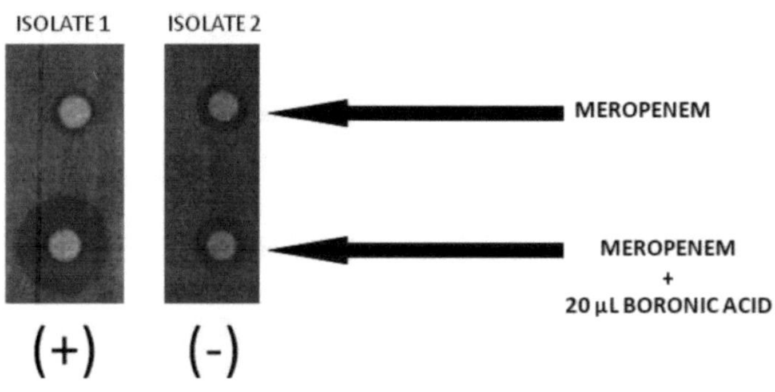

Figure 6. Interpretation of the boronic acid test. (+): Positive; (-): Negative.

3.4. Hodge test

The Hodge test is used to reveal carbapenemase production [32]. This is achieved by inoculating the study isolate together with a carbapenem-susceptible indicator strain and evaluating the distortion of the indicator strain's inhibition zone because of carbapenemase production by the study isolate. Despite its usefulness, this test presents a disadvantage: it detects the presence of carbapenemases only, without being able to discriminate between different carbapenemase types (KPC or MBLs).

3.4.1. Procedure

Step 1: Make a 0.5 McFarland suspension of the indicator strain (for example *E. coli* ATCC 25922).

http://dx.doi.org/10.5772/57582

Step 2: Inoculate with a sterile cotton swab and place a carbapenem disc at the center of the plate.

Step 3: Streak 3-5 colonies of the test isolate from the center to the periphery of the plate (Figure 7).

Step 4: Incubate at 37°C for 18-24h.

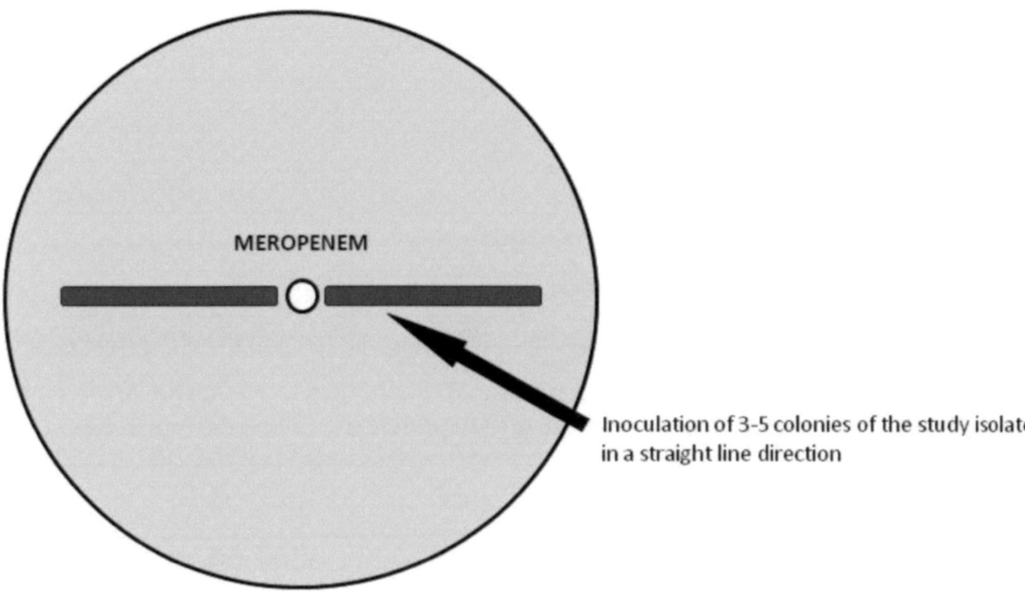

Figure 7. Preparation of the Hodge test.

3.4.2. Interpretation

The presence of a distorted inhibition zone due to growth of the indicator strain toward the carbapenem disc is interpreted as a positive result (Figure 8). This occurs due to carbapenemase production by the study isolate. Uncertain results need to be confirmed by other tests or molecular methods.

3.5. Combination meropenem disc test

This test is a combination of the EDTA and the boronic acid test in a single plate and has been introduced in Greece after the emergence of Gram negative isolates co-producing KPC and MBL carbapenemases [33-37]. The advantage of the test is that it discriminates between carbapenem-susceptible, KPC-producing, MBL-producing and double-carbapenemase-producing bacteria.

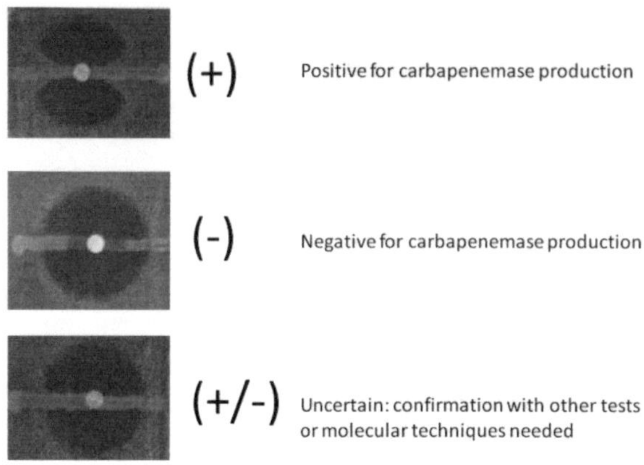

Figure 8. Interpretation of the Hodge test.

3.5.1. Procedure

Step 1: Make a 0.5 McFarland bacterial suspension.

Step 2: Inoculate with a sterile cotton swab and place four meropenem discs (Figure 9).

Step 3: Add 10 μl EDTA 0.1 M on the second disc, 20 μl of phenylboronic acid 20 g/L on the third disc and 20 μl of phenylboronic acid 20 g/L+10 μl EDTA 0.1 M on the fourth disc.

Step 4: Incubate at 37°C for 18-24h.

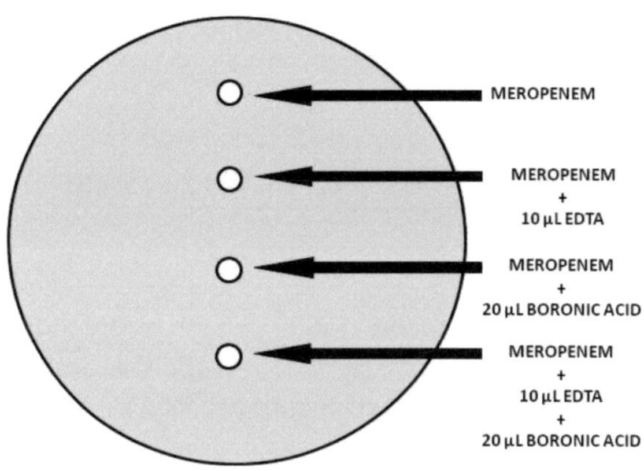

Figure 9. Preparation of the combination meropenem disc test.

3.5.2. Interpretation

The interpretation of the combination meropenem disc test is based on the comparison between the inhibition zones of the four meropenem discs as presented in Figure 10. If no carbapenemase is present, the zone diameters of the discs where inhibitors have been added will not present significant differences (≥5mm) from the meropenem disc alone. In case of KPC production, an increase of ≥5mm in the discs that are supplemented with boronic acid will be observed. MBL production will become evident by an increase of ≥5mm in the discs that are supplemented with EDTA. In case of a KPC+MBL-producer, the fourth disc will present the larger zone diameter of all. The EDTA-supplemented and boronic acid-supplemented discs may or may not have a ≥5mm larger zone diameter than that of the meropenem disc alone.

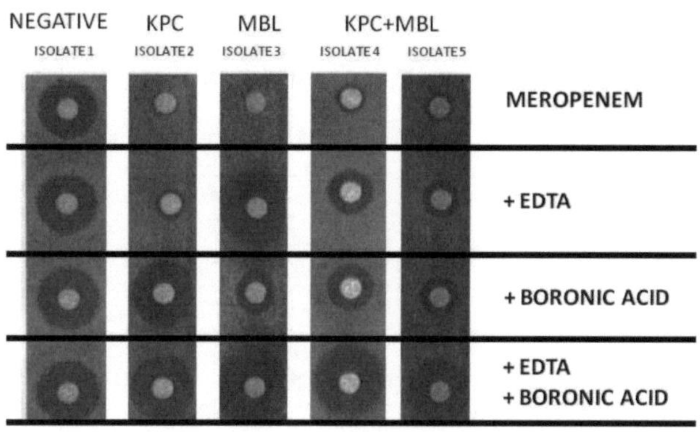

Figure 10. Interpretation of the combination meropenem disc test.

Recently, a novel variation of this test has been proposed [38] for surveillance cultures from rectal swabs. The same principle is generally followed, except that each swab is initially suspended in 1 ml sterile saline by rotating and agitating it to release the microorganisms. Afterwards, the suspension is cultured onto McConkey agar using a different swab. This method allows the identification and differentiation of carbapenemase-producing *Enterobacteriaceae* (Figure 11) directly at patient admission.

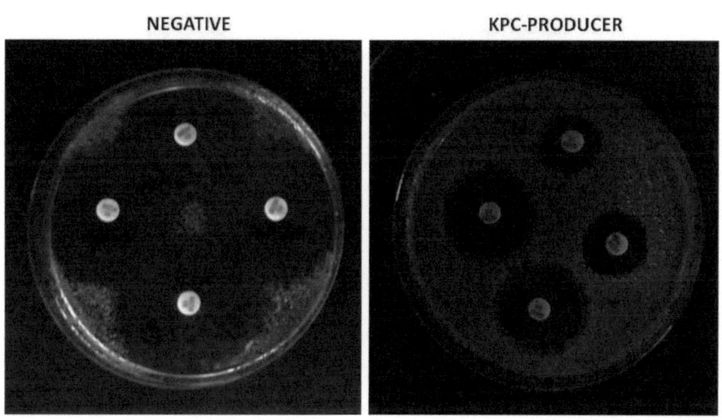

Figure 11. Application of the combination meropenem disc test for the direct differentiation of carbapenemase-producing *Enterobacteriaceae* in rectal swabs.

3.6. D-test

The D-test is used for the detection of inducible AmpC beta-lactamases [39]. An antibiotic is used as an inducer for AmpC production (imipenem or cefoxitin) whereas others are used as substrates (ceftazidime, cefotaxime, piperacillin/tazobactam).

3.6.1. Procedure

Step 1: Make a 0.5 McFarland bacterial suspension.

Step 2: Inoculate with a sterile cotton swab and place an imipenem disc.

Step 3: Place substrate discs (for example ceftazidime and piperacillin/tazobactam) near the imipenem disc as shown in Figure 12.

Step 4: Incubate at 37°C for 18-24h.

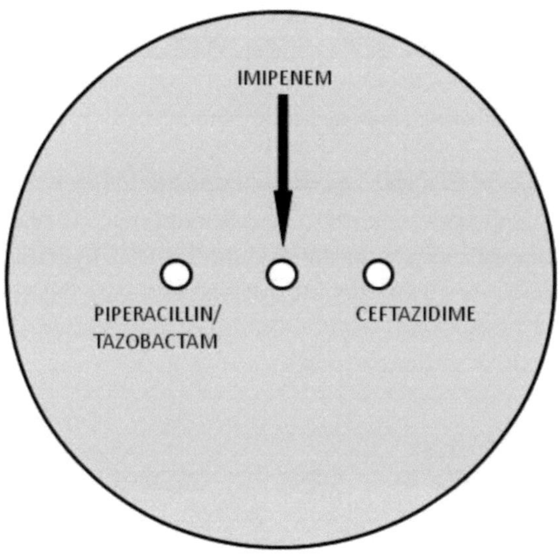

Figure 12. Preparation of a D-test.

3.6.2. Interpretation

The test is positive when a D-shaped inhibition zone is observed for one of the substrate discs (Figure 13) because of the imipenem-mediated induction of the AmpC production and the subsequent inactivation of the substrate antibiotic by the beta-lactamase. An important advantage of the test is that it can be easily incorporated within any routine antibiogram as shown in Figure 14.

http://dx.doi.org/10.5772/57582

3.7. CCCP test

CCCP (Carbonyl cyanide m-chlorophenyl hydrazone) is an efflux pump inhibitor that can be added in Mueller-Hinton agar during its preparation. The test is used to detect efflux pump overexpression that contributes to or determines carbapenem resistance in the study isolate [40].

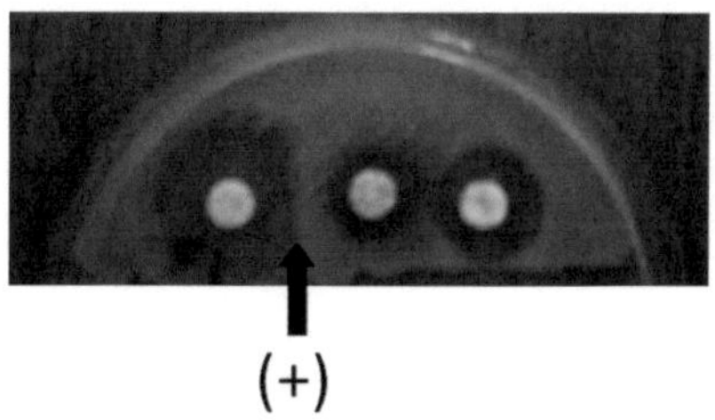

Figure 13. Interpretation of the D-test.

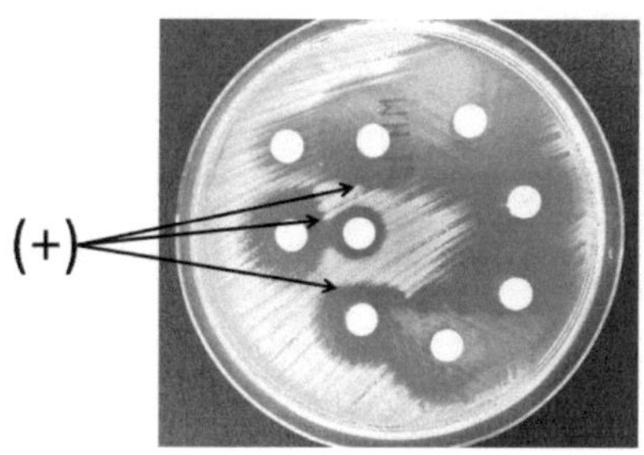

Figure 14. Incorporation of the D-test in a common antibiogram.

3.7.1. Procedure

Step 1: Prepare agar plates containing CCCP at a concentration of 12.5 μM.

Step 2: Make a 0.5 McFarland bacterial suspension.

Step 3: Inoculate with a sterile cotton swab on a CCCP-supplemented plate and in parallel on a CCCP-free plate. For economy reasons, two isolates may be inoculated on the same plate as shown in Figure 15.

Step 4: Place a meropenem disc on both plates for each inoculation.

Step 5: Incubate at 37°C for 18-24h.

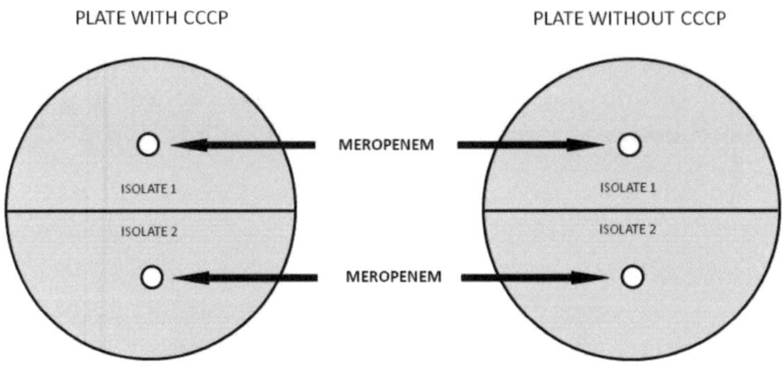

Figure 15. Preparation of the CCCP test.

3.7.2. Interpretation

The test is considered positive when synergy between meropenem and CCCP is observed on the CCCP-supplemented plate (Figure 16).

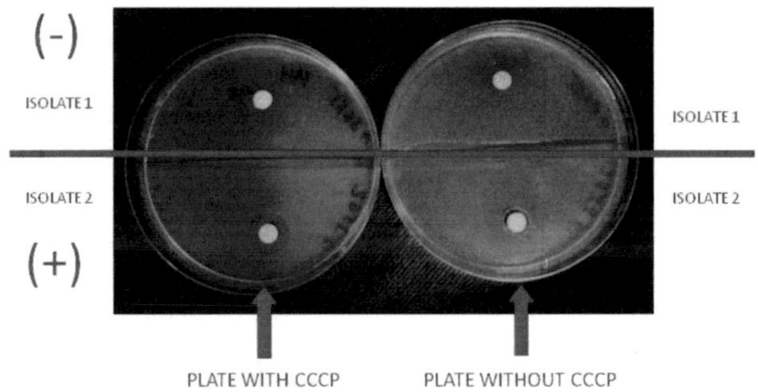

Figure 16. Interpretation of the CCCP test. Isolate 1 is inoculated on the upper side and isolate 2 is inoculated on the lower side of the plates. (+): Positive; (-): Negative.

4. Molecular methods

Genetic methods for the detection of resistance genes are based on nucleic acid hybridization and amplification. Therefore, the knowledge of specific primers (amplification nucleotides) and probes (labeled single-stranded ologonucleotides) is necessary in order to detect the genetic target of interest. The technique used depends on the type of resistance that is suspected. A simple polymerase chain reaction (PCR) may be applied searching for a gene that confers a certain level of resistance when it is expressed. This is the case for example, of genes encoding for antibiotic-inactivating enzymes. In Tables 2 and 3, primers for the detection of aminoglycoside or fluorquinolone resistance-conferring enzymes and beta-lactamases are shown, respectively.

http://dx.doi.org/10.5772/57582

Gene	Primers (5'- 3')	Product size	Reference
aac(6')-Ia	ATGAATTATCAAATTGTG	558 bp	[41]
	TTACTCTTTGATTAAACT		
aac(6')-Ic	CTACGATTACGTCAACGGCTGC	130 bp	[42]
	TTGCTTCGCCCACTCCTGCACC		
aac(3)-Ia	ACCTACTCCCAACATCAGCC	169 bp	[43]
	ATATAGATCTCACTACGCGC		
aac(3)-Ic	GATGATCTCTACTCAAACC	472 bp	[44]
	TTAGGCAGCAGGTTGAGG		
aac(3)-IV	GTTACACCGGACCTTGGA	675 bp	[45]
	AACGGCATTGAGCGTCAG		
aphA-3	GGGACCACCTATGATGTGGAACG	595 bp	[46]
	CAGGCTTGATCCCCAGTAAGTC		
aph(3')-Via	ATACAGAGACCACATACAGT	235 bp	[47]
	GGACAATCAATAATAGCAAT		
aad(2'')-Ia	ATGTTACGCAGCAGGGCAGTCG	188 bp	[48]
	CGTCAGATCAATATCATCGTGC		
aph(3')-IIIa	GGCTAAAATGAGAATATCACCGG	523 bp	[49,50]
	CTTTAAAAAATCATACAGCTCGCG		
ant(4')-Ia	CAAACTGCTAAATCGGTAGAAGCC	294 bp	[49,50]
	GGAAAGTTGACCAGACATTACGAACT		
strA-strB	TATCTGCGATTGGACCCTCTG	519 bp	[51]
	CATTGCTCATCATTTGATCGGCT		
armA	AGGTTGTTTCCATTTCTGAG	590 bp	[52]
	TCTCTTCCATTCCCTTCTCC		
rmtA	CTAGCGTCCATCCTTTCCTC	635 bp	[53]
	TTTGCTTCCATGCCCTTGCC		
rmtB	ATGAACATCAACGATGCCCT	769 bp	[54]
	CCTTCTGATTGGCTTATCCA		
gyrA	AAATCTGCCCGTGTCGTTGGT	343 bp	[55]
(***A. baumannii***)	GCCATACCTACGGCGATACC		
gyrA (*E. coli*)	ACGTACTAGGCAATGACTGG	190 bp	[56]
	AGAAGTCGCCGTCGATAGAAC		
qnrA	TCAGCAAGAGGATTTCTCA	627 bp	[57]
	GGCAGCACTATTACTCCCA		
Qnr	CCGTATGGATATTATTGATAAAG	661 bp	[58]
	CTAATCCGGCAGCACTATTA		

Table 2. Primers used for the detection of aminoglycoside and quinolone resistance determinants.

Gene	Primers (5'- 3')	Product size	Reference
bla$_{SHV}$	GGTTATGCGTTATATTCGCC	867 bp	[59]
	TTAGCGTTGCCAGTGCTC		
bla$_{TEM}$	ATGAGTATTCAACATTTCCG	867 bp	[59]
	CTGACAGTTACCAATGCTTA		
bla$_{CTX-M}$	CGCTTTGCGATGTGCAG	550 bp	[60]
	ACCGCGATATCGTTGGT		
bla$_{CTX-M-2}$	ATGATGACTCAGAGCATTCG	884 bp	[61]
	TTATTGCATCAGAAACCGTG		
bla$_{CTX-M-9}$	GTGACAAAGAGAGTGCAACGG	857 bp	[62]
	ATGATTCTCGCCGCTGAAGCC		
bla$_{CTX-M-10}$	GCTGATGAGCGCTTTGCG	684 bp	[63]
	TTACAAACCGTTGGTGACG		
bla$_{GES/IBC}$	GTTTTGCAATGTGCTCAACG	371 bp	[64]
	TGCCATAGCAATAGGCGTAG		
bla$_{PER-1}$	ATGAATGTCATTATAAAAGC	926 bp	[65]
	AATTTGGGCTTAGGGCAAGAAA		
bla$_{PER-2}$	CGCTTCTGCTCTGCTGAT	469 bp	[66]
	GGCAGCTTCTTTAACGCC		
bla$_{PSE}$	ACCGTATTGAGCCTGATTTA	321 bp	[67]
	ATTGAAGCCTGTGTTTGAGC		
bla$_{TLA-1}$	TCTCAGCGCAAATCCGCG	974 bp	[68]
	CTATTTCCCATCCTTAACTAG		
bla$_{VEB-1}$	CGACTTCCATTTCCCGATGC	643 bp	[69]
	GGACTCTGCAACAAATACGC		
bla$_{KPC}$	TGTCACTGTATCGCCGTC	331 bp	[70]
	TATTTTTCCGAGATGGGTGAC		
bla$_{SME-1}$	AACGGCTTCATTTTTGTTTAG	830 bp	[71]
	GCTTCCGCAATAGTTTTATCA		
bla$_{IMP}$	CTACCGCAGCAGAGTCTTTG	587 bp	[72]
	AACCAGTTTTGCCTTACCAT		
bla$_{IMP-1}$	ATGAGCAAGTTATCTGTATTC	741 bp	[73]
	TTAGTTGCTTGGTTTTGATGG		
bla$_{IMP-2}$	ATGAAGAAATTATTTGTTTTATG	741 bp	[73]
	TTAGTTACTTGGCTGTGATG		

http://dx.doi.org/10.5772/57582

Gene	Primers (5'- 3')	Product size	Reference
bla_{VIM}	TCTACATGACCGCGTCTGTC	748 bp	[74]
	TGTGCTTTGACAACGTTCGC		
bla_{VIM-1}	GTTAAAAGTTATTAGTAGTTTATTG	799 bp	[73]
	CTACTCGGCGACTGAGC		
bla_{VIM-2}	ATGTTCAAACTTTTGAGTAAG	801 bp	[73]
	CTACTCAACGACTGAGCG		
bla_{SPM-1}	CCTACAATCTAACGGCGACC	649 bp	[75]
	TCGCCGTGTCCAGGTATAAC		
bla_{NDM-1}	GGTTTGGCGATCTGGTTTTC	621 bp	[76]
	CGGAATGGCTCATCACGATC		
bla_{OXA-1}	CCAAAGACGTGGATG	540 bp	[77]
	GTTAAATTCGACCCCAAGTT		
bla_{OXA-10}	CGTGCTTTGTAAAAGTAGCAG	652 bp	[78]
	CATGATTTTGGTGGGAATGG		
bla_{OXA-23}	CCTCAGGTGTGCTGGTTATTC	513 bp	[79]
	CCCAACCAGTCTTTCCAAAA		
bla_{OXA-24}	TTCCCCTAACATGAATTTGT	1020 bp	[80]
	GTACTAATCAAAGTTGTGAA		

Table 3. Primers used for the detection of beta-lactamases frequently encountered among Gram negative pathogens.

In cases in which resistance depends upon the expression level (overexpression or downregulation) of the gene, real time Reverse Transcriptase-PCR (rt RT-PCR) is used to detect not only the presence, but also the mRNA expression of the gene. The results are consequently confronted with the expression level of the same gene in a control strain. This technique is useful for the study of the expression of specific porins and efflux pumps (primers and probes for such resistance determinants in *P. aeruginosa* are shown in Table 4).

Gene	Primers (5'- 3')	Reference
ampC	CGCCGTACAACCGGTGAT	[81]
	CGGCCGTCCTCTTTCGA	
probe	[DFAM]TCAGCCTGAAAGGAGAACCGCATTACTTC[DTAM]	
OprD	CTACGGCTACGGCGAGGAT	[81]
	GACCGGACTGGACCACGTACT	
probe	[DFAM]CACCACGAAACCAACCTCGAAGCC[DTAM]	
mexA	AACCCGAACAACGAGCTG	[81]

Gene	Primers (5'- 3')	Reference
	ATGGCCTTCTGCTTGACG	
probe	[DFAM]CATGTTCGTTCACGCGCAGTTG[DTAM]	
mexC	GGAAGAGCGACAGGAGGC	[81]
	CTGCACCGTCAGGCCCTC	
probe	[DFAM]CCGAAATGGTGTTGCCGGTG[DTAM]	
mexE	TACTGGTCCTGAGCGCCT	[81]
	TCAGCGGTTGTTCGATGA	
probe	[DFAM]CGGAAACCACCCAAGGCATG[DTAM]	
mexX	GGCTTGGTGGAAGACGTG	[81]
	GGCTGATGATCCAGTCGC	
probe	[DFAM]CCGACACCCTGCAGGGCC[DTAM]	

Table 4. Primers and probes used in real-time RT PCR for the determination of the expression levels for specific resistance mechanisms in *P. aeruginosa*.

Finally, sequencing [82-84] of the PCR product allows its confrontation with the already known gene sequences that are available in genetic databases. This can lead to the detection of mutations or to the characterization and classification of the gene within a genetic family.

5. Conclusion

There are several benefits and limitations using either phenotypic or molecular methods for the detection of resistance mechanisms in Gram negative pathogens. Phenotypic tests require bacteria in pure culture from a clinical sample thus needing 24-48h to obtain a final result. Molecular techniques on the other hand, can be performed directly with clinical speciments reducing significantly the procedure time.

The detection of low-level resistance is by definition problematic using phenotypic tests thus interpretation problems may appear. In such cases, molecular techniques are an option for clarifying the possible involvement of any known resistance mechanism.

Moreover, genetic detection gives a definite answer for the presence or not of specific resistance determinants within a study isolate (a specific beta-lactamase for example) whereas this is not possible with the phenotypic tests which provide only general information about the resistance mechanisms involved.

Genetic assays however, present also some major limitations: (i) It is possible to screen exclusively for known mechanisms and for one gene at the time (unless a multiplex PCR assay [85-88] can be applied) and; (ii) their cost is high and becomes higher when screening for multiple resistance determinants.

http://dx.doi.org/10.5772/57582

Consequently, the combined and rational use of the available methodologies seems to be the optimal solution for the cost-effective detection of resistance mechanisms in Gram negative pathogens by the Clinical Microbiology laboratory.

Acknowledgements

We are grateful to our teacher, Dr. Danai Sofianou for the knowledge that she has horizontally transferred to us during our collaboration at Hippokration General Hospital of Thessaloniki.

Author details

Meletis Georgios[1,2*], Tzampaz Egki[3] and Sianou Effrosyni[3]

*Address all correspondence to: meletisg@hotmail.com

1 Research Assistant, Aristotle University of Thessaloniki, School of Medicine, Thessaloniki, Greece

2 Clinical Microbiologist, Department of Clinical Microbiology, St. Paul's General Hospital, Thessaloniki, Greece

3 Clinical Microbiologist, Department of Clinical Microbiology, Hippokration General Hospital, Thessaloniki, Greece

References

[1] Meletis G. Editorial: war against multi-drug-resistant pathogens: what is new in the armory? Recent Pat Antiinfect Drug Discov 2012;7. 173-174.

[2] Hanson ND. Editorial: Resistance in gram-negative pathogens: a threat to global health. Curr Pharm Des 2013;19. 163.

[3] Savard P, Perl TM. A call for action: managing the emergence of multidrug-resistant Enterobacteriaceae in the acute care settings. Curr Opin Infect Dis 2012;25. 371-377.

[4] Grundmann H, Klugman KP, Walsh T, et al. A framework for global surveillance of antibiotic resistance. Drug Resist Updat 2011;14. 79-87.

[5] Campbell S. The need for a global response to antimicrobial resistance. Nurs Stand 2007;21. 35-40.

[6] Meletis G, Vavatsi N, Exindari M, et al. Accumulation of carbapenem resistance mechanisms in VIM-2-producing Pseudomonas aeruginosa under selective pressure. Eur J Clin Microbiol Infect Dis 2014;33. 253-258.

[7] Li H, Luo YF, Williams BJ, et al. Structure and function of OprD protein in Pseudomonas aeruginosa: from antibiotic resistance to novel therapies. Int J Med Microbiol 2012;302. 63-68.

[8] Zhang Y, Jiang X, Wang Y, et al. Contribution of β-lactamases and the porin proteins OmpK35 and OmpK36 to carbapenem resistance in clinical isolates of KPC-2-producing Klebsiella pneumoniae. Antimicrob Agents Chemother 2014;58. 1214-1217.

[9] Hong JH, Clancy CJ, Cheng S, et al. Characterization of porin expression in Klebsiella pneumoniae Carbapenemase (KPC)-producing K. pneumoniae identifies isolates most susceptible to the combination of colistin and carbapenems. Antimicrob Agents Chemother 2013;57. 2147-2153.

[10] Zeng ZR, Wang WP, Huang M, et al. Mechanisms of carbapenem resistance in cephalosporin-susceptible Pseudomonas aeruginosa in China. Diagn Microbiol Infect Dis. 2014;78. 268-270.

[11] Perez F, Rudin SD, Marshall SH, et al. OqxAB, a quinolone and olaquindox efflux pump, is widely distributed among multidrug-resistant Klebsiella pneumoniae isolates of human origin. Antimicrob Agents Chemother 2013;57. 4602-4603.

[12] Rodríguez-Martínez JM, Díaz de Alba P, Briales A, et al. Contribution of OqxAB efflux pumps to quinolone resistance in extended-spectrum-β-lactamase-producing Klebsiella pneumoniae. J Antimicrob Chemother 2013;68. 68-73.

[13] Skiada A, Markogiannakis A, Plachouras D, et al. Adaptive resistance to cationic compounds in Pseudomonas aeruginosa. Int J Antimicrob Agents 2011;37. 187-193.

[14] Fu Y, Zhang W, Wang H, et al. Specific patterns of gyrA mutations determine the resistance difference to ciprofloxacin and levofloxacin in Klebsiella pneumoniae and Escherichia coli. BMC Infect Dis 2013;13. 8.

[15] Aldred KJ, McPherson SA, Turnbough CL Jr, et al. Topoisomerase IV-quinolone interactions are mediated through a water-metal ion bridge: mechanistic basis of quinolone resistance. Nucleic Acids Res 2013;41. 4628-4639.

[16] Drlica K, Hiasa H, Kerns R, et al. Quinolones: action and resistance updated. Curr Top Med Chem 2009;9. 981-998.

[17] Gutkind GO, Di Conza J, Power P, et al. β-lactamase-mediated resistance: a biochemical, epidemiological and genetic overview. Curr Pharm Des 2013;19. 164-208.

[18] Ramirez MS, Tolmasky ME. Aminoglycoside modifying enzymes. Drug Resist Updat 2010;13. 151-171.

[19] Labby KJ, Garneau-Tsodikova S. Strategies to overcome the action of aminoglycoside-modifying enzymes for treating resistant bacterial infections. Future Med Chem 2013;5. 1285-1309.

[20] Cornaglia G, Giamarellou H, Rossolini GM. Metallo-β-lactamases: a last frontier for β-lactams? Lancet Infect Dis 2011;11. 381-393.

[21] Munoz-Price LS, Poirel L, Bonomo RA, et al. Clinical epidemiology of the global expansion of Klebsiella pneumoniae carbapenemases. Lancet Infect Dis 2013;13. 785-796.

[22] Queenan AM, Bush K. Carbapenemases: the versatile beta-lactamases. Clin Microbiol Rev. 2007;20. 440-458.

[23] Falagas ME, Karageorgopoulos DE. Extended-spectrum beta-lactamase-producing organisms. J Hosp Infect. 2009;73. 345-354.

[24] Bradford P. Extended-Spectrum-β-Lactamases in the 21st century: Characterization, epidemiology, and detection of this important resistance threat. Clin Microbiol Rev 2001;14. 933-951.

[25] Jacoby GA. AmpC beta-lactamases. Clin Microbiol Rev. 2009;22. 161-182.

[26] Brown S, Amyes S. OXA (beta)-lactamases in Acinetobacter: the story so far. J Antimicrob Chemother. 2006;57. 1-3.

[27] Jiang X, Zhang Z, Li M, et al. Detection of extended-spectrum beta-lactamases in clinical isolates of Pseudomonas aeruginosa. Antimicrob Agents Chemother 2006;50. 2990-2995.

[28] Lee K, Lim YS, Yong D, et al. Evaluation of the Hodge test and the imipenem-EDTA double-disk synergy test for differentiating metallo-beta-lactamase-producing isolates of Pseudomonas spp. and Acinetobacter spp. J Clin Microbiol 2003;41. 4623-4629.

[29] Pournaras S, Poulou A, Tsakris A. Inhibitor-based methods for the detection of KPC carbapenemase-producing Enterobacteriaceae in clinical practice by using boronic acid compounds. J Antimicrob Chemother 2010;65. 1319-1321.

[30] Tsakris A, Kristo I, Poulou A, et al. Evaluation of boronic acid disc tests for differentiating KPC-possessing Klebsiella pneumoniae isolates in the clinical laboratory. J Clin Microbiol 2009;47. 362–367.

[31] Tsakris A, Poulou A, Themeli-Digalaki K, et al. Use of boronic acid disc tests to detect extended-spectrum b-lactamases in clinical isolates of KPC carbapenemase-possessing Enterobacteriaceae. J Clin Microbiol 2009;47. 3420–3426.

[32] Pasteran F, Veliz O, Rapoport M, et al. Sensitive and specific modified Hodge test for KPC and metallo-beta-lactamase detection in Pseudomonas aeruginosa by use of a

novel indicator strain, Klebsiella pneumoniae ATCC 700603. J Clin Microbiol 2011;49. 4301-4303.

[33] Giakkoupi P, Pappa O, Polemis M, et al. Emerging Klebsiella pneumoniae isolates coproducing KPC-2 and VIM-1 carbapenemases. Antimicrob Agents Chemother 2009;53. 4048–4050.

[34] Meletis G, Tzampaz E, Protonotariou E, et al. Emergence of Klebsiella pneumoniae carrying bla(VIM) and bla(KPC) genes. Hippokratia 2010;14. 139 –140.

[35] Papagiannitsis CC, Giakkoupi P, Vatopoulos AC, et al. Emergence of Klebsiella pneumoniae of a novel sequence type (ST383) producing VIM-4, KPC-2 and CMY-4 beta-lactamases. Int J Antimicrob Agents 2010;36. 573–574.

[36] Pournaras S, Poulou A, Voulgari E, et al. Detection of the new metallo-beta-lactamase VIM-19 along with KPC-2, CMY-2 and CTX-M-15 in Klebsiella pneumoniae. J Antimicrob. Chemother 2010;65. 1604 –1607.

[37] Zioga A, Miriagou V, Tzelepi E, et al. The ongoing challenge of acquired carbapenemases: a hospital outbreak of Klebsiella pneumoniae simultaneously producing VIM-1 and KPC-2. Int J Antimicrob Agents 2010;36. 190–191.

[38] Pournaras S, Zarkotou O, Poulou A, et al. A combined disk test for direct differentiation of carbapenemase-producing enterobacteriaceae in surveillance rectal swabs. J Clin Microbiol 2013;51. 2986-2990.

[39] Dunne WM Jr, Hardin DJ. Use of several inducer and substrate antibiotic combinations in a disk approximation assay format to screen for AmpC induction in patient isolates of Pseudomonas aeruginosa, Enterobacter spp., Citrobacter spp., and Serratia spp. J Clin Microbiol 2005;43. 5945-5949.

[40] Pournaras S, Maniati M, Spanakis N, et al. Spread of efflux pump-overexpressing, non-metallo-beta-lactamase-producing, meropenem-resistant but ceftazidime-susceptible Pseudomonas aeruginosa in a region with blaVIM endemicity. J Antimicrob Chemother 2005;56. 761-764.

[41] Ploy MC, Giamarellou H, Bourlioux P, et al. Detection of aac(6')-I genes in amikacin-resistant Acinetobacter spp. by PCR. Antimicrob Agents Chemother 1994;38. 2925-2928.

[42] Hannecart-Pokorni E, Depuydt F, de wit L, et al. Characterization of the 6'-N-aminoglycoside acetyltransferase gene aac(6')-Im [corrected] associated with a sulI-type integron. Antimicrob Agents Chemother 1997;41. 314-318.

[43] Van de Klundert JM, Vliegenthart JS. PCR detection of genes coding for aminoglycoside-modifying enzymes, p. 547-552. In: Diagnostic Molecular Microbiology: Principles and Applications. American Society for Microbiology, Washington, D.C.

http://dx.doi.org/10.5772/57582

[44] Riccio ML, Docquier JD, Dell'Amico E, et al. Novel 3-N-aminoglycoside acetyltransferase gene, aac(3)-Ic, from a Pseudomonas aeruginosa integron. Antimicrob Agents Chemother 2003;47. 1746-1748.

[45] Guerra B, Soto SM, Argüelles JM, et al. Multidrug resistance is mediated by large plasmids carrying a class 1 integron in the emergent Salmonella enterica serotype [4,5,12:i:-]. Antimicrob Agents Chemother 2001;45. 1305-1308.

[46] Gibreel A, Sköld O, Taylor DE. Characterization of plasmid-mediated aphA-3 kanamycin resistance in Campylobacter jejuni. Microb Drug Resist 2004;10. 98-105.

[47] Vila J, Ruiz J, Navia M, et al. Spread of amikacin resistance in Acinetobacter baumannii strains isolated in Spain due to an epidemic strain. J Clin Microbiol 1999;37. 758-761.

[48] Vanhoof R, Content J, Van Bossuyt E, et al. Identification of the aadB gene coding for the aminoglycoside-2"-O-nucleotidyltransferase, ANT(2"), by means of the polymerase chain reaction. J Antimicrob Chemother 1992;29. 365-374.

[49] Sundsfjord A, Simonsen GS, Haldorsen BC, et al. Genetic methods for detection of antimicrobial resistance. APMIS 2004;112. 815-837.

[50] Vakulenko SB, Donabedian SM, Voskresenskiy AM, et al. Multiplex PCR for detection of aminoglycoside resistance genes in enterococci. Antimicrob Agents Chemother 2003;47. 1423-1426.

[51] Sunde M, Norström M. The genetic background for streptomycin resistance in Escherichia coli influences the distribution of MICs. J Antimicrob Chemother 2005;56. 87-90.

[52] Yamane K, Wachino J, Doi Y, et al. Global spread of multiple aminoglycoside resistance genes. Emerg Infect Dis 2005;11. 951-953.

[53] Yokoyama K, Doi Y, Yamane K, et al. Acquisition of 16S rRNA methylase gene in Pseudomonas aeruginosa. Lancet 2003;362. 1888-1893.

[54] Yan JJ, Wu JJ, Ko WC, et al. Plasmid-mediated 16S rRNA methylases conferring high-level aminoglycoside resistance in Escherichia coli and Klebsiella pneumoniae isolates from two Taiwanese hospitals. J Antimicrob Chemother 2004;54. 1007-1012.

[55] Vila J, Ruiz J, Goñi P, et al. Mutation in the gyrA gene of quinolone-resistant clinical isolates of Acinetobacter baumannii. Antimicrob Agents Chemother 1995;39. 1201-1203.

[56] Everett MJ, Jin YF, Ricci V, et al. Contributions of individual mechanisms to fluoroquinolone resistance in 36 Escherichia coli strains isolated from humans and animals. Antimicrob Agents Chemother 1996;40. 2380-2386.

[57] Robicsek A, Sahm DF, Strahilevitz J, et al. Broader distribution of plasmid-mediated quinolone resistance in the United States. Antimicrob Agents Chemother 2005;49. 3001-3003.

[58] Mammeri H, Van De Loo M, Poirel L, et al. Emergence of plasmid-mediated quinolone resistance in Escherichia coli in Europe. Antimicrob Agents Chemother 2005;49. 71-76.

[59] Rasheed JK, Jay C, Metchock B, et al. Evolution of extended-spectrum beta-lactam resistance (SHV-8) in a strain of Escherichia coli during multiple episodes of bacteremia. Antimicrob Agents Chemother 1997;41. 647-653.

[60] Bonnet R, Dutour C, Sampaio JL, et al. Novel cefotaximase (CTX-M-16) with increased catalytic efficiency due to substitution Asp-240-->Gly. Antimicrob Agents Chemother 2001;45. 2269-2275.

[61] Petroni A, Corso A, Melano R, et al. Plasmidic extended-spectrum beta-lactamases in Vibrio cholerae O1 El Tor isolates in Argentina. Antimicrob Agents Chemother 2002;46. 1462-1468.

[62] Sabaté M, Tarragó R, Navarro F, et al. Cloning and sequence of the gene encoding a novel cefotaxime-hydrolyzing beta-lactamase (CTX-M-9) from Escherichia coli in Spain. Antimicrob Agents Chemother 2000;44. 1970-1973.

[63] Oliver A, Pérez-Díaz JC, Coque TM, et al. Nucleotide sequence and characterization of a novel cefotaxime-hydrolyzing beta-lactamase (CTX-M-10) isolated in Spain. Antimicrob Agents Chemother 2001;45. 616-620.

[64] Weldhagen GF, Prinsloo A. Molecular detection of GES-2 extended spectrum Beta-lactamase producing Pseudomonas aeruginosa in Pretoria, South Africa. Int J Antimicrob Agents 2004;24. 35-38.

[65] Vahaboglu H, Hall LM, Mulazimoglu L, et al. Resistance to extended-spectrum cephalosporins, caused by PER-1 beta-lactamase, in Salmonella typhimurium from Istanbul, Turkey. J Med Microbiol 1995;43. 294-299.

[66] Bauernfeind A, Stemplinger I, Jungwirth R, et al. Characterization of beta-lactamase gene blaPER-2, which encodes an extended-spectrum class A beta-lactamase. Antimicrob Agents Chemother 1996;40. 616-620.

[67] Bert F, Branger C, Lambert-Zechovsky N. Identification of PSE and OXA beta-lactamase genes in Pseudomonas aeruginosa using PCR-restriction fragment length polymorphism. J Antimicrob Chemother 2002;50. 11-18.

[68] Alcantar-Curiel D, Tinoco JC, Gayosso C, et al. Nosocomial bacteremia and urinary tract infections caused by extended-spectrum beta-lactamase-producing Klebsiella pneumoniae with plasmids carrying both SHV-5 and TLA-1 genes. Clin Infect Dis 2004;38. 1067-1074.

[69] Naas T, Poirel L, Karim A, et al. Molecular characterization of In50, a class 1 integron encoding the gene for the extended-spectrum beta-lactamase VEB-1 in Pseudomonas aeruginosa. FEMS Microbiol Lett 1999;176. 411-419.

[70] Yigit H, Queenan AM, Anderson GJ, et al. Novel carbapenem-hydrolyzing beta-lactamase, KPC-1, from a carbapenem-resistant strain of Klebsiella pneumoniae. Antimicrob Agents Chemother 2001;45. 1151-1161.

[71] Queenan AM, Torres-Viera C, Gold HS, et al. SME-type carbapenem-hydrolyzing class A beta-lactamases from geographically diverse Serratia marcescens strains. Antimicrob Agents Chemother 2000;44. 3035-3039.

[72] Senda K, Arakawa Y, Ichiyama S, et al. PCR detection of metallo-beta-lactamase gene (blaIMP) in gram-negative rods resistant to broad-spectrum beta-lactams. J Clin Microbiol 1996;34. 2909-2913.

[73] Gutiérrez O, Juan C, Cercenado E, et al. Molecular epidemiology and mechanisms of carbapenem resistance in Pseudomonas aeruginosa isolates from Spanish hospitals. Antimicrob Agents Chemother 2007;51. 4329-4335.

[74] Poirel L, Naas T, Nicolas D, et al. Characterization of VIM-2, a carbapenem-hydrolyzing metallo-beta-lactamase and its plasmid-and integron-borne gene from a Pseudomonas aeruginosa clinical isolate in France. Antimicrob Agents Chemother 2000;44. 891-897.

[75] Sader HS, Reis AO, Silbert S, et al. IMPs, VIMs and SPMs: the diversity of metallo-beta-lactamases produced by carbapenem-resistant Pseudomonas aeruginosa in a Brazilian hospital. Clin Microbiol Infect 2005;11. 73-76.

[76] Nordmann P, Poirel L, Carrër A, et al. How to detect NDM-1 producers. J Clin Microbiol 2011;49. 718-721.

[77] Siu LK, Lo JY, Yuen KY, et al. beta-lactamases in Shigella flexneri isolates from Hong Kong and Shanghai and a novel OXA-1-like beta-lactamase, OXA-30. Antimicrob Agents Chemother 2000;44. 2034-2038.

[78] Steward CD, Rasheed JK, Hubert SK, et al. Characterization of clinical isolates of Klebsiella pneumoniae from 19 laboratories using the National Committee for Clinical Laboratory Standards extended-spectrum beta-lactamase detection methods. J Clin Microbiol 2001;39. 2864-2872.

[79] Brown S, Young HK, Amyes SG. Characterisation of OXA-51, a novel class D carbapenemase found in genetically unrelated clinical strains of Acinetobacter baumannii from Argentina. Clin Microbiol Infect 2005;11. 15-23.

[80] Bou G, Oliver A, Martínez-Beltrán J. OXA-24, a novel class D beta-lactamase with carbapenemase activity in an Acinetobacter baumannii clinical strain. Antimicrob Agents Chemother 2000;44. 1556-1561.

[81] Quale J, Bratu S, Gupta J, et al. Interplay of efflux system, ampC, and oprD expression in carbapenem resistance of Pseudomonas aeruginosa clinical isolates. Antimicrob Agents Chemother 2006;50. 1633-1641.

[82] Franca LT, Carrilho E, Kist TB. A review of DNA sequencing techniques. Q Rev Biophys 2002;35. 169-200.

[83] Diene SM, Rolain JM. Investigation of antibiotic resistance in the genomic era of multidrug-resistant Gram-negative bacilli, especially Enterobacteriaceae, Pseudomonas and Acinetobacter. Expert Rev Anti Infect Ther 2013;11. 277-296.

[84] Fournier PE, Drancourt M, Raoult D. Bacterial genome sequencing and its use in infectious diseases. Lancet Infect Dis 2007;7. 711-723.

[85] Woodford N. Rapid characterization of beta-lactamases by multiplex PCR. Methods Mol Biol 2010;642. 181-192.

[86] Bisiklis A, Papageorgiou F, Frantzidou F, et al. Specific detection of blaVIM and blaIMP metallo-beta-lactamase genes in a single real-time PCR. Clin Microbiol Infect 2007;13. 1201-1203.

[87] Poirel L, Walsh TR, Cuvillier V, et al. Multiplex PCR for detection of acquired carbapenemase genes. Diagn Microbiol Infect Dis 2011;70. 119-123.

[88] Huang XZ, Cash DM, Chahine MA, et al. Development and validation of a multiplex TaqMan real-time PCR for rapid detection of genes encoding four types of class D carbapenemase in Acinetobacter baumannii. J Med Microbiol 2012;61. 1532-1537.

Chapter 7

Trends in Research and Technology Development Related to Zoonosis Control Based on Bibliometric and Patent Analyses–Taking Rabies as an Example

Hiromi Takahashi-Omoe and Katsuhiko Omoe

Additional information is available at the end of the chapter

http://dx.doi.org/10.5772/57566

1. Introduction

Infectious diseases, particularly zoonoses, are recognized as the sources of serious problems that affect public and animal health around the world. Emerging infectious diseases have been reported at an unprecedented rate since the 1970s and a large proportion of these diseases are considered to be zoonoses [1]. However, reemerging zoonoses are also affecting public health around the world, in particular rabies, a classic zoonosis that is problematic in Africa and Asia, while new outbreaks have occurred in areas that were previously free of this disease, such as the islands of Flores and Bali in Indonesia [2].

Thus, research and technology development have been promoted for controlling emerging and reemerging zoonoses in developed countries. In the case of rabies, the research and technology developed to prevent this disease has been advancing. Rabies is a vaccine-preventable disease, so a vaccine has been developed. The type of vaccine produced using animal nervous tissues has been progressively replaced by safer and more immunogenic vaccines, which are purified from cell culture supernatants. In addition, new replicative vaccines have been developed for the oral vaccination of wildlife, which are either attenuated rabies vaccines or recombinant vaccines where different viruses express the rabies glycoprotein [3]. Moreover, user-friendly diagnostic methods have been developed, e.g., a rapid immunochromatographic test kit and a simple enzyme-linked immunosorbent assay (ELISA) [4,5]. Understanding the current trends in research and technology development related to rabies control may provide a useful reference regarding the technological needs encountered in the field of zoonoses.

Bibliometric analysis is considered to be an effective method for identifying research trends in infectious disease control. Quantitative surveys of research articles (hereafter referred to as article) based on bibliometric studies have been reported in the field of infectious diseases, such as human immunodeficiency virus (HIV)/acquired immune deficiency syndrome (AIDS) [6], tuberculosis research in India and China [7], and various forms of infectious disease research in different regions of the world [8], Asia [9], and around the world [10]. In particular, we have surveyed Asian and worldwide research trends, while ensuring that we avoided underestimating the number of articles in non-English and regional journals, rather than simply surveying journals registered in the "Infectious Disease Category" of the Science Citation Index Expanded™ [9,10].

Patent analysis is also considered to be an effective method for technology development trend analysis. Patents are examined and granted by patent offices, and they are considered to be objective indicators of technology development activities. In addition, patents have significant advantages in terms of database availability, the variety of information included, and their systematic classification according to standardized schemes, e.g., the international patent classification (IPC) supports the detailed analysis of specific technological aspects. For these reasons, patent data are used intensively for strategic technology management by companies [11], as well as for science and technology (S&T) measurement in policy-making processes and academic research in various fields [12]. Indeed, patent analyses have been reported in the field of infectious diseases, such as hepatitis B vaccines [13] and influenza [14,15].

Research and technology development for rabies control is considered to be important for future public and animal health throughout the world, as described above. However, to the best of our knowledge, bibliometric and patent analyses of rabies have not been reported yet. Therefore, in this chapter, we report the current trends in research and technology development for rabies control in the US, the EU, and Asia based on analyses of articles and patent applications. We targeted patent applications because publication of a patent application is invariably the earliest point when relevant technology information becomes available to the public because it is the first set of detailed and up-to-date published information. Furthermore, the number of patent applications in particular technological areas is considered to indicate the volume of resources allocated [16].

The trends in research and technology development for rabies control will be summarized using the following indicators.

- Number of articles and patent applications during each year and by each country
- Number of authors and applicants by nationality
- Number of articles by organization
- Major research areas of articles and the technical areas of patent applications
- Top 10 cited articles and patent applications

Based on this analysis, we discuss the future directions of research and technology development for rabies control. Moreover, we propose the development of a survey method for zoonosis control, research and technology development.

http://dx.doi.org/10.5772/57566

2. Trends in rabies research based on articles

We used a two-tiered approach to analyze research related to rabies control. First, we performed a quantitative analysis of all articles about rabies. Subsequently, we analyzed the top 10 cited articles, irrespective of whether they were related to rabies control.

2.1. Method of analysis

The Web of Science® [17] was used to survey articles about rabies, which covers over 12,000 journals worldwide, including open access journals. Using the Web of Science®, keyword and title search of articles was performed using the terms "Rabies" OR "Lyssa" (to include virus species related to rabies virus) NOT "Rabi" (to exclude articles in the field of optics, e.g., articles related to "Rabi oscillations") on June 24, 2013. The publication period of articles ranged from January 1, 2001 to December 31, 2011.

We focused on articles and excluded reviews, proceedings papers, and other types of publications. This is because articles are high quality because they have been peer reviewed and are directly linked to the outputs of the latest research.

Other articles in the field of infectious diseases retrieved by the Web of Science® were also analyzed to identify the characteristics of articles related to rabies.

2.2. Leading countries based on the number of articles

The total number of articles related to rabies published throughout the world during 2001–2011 was 2,565. We regrouped the articles by country to identify any possible differences in research output among countries. The US was the leading country, with the highest percentage of total articles, i.e., 32.5% of the total (833 articles). There was a big gap for the second placed country, France, with 10.6% of the total (273 articles). The UK, Brazil, and Germany followed with 10.1% (258 articles), 8.6% (220 articles), and 7.2% (185 articles), respectively (Figure 1).

As shown in Table 1, the US, France, the UK, and Germany were the top four countries with most articles related to rabies, and they were also the leading countries for all articles about infectious diseases. However, Brazil ranked in the top five with most articles related to rabies. This showed that rabies research was a particular focus in Brazil.

2.3. Annual changes in the number of articles

As shown in Figure 2, the total number of articles related to rabies increased during 2001–2011. However, the US did not show a remarkable change, although it produced the highest output. Other countries such as the UK, France, Brazil, and Germany also had stable outputs. Thus, the overall increase in articles was considered to be attributable to other countries that were not surveyed in this study.

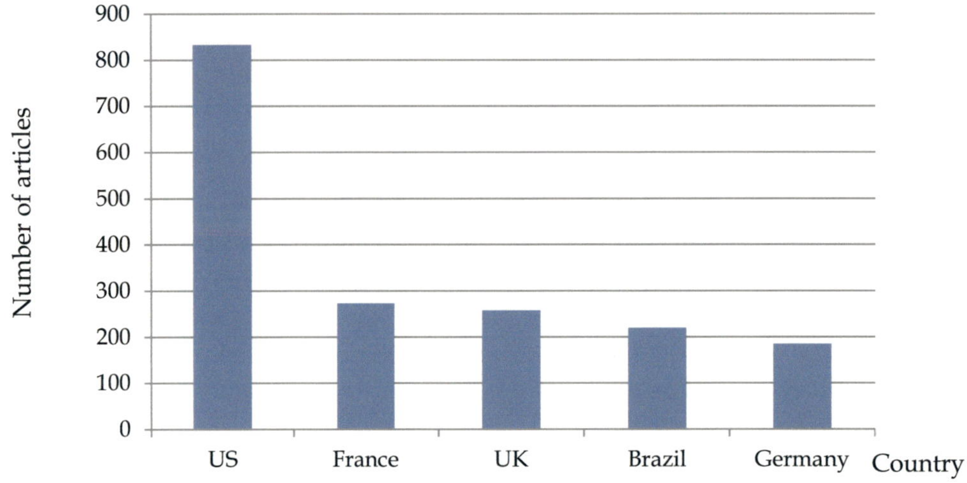

Figure 1. Number of articles related to rabies by country during 2001–2011

Number of articles about rabies

Rank	Country	Number of articles	Relative to the total number of articles (%)
1	US	833	32.5
2	France	273	10.6
3	UK	258	10.1
4	Brazil	220	8.6
5	Germany	185	7.2

Search condition
Keywords: Rabies OR Lyssa NOT Rabi
Document type: Article
Total number of articles: 2,565 articles

Number of articles in the field of infectious diseases

Rank	Country	Number of articles	Relative to the total number of articles (%)
1	US	35,488	38.5
2	UK	9,437	10.2
3	France	7,625	8.3
4	Germany	4,908	5.3
5	Spain	4,906	5.3

Search condition
Research field: infectious diseases
Document type: Article
Total number of articles: 92,113 articles

Table 1. Comparison of the rankings for articles related to rabies and all infectious disease articles during 2001–2011

2.4. Number of articles by organization

US Centers for Disease Control and Prevention (US CDC) published most articles related to rabies (198 articles) during 2001–2011. Institut Pasteur (France) and Thomas Jefferson University (US) published the second and third highest numbers of articles (141 and 87 articles, respectively) (Figure 3).

http://dx.doi.org/10.5772/57566

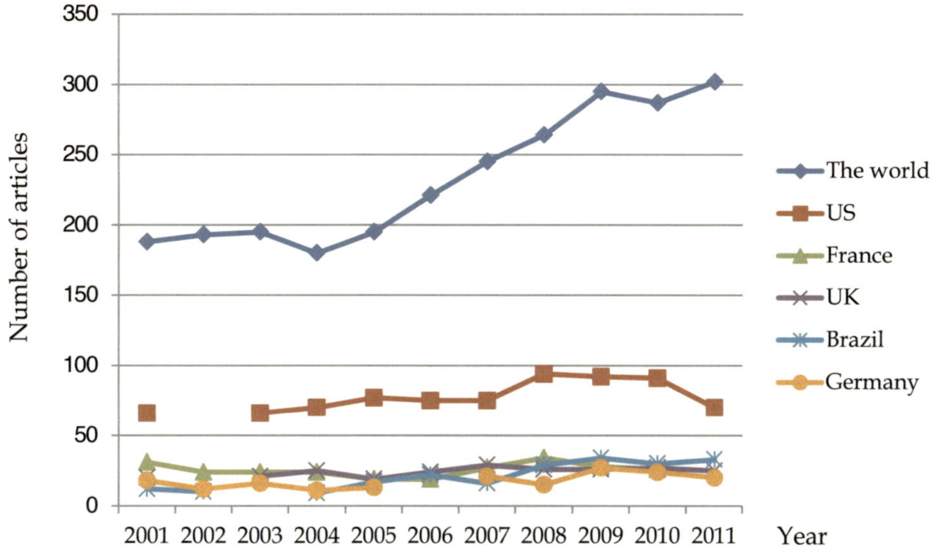

Figure 2. Number of articles related to rabies by year during 2001–2011

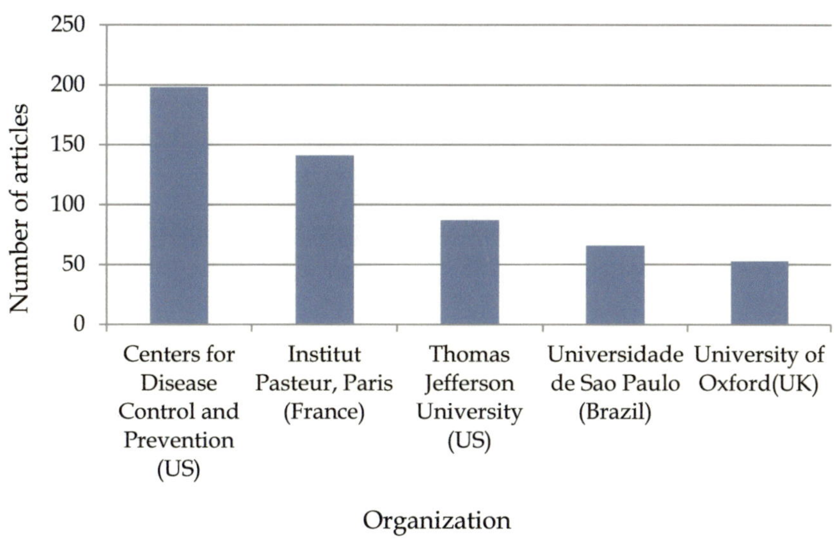

Figure 3. Number of articles related to rabies by organization during 2001–2011

2.5. Major research areas

Figure 4 shows the number of articles related to rabies for each research field, which showed that the main field of rabies research was veterinary sciences. Research was also conducted in basic sciences, such as virology and immunology. It is considered that virological and immunological research on rabies contributes to the development of vaccines and diagnostic methods.

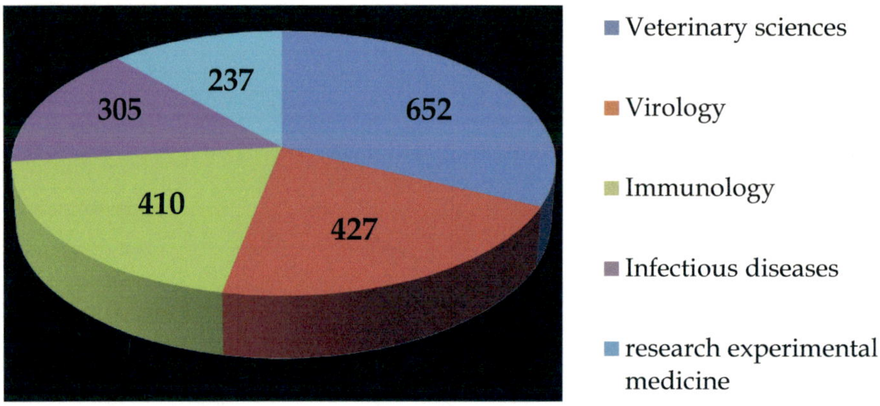

The values are the number of articles.

Figure 4. Number of articles related to rabies by research field during 2001–2011

2.6. Top 10 cited articles

Table 2 shows top 10 most cited articles related to rabies. Of these articles, two reported and discussed methods for rabies control [18,19]. It was interesting that the two articles were based on new research areas, i.e., agent-based modeling and economic analysis. These studies were not categorized in the major research areas described in Section 2.5.

Three articles reported rabies virus as the delivery of a substance to the brain, i.e., a neuronal tracer, and a vector [20–22]. This shows that research on rabies may contribute to neuroscience research.

3. Trends in technology development related to rabies control based on patent applications

Subsequently, we performed quantitative and qualitative analyzes of patent applications related to rabies control, e.g., technologies related to vaccines, screening, and the diagnosis of rabies.

3.1. Method of analysis

The survey of patent applications comprised the following four steps.

http://dx.doi.org/10.5772/57566

Rank	Cited number	Title	Author(s)	Journal	Volume, Page, Year	Contribution to rabies control
1	400	Pattern-oriented modeling of agent-based complex systems: Lessons from ecology	Grimm, V. et al.,	SCIENCE	310, 987-991, 2005	Yes (rabies prevalence simulation)
2	377	Transvascular delivery of small interfering RNA to the central nervous system	Kumar, P. et al.,	NATURE	448, 39-43, 2007	No (usage of viral peptide as delivery to the brain)
3	339	Cerebellar loops with motor cortex and prefrontal cortex of a nonhuman primate	Kelly, R.M. et al.,	JOURNAL OF NEUROSCIENCE	23, 8432-8444, 2003	No (usage of virus as neuronal tracer)
4	314	Efficacy of RTS,S/ASO2 malaria vaccine against Plasmodium falciparum infection in semi-immune adult men in The Gambia: a randomised trial	Bojang, K.A. et al.,	LANCET	358, 1927-1934, 2001	No (usage of rabies vaccine as a control of malaria vaccine)
5	288	Re-evaluating the burden of rabies in Africa and Asia	Knobel, D.L. et al.,	BULLETIN OF THE WORLD HEALTH ORGANIZATION	83, 360-368, 2005	Yes (study to quantify public health and economic burden)
6	261	Small world effect in an epidemiological mode	Kuperman, M. et al.,	PHYSICAL REVIEW LETTERS	86, 2909-2912, 2001	No (epidemiological model based on the structure of a population)
7	249	Cannabinoid-based drugs as anti-inflammatory therapeutics	Klein, T.W.	NATURE REVIEWS IMMUNOLOGY	5, 400-411, 2005	No (therapeutic usefulness of these drugs in chronic inflammatory diseases)
8	239	Diseases of humans and their domestic mammals: pathogen characteristics, host range and the risk of emergence	Cleaveland, S. et al.,	PHILOSOPHICAL TRANSACTIONS OF THE ROYAL SOCIETY OF LONDON SERIES B-BIOLOGICAL SCIENCES	356, 991-999, 2001	Indirectly yes (database analysis of multihost pathogens)
9	214	Rabies virus glycoprotein pseudotyping of lentiviral vectors enables retrograde axonal transport and access to the nervous system after peripheral delivery	Mazarakis, N,D. et al.,	HUMAN MOLECULAR GENETICS	10, 2109-2121, 2001	No (usage of virus protein as a virus vector)
10	208	Population biology of multihost pathogens	Woolhouse, M.E.J. et al.,	SCIENCE	292, 1109-1112, 2001	Indirectly yes (database analysis of multihost pathogens)

Table 2. Top 10 cited articles related to rabies during 2001–2011

3.1.1. Step 1-Collection of data sources for patent applications

The Derwent Patent Index® (DWPI) and the Derwent Patent Citation Index® (DPCI) [23,24] were used to survey patent applications related to rabies control using the search strategy described below.

DWPI is one of the largest and most user-friendly patent databases in the world, which contains over 21.85 million patent families that cover over 45.2 million patent documents. It includes coverage of over 47 worldwide patent authorities with enhanced patent titles and abstracts prepared by subject experts to facilitate the survey of patent documents. Additionally the DWPI assembles all of the patent documents relating to an invention into a single database record as a "patent family". A single "patent family" is a set of either patent applications or publications taken in multiple countries to protect a single invention by a common inventor(s) [25]. DPCI provides patent citation information from 10 organizations, including the EPO and the WIPO.

To survey the number of applicants by nationality, we used the FAMPAT® [26], which is a comprehensive worldwide patent family database. We used the FAMPAT® because the DWPI does not include the nationalities of applicants.

3.1.2. Step 2-Screening and selection of patent applications

Using the DWPI, we surveyed Asian, US, and European patent applications related to rabies control by patent family, as well as patent applications filed under the International Patent Cooperation Treaty [27] for 2001–2011 (the year when priority was claimed based on the patent application) on December 21, 2012. In this study, one should note that the data of "patent applications" represented the data of "patent families" assembled uniquely by the DWPI. The countries targeted for analysis are shown in Table 3 and they were selected based on our previous study, i.e., the countries that published more infectious disease research articles than other countries [10].

We screened patent applications using search formulae 1–7 as shown in Table 3, which were based on keywords and the IPC. Patent applications were selected that contained the keywords in the titles or abstracts and that belonged to the IPC categories. To ensure the complete capture of all relevant patent applications, we used "Rabies" and inflected forms of the keywords such as "Rabic" and "Rabid", and "Lyssa." We also used the IPC categories that included antigens, antibodies, amino acids, chemical compounds, and anti-infectives related to the *Rhabdoviridae* family or RNA viruses, which include the rabies virus and lyssaviruses.

After screening the patent applications, we selected patent applications related to rabies control. We reviewed all the abstracts and claims for patent applications to identify applications related to the prevention and diagnosis of rabies.

We primarily focused on patent applications that claimed technologies for preventive and diagnostic uses related to rabies genes and proteins, but we also included applications related to technologies for producing vaccine adjuvants and for stabilization, as well as other pertinent items within the search scope. For example, a patent application was included that claimed a recombinant adenovirus as a rabies vaccine carrier. However, we excluded patent applications related to research and therapeutic tools for other diseases, e.g., the synthesis of rabies virus proteins for human neurodegenerative disorder therapy and the development of a rabies virus vector for expressing other viral proteins.

3.1.3. Step 3-Analysis of patent applications

The patent applications selected in Step 2 were analyzed with respect to the following items; patenting activity (the number of patent applications per application year and for each country, and the number of applicants by nationality), major technical areas of patent applications, and the most cited patent applications. We used citation analysis as an indicator of important technological progress, upon which many later patents may rely [28].

3.2. Total number of patent applications

The screening of patent applications related to rabies control retrieved 354 candidates. The candidates included keywords related to rabies in the titles or abstracts and belonged to the IPC categories A61K-039/205, C07K-014/145, A61P-031/12, A61P-031/14, or G01N-033/569 (Table 3). Subsequently, we selected 237 of 354 patent applications by reviewing all the

http://dx.doi.org/10.5772/57566

	Search formula	Number of patent applications retrieved*	Survey content
1	PRD = 2001:2011	11,315,347	Priority year
2	(US OR EP OR GB OR DE OR ES OR FR OR IT OR NL OR JP OR CN OR KR OR IN)/PC	20,081,126	Country or patent administration office (the US, the European Patent Office, the UK, Germany, Spain, France, Italy, the Netherlands, Japan, China, Korea, and India)
3	(RABIES OR RABIC OR RABID OR LYSSA)/TI/AB/EAB	1,317	Keywords related to rabies
4	(A61K-039/205 OR C07K-014/145)/IC	601	IPC for medical preparations containing antigens or antibodies against *Rhabdoviridae* (A61K-039/205) or peptides with more than 20 amino acids from *Rhabdoviridae* (C07K-014/145)
5	(A61P-031/12 OR A61P-031/14)/IC	25,706	IPC for the specific therapeutic activity of chemical compounds or medicinal preparations for antiinfectives (A61P-031/12) or RNA viruses (A61P-031/14)
6	(G01N-033/569)/IC	11,177	IPC for investigating or analyzing materials by determining the chemical or physical properties of micro-organisms
7	1 AND 2 AND 3 AND (4 OR 5 OR 6)	354	Targeted patent applications

IPC: International Patent Classification

*The number of patent applications was calculated by patent family. In some cases, a patent family contains a number of relevant patent applications.

Table 3. Table 3 Search formula and the number of patent applications retrieved

abstracts and claims to identify patent applications related to rabies control. The following analysis was based on results, which included 237 patent applications.

3.3. Annual change in the number of patent applications by country

We regrouped the patent applications and applicants for each country to identify possible differences in technology development among various countries. The numbers of PCT applications and applications in each country were stable during 2001–2011, except in China where the number increased relatively. The US had the most patent applications until 2007, but was overtaken by China in 2008. We found that China had a remarkable increase in patent applications after 2002. Japan had a downward trend after 2009 and fell behind India during 2009–2010 (Figure 5).

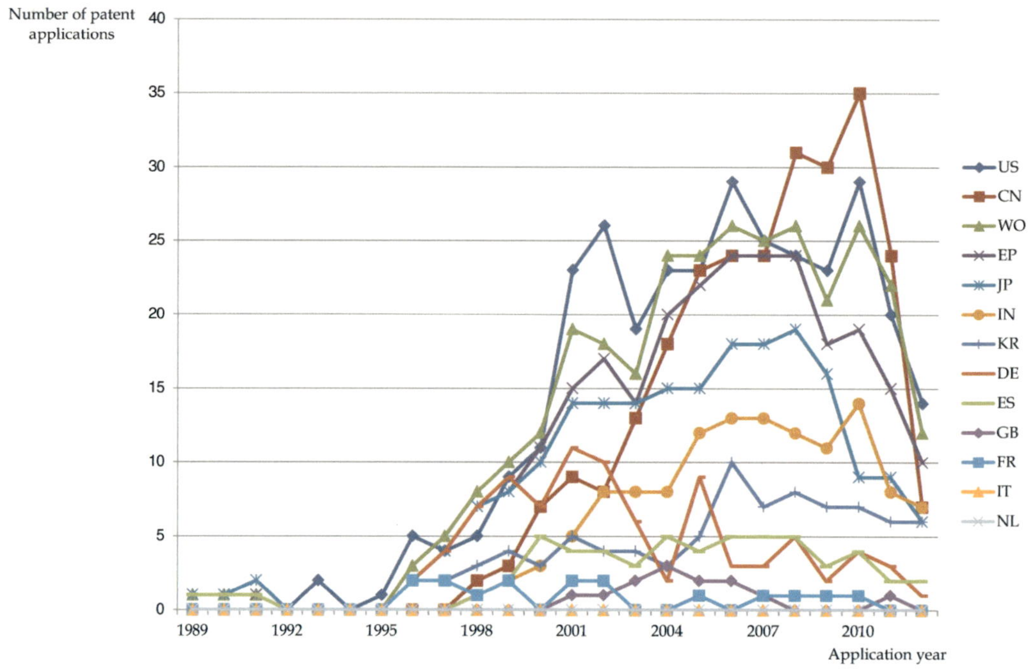

Figure 5. Number of patent applications related to rabies control by country during 2001–2011

The number of patent applications was calculated by patent family. In some cases, a patent family contains a number of relevant patent applications. US: United States, CN: China, WO: PCT, EP: European Patent Office, JP: Japan, IN: India, KR: Korea, DE: Germany, ES: Spain, GB: UK, FR: France, IT: Italy, NL: the Netherlands

3.4. Number of patent applicants by country

The US had the most applicants, but was overtaken by China in 2008–2009. China had a remarkable increase in applicants after 2003, while it decreased temporarily in 2006. Germany, Japan, and France had ≤5 patent applications per year during 2001–2011 (Figure 6).

3.5. Major technological fields of patent applications

The technological types of 237 patent applications related to rabies control were determined in the contexts of prevention, diagnosis, and treatment. As shown in Table 4, the patent applications were classified into seven technological fields: recombinant virus, protein, peptide, organic active ingredient, natural product, fabrication method, and mutant. Patent applications related to recombinant viruses were the most frequent and they primarily claimed

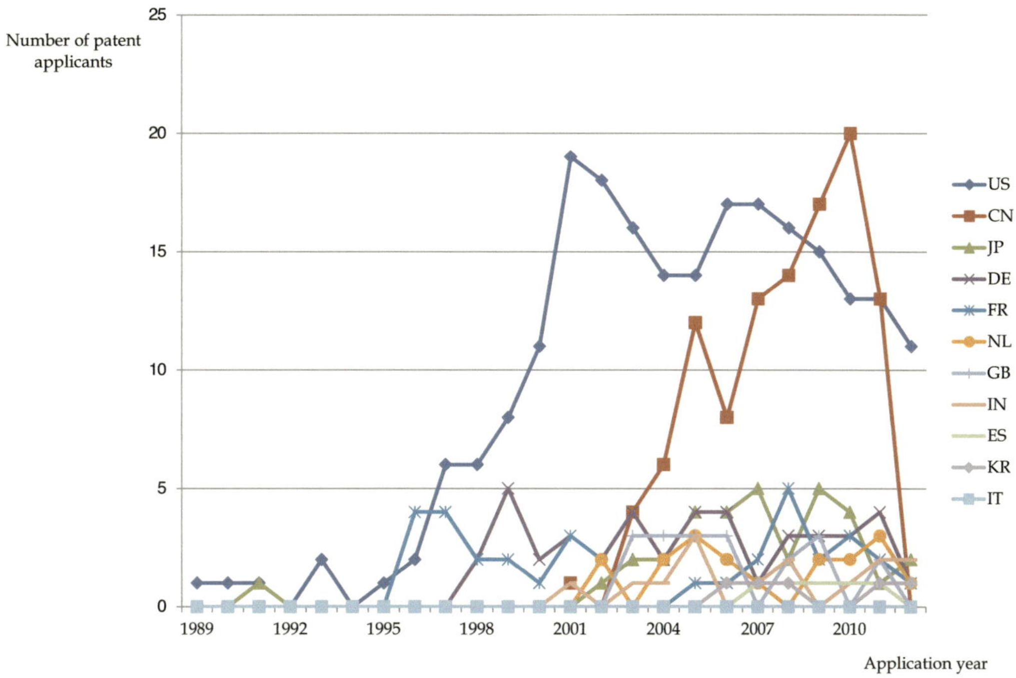

US: United States, CN: China, JP: Japan, DE: Germany, FR: France, NL: the Netherlands, GB: UK, IN: India, ES: Spain, KR: Korea, IT: Italy

Figure 6. Number of patent applicants related to rabies control by country during 2001–2011

uses for the prevention and treatment of rabies. Patent applications related to organic active ingredients used for treatments, fabrication methods for prevention (primarily vaccines), and natural products and Chinese herbal extracts for treatment were more frequent than other patent applications. Patent applications related to natural products and Chinese herbal extracts were primarily from China.

The number of patent applications was calculated by patent family. In some cases, a patent belonged to two or more technology fields, so the total number of applications exceeded 237.

3.6. Top 10 most cited patent applications

Table 5 shows the top 10 most cited patent applications related to rabies. All the patent applications were related to diagnostic or therapeutic methods for rabies, such as immuno-conjugates (US 5332567, WO200454622), a vaccine carrier (US 6019978), and a monoclonal antibody production system (WO200476677). It was interesting that all the patent applications were applicable to various pathogens, such as bacteria, viruses, and mycoplasma, whereas none were specifically applicable to the rabies virus.

	Prevention (primarily vaccine)	Diagnosis (detection of virus, antibodies)	Treatment (medical drugs for post-exposure prophylaxis etc.)	Other
Recombinant virus (e.g. replication-defective adenovirus recombinant as a rabies vaccine carrier)	60	12	42	9
Protein (e.g. chimeric rabies G protein)	18	13	15	0
Peptide (e.g. antigenic peptide of rabies virus)	10	8	14	0
Organic active ingredient (e.g. organophosphorous compound for producing medicaments for therapeutic treatment of infections caused by virus)	17	2	36	0
Natural product, Chinese herbal extract (e.g. red bean-derived antiviral agent)	9	0	24	2
Fabrication method (e.g. preparation method of rabies vaccine)	31	7	15	8
Mutant (e.g. attenuated recombinant rabies virus mutant for live vaccines)	10	1	5	0
Other	10	14	5	2

Table 4. Technology fields of patent applications related to rabies control during 2001–2011

Rank	Cited number	patent number	applicants	Title	Contribution to rabies control
1	101	US5332567	IMMUNOMEDICS	Detection and treatment of infections with immunoconjugates	Yes (method of targeting a polyspecific diagnostic agent for virus infection including rabies)
2	57	WO200366005	CONFORMA THERAPEUTICS	Ansamycins having improved pharmacological and biological properties	Yes (method of treating or preventing infection including rabies)
3	45	WO200464759	CHIRON	Use of tryptanthrin compounds for immune potentiation	Yes (enhancement of the immune response to infections including rabies)
4	40	WO200476677	INSTITUTE FOR RESEARCH BIOMEDICINE	Monoclonal antibody production by EBV transformation of B cells	Yes (providing a neutralizing monoclonal human antibodies that recognizes antigens from various pathogens including rabies virus)
5	37	US20060228300	IBC PHARMACEUTICALS	Stably tethered structures of defined compositions with multiple functions or binding specificities	Yes (useful for treating subjects infected with various pathogens including rabies virus)
6	32	US6019978	WISTAR INSTITUTE OF ANATOMY & BIOLOGY UNIVERSITY OF PENNSYLVANIA	Replication-defective adenovirus human type 5 recombinant as a vaccine carrier	Yes (more efficacious method in comparison with the currently used vaccinia rabies vaccine)
7	31	WO9800166	RHONE MERIEUX	Recombinant canine adenovirus (CAV) containing exogenous DNA	Yes (vector for cloning heterologous DNA encodes epitopes of interests from antigens of veterinary pathogens including rabies)
8	31	US6180111	MARYLAND UNIVERSITY OF	Vaccine delivery system	Yes (useful for the diagnosis of viral diseases including rabies)
9	29	WO200775270	IBC PHARMACEUTICALS	Multivalent immunoglobulin-based bioactive assemblies	Yes (useful for treating infection with various pathogens including rabies virus)
10	29	WO200454622	IMMUNOMEDICS MCCALL JOHN DOUGLAS	Immunoconjugates with an intracellularly-cleavable linkage	Yes (useful for therapeutic conjugates against pathogens including rabies virus)

Table 5. Top 10 most cited patent applications related to rabies control during 2001–2011

http://dx.doi.org/10.5772/57566

4. General overview of research and technology development related to rabies control based on bibliometric and patent analyses

Our bibliometric and patent analyses using the Web of Science®, DWPI, and DPCI highlighted five main features of the trends in research and technology development related to rabies control during 2001–2011.

4.1. Research and technology developments related to rabies control were diverse and polyspecific

Given that the major research areas were veterinary sciences, virology, and immunology (Figure 4), and that the two most cited articles related to rabies control belonged to interdisciplinary research regions, i.e., agent-based modeling and economic analysis (Table 2), it is apparent that rabies research has diversified from classical to novel research areas. In particular, new research is prospective and aims to accelerate the development of domestic and international management frameworks for rabies.

However, the methods used for rabies diagnosis and vaccine development are progressing if we take patent US 5332567 and US 6019978 as examples of the top 10 most cited patent applications (Table 5). These methods were characterized as being applicable to various other pathogens and were polyspecific. Given that current rabies vaccines aim to introduce new functions, e.g., animal rabies vaccines combined with other antigens [3], these polyspecific methods would contribute to further vaccine development.

4.2. Gap between research and technology development for rabies control

We found that the number of articles related to rabies increased throughout the world, but the number of patent applications directed at rabies control was stable according to PCT and in each country. Given that only two of the top 10 most cited articles were directly related to rabies control, as shown in Table 2, and that none of the top 10 patent applications were specifically for rabies control, as shown in Table 5, it was not clear whether the articles were directly linked to the patent applications for rabies. Thus, it is not necessarily that research on rabies leads to technological developments related to rabies control.

4.3. The US, France, and the UK are the leading countries for rabies research

The survey demonstrated that the US led rabies research because it had the highest percentage of total articles related to rabies, i.e., 32.5% of the total. France ranked second (10.6%) but there was a big difference compared with the US. These two countries and the UK were also the top three producers of articles in the area of infectious diseases (Table 1). Four of the top five organizations that published articles related to rabies were also in these three countries. These results showed that the US, France, and the UK were the undisputed leaders in research on rabies and all infectious diseases.

4.4. Brazil was a particularly productive country for rabies research

Like the US, France, and the UK, Brazil was considered to be a productive country for rabies research because it published the fourth highest number of articles (Table 1). The Universidade de Sao Paulo was ranked fourth among the top five organizations (Figure 3) and it played a leading role in rabies research in Brazil.

Brazil may have a high level of rabies research because this country has initiated nationwide public campaigns to vaccinate dogs and cats against rabies, which have demanded studies to assess the antibody levels in vaccinated animals [29]. Moreover, research on rabies control has been active because the population has a serious risk of infection given the close relationships between these potential zoonosis-transmitting animals and humans [29].

4.5. Development of patent applications for rabies control in China

China exhibited a remarkable increase in patent applications (Figure 5). It was significant that China overtook the US with respect to the number of patent applications after 2007. From a technological perspective, patent applications related to natural products and Chinese herbal extracts increased greatly, as described in section 3.5.

The Chinese statistics showed that 1,633,000 patent applications (the total number of invention patents, design patents, and utility models) were filed with the State Intellectual Property Office (SIPO) by 2011, with a greater than threefold increase during 2005 alone [30]. This remarkable increase in the overall volume of patent applications in China may be attributable to the subsidization policy specified by the China Elements of Strategy for Intellectural Property Right, which facilitated the creation, application, protection, and management of intellectual property rights in 2008. Thus, the notable increase in overall patent applications after the change in China's policy may have led to the increased number of patent applications related to rabies control.

5. Conclusion

This chapter describes the trends in research and technology development related to rabies control during 2001–2011, which illustrate the measures introduced to control zoonoses. We found that the research and technology development activities differed among countries, which were characterized as diverse and polyspecific. The methods used for rabies diagnosis and vaccine development were found to be progressing.

The highly cited research on agent-based modeling and economic impact analysis shows that new interdisciplinary studies of rabies are being conducted. These studies are aimed to accelerate the development of domestic and international management frameworks for rabies.

This bibliometric and patent analysis did not demonstrate that articles (indicators of research outputs) were closely linked to patent applications (indicators of technology development). Our method aimed to measure science linkage to analyze the effects of science and research

http://dx.doi.org/10.5772/57566

on technology development. Science linkage is an indicator of technological innovation, which is based on calculating the number of non-patent references such as articles, which are an indicator of the degree of science related to patents, i.e., the number of articles cited per patent [31]. There are technological limitations to science linkage, but many studies have aimed to measure the linkage of patents filed in the US and Europe [31]. From this perspective, measuring science linkage may be a challenge during future surveys of the trends in research and technology development related to rabies control. This challenge will also apply to zoonoses in general.

Acknowledgements

The study described in this chapter was supported by a Japanese Grant-in-Aid for Scientific Research (KAKENHI) (research project number 23580435). We thank Mr. Mitsuaki Baba (Property Co., Ltd.) for his technical support to survey patents.

Author details

Hiromi Takahashi-Omoe[1*] and Katsuhiko Omoe[2]

*Address all correspondence to: omoe@nistep.go.jp

1 National Institute of Science and Technology Policy (NISTEP), Japan

2 Iwate University, Japan

References

[1] Jones KE, Patel NG, Levy MA, Storeygard A, Balk D, Gittleman JL, Daszak P. Global trends in emerging infectious diseases. Nature 2008; 451 990-994.

[2] Lembo T, Hampson K, Kaare MT, Ernest E, Knobel D, Kazwala RR, Haydon DT, Cleaveland S. The feasibility of canine rabies eliminations in Africa: Dispelling doubts with data. PLOS Neglected Tropical Diseases 2010; 4 e626. http://www.plosntds.org/article/info%3Adoi%2F10.1371%2Fjournal.pntd.0000626 (accessed 15 August 2013)

[3] Tordo N. New developments in rabies vaccines. OIE Global Conference on Rabies Control, 7-9 September 2011, Seoul, Republic of Korea. http://www.oie.int/eng/A_RABIES/Abstracts_rabiesConf/abstract1-6/S2/Tordo.pdf (accessed 15 August 2013)

[4] Nishizono A, Khawplod P, Ahmed K, Goto K, Shiota S, Mifune K, Yasui T, Takayama K, Kobayashi Y, Mannen K, Tepsumethanon V, Mitmoonpitak C, Inoue S, Morimoto K. A simple and rapid immunochromatographic test kit for rabies diagnosis. Microbiology and Immunology 2008; 52 243-249.

[5] Xu G, Weber P, Hu Q, Xue H, Audry L, Li C, Wu J, Bourhy H. WELYSSA: a simple tool using mouse monoclonal antibodies for the detection of lyssavirus nucleocapsid in rabies suspecyed speciments. Developments in biologicals 2008; 131 555-561.

[6] Falagas ME, Bliziotis IA, Kondilis B, Soteriades ES. Eighteen years of research on AIDS: contribution of and collaborations between different world regions. AIDS Research and Human Retroviruses 2006; 22 1199-1205.

[7] Arunachalam S, Gunasekaran S. Tuberculosis research in India and China: From bibliometrics to research policy. Current Science 2002, 82 933-947.

[8] Bliziotis IA, Paraschakis K, Vergidis PI, Karavasiou AI, Falagas ME. Worldwide trends in quantity and quality of published articles in the field of infectious diseases. BMC Infectious Diseases 2005; 5 16. http://www.biomedcentral.com/1471-2334/5/16 (accessed 15 August 2013)

[9] Takahashi-Omoe H, Omoe K, Okabe N. New journal selection for quantitative survey of infectious disease research: application for Asian trend analysis. BMC Medical Research Methodology 2009; 9 67. http://www.biomedcentral.com/1471-2288/9/67 (accessed 15 August 2013)

[10] Takahashi-Omoe H, Omoe K. Worldwide trends in infectious disease research revealed by a new bibliometric method. Rijeka, In Tech; 2012. http://www.intechopen.com/books/insight-and-control-of-infectious-disease-in-global-scenario/worldwide-trends-in-infectious-disease-research-revealed-by-bibliometrics (accessed 15 August 2013)

[11] Ernst, H. Patent information for strategic technology management. World Patent Information 2003; 25 233-242.

[12] Organizsation for Economic Co-operation and Development. Patent statistics manual.

[13] http://www.oecd.org/science/innovationinsciencetechnologyandindustry/oecdpatentstatisticsmanual.htm (accessed 15 August 2013)

[14] Sanyal G, Shi L. A review of multiple approaches towards an improved hepatitis B vaccine. Expert Opinion on Therapeutic Patents 2009; 19 59-72.

[15] World Intellectual Property Organization. WIPO patent search report on pandemic influenza preparedness (PIP)-related patents and patent applications. WIPO; 2011. http://www.wipo.int/export/sites/www/patentscope/en/programs/patent_landscapes/documents/patent_landscapes/influenza_full_report_01_04_2011.pdf (accessed 15 August 2013)

[16] Dou H, Bai Y.. A rapid analysis of avian influenza patens in the Esp@cenet database – R&D strategies and country comparisons. World Patent Information 2007; 29 26-32.

[17] Wang SJ. Candida vaccines development from point view of US patent application. Human Vaccines 2011,7 1165-1171.

[18] Thomson Reuters. Web of Science. http://thomsonreuters.com/web-of-science/ (accessed 15 August 2013)

[19] Grimm V, Revilla E, Berger U, Jeltsch F, Mooij WM, Railsback SF, Thulke HH, Weiner J, Wiegand T, DeAngelis DL. Pattern-oriented modeling of agent-based complex systems: Lessons from ecology. Science 2005; 310 987-991.

[20] Knobel DL, Cleaveland S, Coleman PG, Fèvre EM, Meltzer MI, Miranda ME, Shaw A, Zinsstag J, Meslin FX. Re-evaluating the burden of rabies in Africa and Asia. Bulletin of the World Health Organization 2005; 83 360-368.

[21] Mazarakis ND, Azzouz M, Rohll JB, Ellard FM, Wilkes FJ, Olsen AL, Carter EE, Barber RD, Baban, DF, Kingsman SM, Kingsman AJ, O'Malley K, Mitrophanous KA. Rabies virus glycoprotein pseudotyping of lentiviral vectors enables retrograde axonal transport and access to the nervous system after peripheral delivery. Human Molecular Genetics 2001; 10 2109-2121.

[22] Kelly RM, Strick PL. Cerebellar loops with motor cortex and prefrontal cortex of a nonhuman primate. Journal of Neuroscience 2003; 23 8432-8444.

[23] Kumar P, Wu H, McBride JL, Jung KE, Kim MH, Davidson BL, Lee SK, Shankar P, Manjunath N. Transvascular delivery of samll interfering RNA to the central nervous system. Nature 2007; 448 39-43.

[24] Thomson Reuters. Derwent World Patents Index. http://thomsonreuters.com/derwent-world-patents-index/ (accessed 15 August 2013)

[25] Thomson Reuters. Patent Citation Index. http:// http://ip-science.thomsonreuters.com/support/patents/userguides/pciguides/ (accessed 15 August 2013)

[26] Questel. FamPat-The invention at the heart of family. http://www.questel.orbit.com/prodsandservices/FamPat.htm (accessed 15 August 2013)

[27] World Intellectual Property Organization. PCT. The International Patent System. http://www.wipo.int/pct/en/ (accessed 15 August 2013)

[28] Smith VM. Who's who in additives-a technological approach. Chemical Week 1993; 38 137-142.

[29] Albas A, Picolo MR, Soares CN, Bachega HV, Tarumoto MH. Humoral immune response in dogs and cats vaccinated against rabies in southeastern Brazil. Journal of Venomous Animals and Toxins including Tropical Diseases 2013;19 17.

[30] Nishiuchi, S. Analysis of the trend on intellectual property in China. http://monoist.atmarkit.co.jp/mn/articles/1207/23/news009.html (accessed 15 August 2013)

[31] Tamada S. Measureing science linkage in four priority technology categories. Research & Review, Research Institute of Economy, Trade & Industry, IAA; 2004. http://www.rieti.go.jp/en/papers/research-review/020.html (accessed 15 August 2013)

Section 4

Infectious Diseases Epidemiology & Surveillance

Chapter 8

Unearthing the Complexities of Mathematical Modeling of Infectious Disease Transmission Dynamics

Sutapa Biswas Majee and Gopa Roy Biswas

Additional information is available at the end of the chapter

http://dx.doi.org/10.5772/57387

1. Introduction

Epidemiology is considered as the study of causes of occurrence and transmission of diseases in human population. It deals with the properties of epidemics in the equilibrium or long-time steady state. It involves prediction and monitoring of the spread of both naturally occurring infection and infection caused by bioterrorism, within a population based on the data regarding course of infection in a single isolated individual. It enables identification of measures for improving the health of the community as a whole. Epidemics can pass through the population at an extremely fast rate, may persist for a long time at low levels, may show cyclic patterns or there may be sudden flare-ups. Therefore, meaningful data collection and data interpretation are the essential components of epidemiology. These data can be exploited to identify trends, make general predictions and assess shortcomings of those predictions. Such prediction can be highly erroneous unless derived mathematically and here lies the utility of mathematical modeling. Moreover, age, clinical status and socio-economic status of the patient, environmental condition, demographic data, meta-population structure, geographical location etc are of great relevance to the disease occurrence, prevalence, persistence and ultimately eradication from a heterogeneous population.

For an in-depth and complete understanding of the unpredictable behavior and pattern of transmission of infectious diseases, both in time and space, epidemiological modeling proves to be a very powerful tool. It enables the epidemiologist to think rigorously and frame policies for protection and treatment of the unaffected and affected population respectively from the invasion by the pathogen. The use of mathematical model in the study of infectious diseases is being envisaged as an insightful alternative to ethically challenging, expensive and at times, practically impossible in vivo and in vitro detailed experimentation and subsequent complicated interpretation. There are instances when the models and the experimental data exist in a symbiotic relationship and improve our quantitative understanding of the infection dynamics. These models are used to hypothetically disrupt or neutralize genes and simulate infections within a few seconds. Latent infections that can be maintained for decades in a host can be mathematically reactivated to determine the effect on an outbreak. Sometimes, the concept of modeling has been enriched by introduction of an idea from a related field of science as in the case of HIV quasi-species model inspired by molecular quasi-species model in chemistry [1].

Interpretation of variables associated with mathematical modeling helps in estimation of parameters of biological significance and deduction of concepts not directly perceptible from the data. These concepts prove invaluable in giving rise to the observed patterns as also unearthing the complexities underlying the infection. Concept-building, as derived from the framework of mathematical model, gives lead-time to the medical fraternity and the government policy-makers in designing and implementing timely intervention measures for prevention and control of spread of a communicable disease.

Daniel Bernoulli is regarded as the father of epidemiological modeling since he investigated the influence of variolation on life expectancy as early as 1760. One of the fundamental principles of epidemiology, the threshold theorem was established by Kermack and McKendrick in 1927 to establish the dynamics of bubonic plague. Disease persistence in large host population was determined by Barlett.

2. Basis of infectious disease

Spread of an infectious disease depends on several factors like factors related to the pathogen, environmental factors, population factors and finally, social structure and behavior of the contagion. Natural birth and death rates of the population are independent of the pathogen. The rate of transmission may differ in different age groups where incubation period may vary. Type and mode of contact or incidence function and immunity duration are known to govern the spread. Geographical location and seasonality are other factors affecting the spread of an infection [2-4].

Complete understanding of infectious diseases requires knowledge of the various processes involved in host-parasite interactions. The two most important processes in these interactions are the epidemiological process associated with disease transmission within the population and immunological process involved in the disease dynamics within the host. Modeling of host-pathogen interactions helps in identification of key factors that may have a major impact on the outcome of an infection. In dynamic models of viral diseases, epidemiological modeling is based on the interaction between the susceptible and infected classes of the population and within-host dynamics is usually overlooked [5]. In any viral or bacterial infection, one of the key determinants of the disease progression within the host is the immunological status which is governed by dynamic interaction between different groups of cells and various signaling molecules [1].

Some of the terminologies associated with infectious disease are (a) infectivity or secondary attack rate, which is defined as the ratio of number infected and number exposed, (b) patho-

http://dx.doi.org/10.5772/57387

genicity or illness rate, which is expressed as the ratio of number with symptoms and number infected and lastly, (c) virulence which may be written as the ratio of number of severe/fatal cases and total number of cases. For example, chicken pox and measles are characterized by high infectivity, high pathogenicity and low virulence whereas, smallpox is recognized by high levels of all the three variables and tuberculosis is found to possess low infectivity, low pathogenicity and high degree of virulence.

3. Categories of infectious diseases

The etiological agents of micro-parasitic infections are viruses, bacteria, protozoa or prions, all of which are usually unicellular and of microscopic size and can reproduce very fast. High degree of prevalence of this class of infections among the children worldwide is a matter of great concern to the parents, school authorities and the government. They include measles, rubella, chickenpox, mumps, whooping cough etc. Usual route of transmission is by direct contact through air-borne droplets. These diseases are characterized by high infectivity, short disease generation length and low mean age at infection, on one hand and lifelong acquired immunity following recovery on the other hand.

Macroparasitic infections, caused by parasites, visible to the naked eye (e.g. helminthes, arthropods) are characterized by short duration of immunity following recovery. The number of parasites per host is a critical factor in epidemiology of this category of infections [6].

Microparasitic or macroparasitic infections can occur by either direct or indirect transmission. Usually microparasitic infections are transmitted by direct contact between two individuals as in the case of influenza, HIV, measles etc. The pathogen cannot survive outside the host body. Macroparasites, on the other hand, are indirectly transmitted and they spend a part of their lifecycle outside the host system, freely in the environment. There is a third category of diseases or vector-borne diseases where the causative organism is passed from primary host to the vector and from vector to another primary host as found in case of malaria, filariasis, sleeping sickness etc. [7].

Variation in the characteristics of the infectious agent is manifested as difference in traits and thus arises the need of different dynamics.

4. Mathematical model

Mathematical models help in generating and clarifying hypotheses, assessing quantitative conjectures, finding answers to specific questions, determining sensitivities to changes in parameter values and estimating parameters from data in absence and presence of preventive and therapeutic interventions. Therefore, according to input-output approach, mathematical model may be viewed as a system where the facts about the disease serve as the inputs and prediction about the number of infected and uninfected people over time is regarded as the output. A model is usually expressed in terms of variables which are related to experimentally measurable quantities.

A mathematical model helps in establishment of links between sets of epidemiological data through well-understood mathematical relationships. This is facilitated only through a thorough understanding of various factors associated with the disease like, incubation, transmission and mortality and also factors associated with the vector. Models may also help to characterize and integrate the cellular network and molecular data operating within the different compartments of the host immunity system for disease progression. At a mechanistic level, they help in finding answers to several biological questions which cannot be addressed experimentally. Different conceptual qualitative results and threshold values of paramount importance like basic reproduction ratio, contact numbers, replacement numbers and herd immunity, are derived from mathematical models, since the quantity and diversity of available data is limited. Conditions for local and global stability of various equilibria, relationships among these stability conditions and endemicity are also derived from the epidemiological models. Prediction and recommendations for control of an epidemic outbreak are therefore, the most important outcomes of mathematical modeling of a communicable disease and then they are known as decision models. These models facilitate economic evaluation of different courses of action for mitigation of a particular infection and finally help in selection of optimal control measure [8].

Spatio-temporal progression and temporal development of communicable diseases can be explained by compartmental, agent-based or contact network-based model. In the compartmental model, the host population is divided into different states or compartments, depending on the level of infection in them. Rates of transfer e.g. transmission rate, removal rate between compartments are expressed as derivatives of the sizes of the compartments with respect to time and are assumed to be constant. Ordinary differential equations form the basic framework of compartmental models. In agent-based model, the region of interaction of people in a population is considered as a system of software agents interacting in time and space. It is a high fidelity model and involves complex parameterization and extensive computation. Modern concepts of network theory are employed in dissecting the transmission dynamics within heterogeneous population in a contact network model. Social networking among the individuals influence the possibility, extent and speed of epidemic spreading. This model is intermediate between compartmental model and agent-based model. In this model, the pathogen and the social network within the population are closely intertwined and represented by a node for each individual. The framework of contact network highly depends on the mode of transmission of the disease [2], [9].

Accuracy, transparency and flexibility are the key elements which should be balanced to develop a mathematical model of high quality. For development of any type of mathematical model, mathematical modelers formulate a set of equations by feeding into them various type of factors like the length of time one is ill, the length of time one can infect others, the level of contagiousness of the disease, the number of uninfected individuals who can contract the disease, human behavior and any such known component of disease dynamics. Once a model with biological significance and relevance has been formulated, the model can be fitted to the

http://dx.doi.org/10.5772/57387

experimental data to obtain estimates for the kinetic parameters associated with the system, which are otherwise difficult to obtain experimentally.

Qualitative fitting of the data enables deeper understanding of the disease dynamics and quantitative fitting helps in designing and implementing control measures [7]. Apart from constructing a set of equations, data fitting and estimation of parameters, mathematical model also uses some graphical tools for characterization of dynamical systems. Phase plane technique like, linearization approximation is a graphical tool used to analyze the system dynamics of one state variable as a function of another state variable. In such plot, time dimension is not present but the trajectory of the dynamics is shown by arrows. The second technique is bifurcation diagram reserved for visualization of relatively complex dynamics. Bifurcation diagram is a summary of the asymptomatic dynamics of a dynamical system as a function of a bifurcation parameter [6].

5. Compartmental mathematical models

These models can be either Susceptible-Infectious-Recovered (SIR), Susceptible-Infectious-Recovered-Susceptible (SIRS), Susceptible-Exposed-Infectious-Recovered (SEIR), Susceptible-Infected (SI) or Susceptible-Infectious-Susceptible (SIS). Number of compartments in the model depend on the disease being studied and the objective of the study. In this approach, the progress of the disease is defined in terms of level of pathogen within the host.

5.1. SIR model

Number or density of individuals in each stage of infection is more important than the load of the pathogen per person in modeling of microparasitic infections. In the SIR model in order to emulate epidemics, population is classified as Susceptible, currently Infectious and Recovered. The total size of the host population is the summation of the three classes. When an individual is concerned, he is assumed to exist in either of the three states. Susceptible means that the individual has never had the disease and is susceptible to contraction of the disease by an infected individual, at random from the population. The mode of transmission of infection depends on the type of the pathogen. Depending on the relative magnitude of the latent period of the infection, the infected host can infect others and then it becomes Infectious. The total time spent in the infected state by an individual is a geometric random variable. When the infectious agent is removed from the system of the infected class or death occurs, they become Recovered with immunity and will never be infected again. In case of a dead individual, he cannot get infected or cannot infect anybody and thus is equivalent to a recovered individual with acquired immunity. Then, it can be assumed that the number of infected individuals tends to decrease towards zero and finally disappears from the network permanently. In the study of disease dynamics, six distinct and well-defined events can be assumed to occur : birth, death of a susceptible individual, death of an infected individual, death of a recovered individual, infection and recovery. Epidemic data supports the assumption that the per capita rate at which a given susceptible individual becomes infected is proportional to the prevalence of infection in the population. Therefore, according to SIR model, number of cases increases exponentially initially till there has been a sufficient decrease in the proportion of susceptible when the growth rate slows; this process goes on until the epidemic can no longer be maintained and the number of cases goes below a threshold level resulting in disease eradication. Human behavior can affect the disease dynamics in an individual as also in the whole population because it may influence the disease state of an individual, rate of infection or recovery rate and the contact network structure. Therefore, behavioral responses should be considered as an integral part of the study of dynamics of infectious diseases. An intriguing feature of childhood microparasitic infections is that the children are born in the susceptible category as there is no vertical transmission. Birth rate and vaccination affect the recruitment to the susceptible compartment. Moreover, in case of common cold, there is no permanent removal state because the individual enters the susceptible class soon after recovery. This widely used model is applicable for diseases which are contracted by an individual only once in its lifetime and either acquired lifelong immunity develops or death occurs as in case of measles, mumps, SARS, influenza. An important drawback of the model is that it ignores the random effects, specially at early stages of infection, when the number of both susceptible and infected classes is low. This model is unable to describe the spatial aspects of the spread of the disease. Moreover, in this modeling approach it is assumed that each individual has the same amount of contacts as every other individual. Therefore, if the rate of contact varies during course of infection, it cannot be appropriately included in the simple SIR model. Precision in prediction can be improved by incorporating realistic contact patterns or by using modeling approaches possessing higher fidelity.

The SIR model can also be expressed by a stochastic version where the future course of the infection is independent of the past, if present is known completely [2], [6], [9-10].

5.2. SIRS

This model assumes that after recovery, the person becomes susceptible again as immunity wanes, i.e. recovered individuals possess short-term immunity [4], [14].

5.3. SEIR

It is an extended SIR model where a new compartment or state is added. It is known as Exposed or E which is positioned between the susceptible and infectious compartments. The Exposed individual is infected but not infectious, i.e. the disease remains in latent state [15].This concept can also be explained on the basis of the level of pathogen within the host and immunological status of the host. When the host is susceptible, it indicates that no pathogen is present and only a low level of non-specific immunity exists within the host. As soon as the susceptible encounters an infectious individual, he becomes infected. The pathogen increases in number and the infected host may not show any signs of infection and thus he enters the Exposed compartment. As soon as the pathogen burden is sufficiently high, the Exposed host becomes Infectious and disease is transmitted to another susceptible individual. When the Infectious individual can no longer transmit infection as the pathogen is cleared from his immunity system, he belongs to the Recovered category. The class distinction between Exposed-

http://dx.doi.org/10.5772/57387

Infectious and Infectious-Recovered is not very distinct because of variability in responses between different individuals and variability in pathogen levels over the infectious period [7].

5.4. SI model

This modeling approach is unrealistic in case of animal or human infections because here it is assumed that an infected individual remains in this state forever. Hence, the ultimate consequence of the presence of one infected individual in the population is the infection of the entire population. In the early stages of an infection, when the count of infected cases is low, the SI and SIR models behave in a similar fashion as there is limited number of recovered individuals.

5.5. SIS model

In this model, individuals run stochastically through the cycle of Susceptible-Infected – Susceptible. Thus, here exist only two states because the infected individual, after recovery, again becomes susceptible to infection. Removal due to death or acquired immunization is not considered. Therefore, the number of infected individuals increases up to a stationary non-zero constant value as observed in case of sexually transmitted diseases [10]. The renewed susceptibility of an individual is due to vast antigenic variation associated with gonorrhea and other similar sexually transmitted diseases [7]. This model is based on assumptions like, different contagion probabilities between different pairs of people, probabilistic recovery from the disease and multiple stages of infection, with varying disease properties [9].

6. Deterministic and Stochastic approach to mathematical modeling

If the objective of the study is to model disease propagation in a large population, with continuous variations of population sizes, deterministic model is the most appropriate one. Such model indicates same output or same fate of individuals subjected to same possible events with identical probabilities [6]. For a given set of parameter values, the deterministic model has one solution which can be fitted to data using various methods. The most common method minimizes the sum of squares of differences between observed data and model prediction.

Natural and biological discrete events of random occurrence in a small population cannot be explained by deterministic and continuous modeling and here comes the utility of stochastic modeling. Stochastic models capture the randomness of birth and death rates associated with disease dynamics and also the variability among disease strains. The earliest stages of an infection are stochastic. This occurs because encounter with a pathogen may either lead to an infection or elimination from the system. Stochasticity decreases as the number of cases increases. Emergent behaviors that have neither been defined nor expected are simulated in this modeling approach. Probability distributions associated with such systems are typically memory-less. If the objective of modeling of disease dynamics is to establish the conditions for disease eradication, or if irregular epidemics are to be modeled, stochastic model is the choice. Stochasticity can induce chance extinctions of the disease and it introduces variances and covariances that can influence the deterministic behavior. Stochastic simulations are computationally intensive.

In stochastic modeling of HIV dynamics, it is assumed that the viral population is governed by the availability of target cells that can be infected and does not take into account the contribution of the immune responses in the control of virus load.

Stochastic extinction or disease eradication by chance occurs when an infected individual fails to reproduce and transmit the infection and ultimately the pathogen dies out.

An interesting thing to note at this juncture is that deterministic model can be transformed to the corresponding stochastic model by conversion of deterministic rates into the probabilistic ones on the basis of a fixed reference volume of the model. This has been done in the analysis of dynamics of HIV and the opportunistic co-infection TB by incorporation of the response of cytotoxic T-lymphocytes in absence and presence of HAART therapy by altering the model's parameters. Evolution of drug resistant strains can also be assumed to exhibit a stochastic pattern.

A combination of deterministic and stochastic approaches will be the most effective one because of their complementary features, although it may be time-consuming and may exploit more resources [1], [7], 12, [16-18].

As no element of chance or uncertainty is involved in the development of deterministic models, they account for the mean trend of a process only. However in addition to the above feature, stochastic model also accounts for the variance component around the process. Initial epidemic growth of an infection cannot be properly approximated by deterministic SIR model. This occurs because at this stage only a seed of infection is introduced in contrast to the large population at later stages. Probability that an infection will occur is governed by demographic stochasticity. In case of stochastic models, some parameters are characterized by a probability distribution, instead of a fixed constant value, as observed with the deterministic models [6]. Given a stochastic transmission model, most inferential methods rely on likelihood. Given a likelihood, inference can proceed along conventional lines, using tools such as maximum likelihood estimation, expectation maximization algorithm, rejection sampling and Markov chain Monte Carlo methods.

7. Insights into conceptual results from mathematical model

Two approaches can be used to determine the time-scale of disease transmission by utilizing data on individual-to-individual chains of transmission. Estimation of disease generation time (T) is one approach. It may be defined as the expected length of time between infection of an index case and infection of his or her secondary cases. It is the duration of latency plus infectiousness. The generation time of measles is approximately 14 days. A short generation time indicates rapid transmission whereas a longer T suggests slower spread but longer carriage. The duration of carriage of pathogens represents an upper limit on T and it can be concluded that directly transmitted acute infections have T < 1 month and chronic infections

http://dx.doi.org/10.5772/57387

have T values in the order of months or years [19]. But, determination of generation time becomes complicated if the disease possesses asymptomatic periods of infection of variable or unknown duration. Another quantity that is estimated is the serial interval. It is the time between clinical onset of symptoms in the index case and the clinical onset of symptoms in the average secondary case [2].

In a system of differential equations, an equilibrium point is a point at which all the equations equal zero. This indicates that the state of the system is not changing. In a mathematical model, a disease-free equilibrium (DFE) and one or more endemic equilibria are present. The DFE indicates that the entire population is susceptible since not a single infective exists in the population. Endemic equilibrium is steady-state equilibrium produced by spread of infection. If the solutions of the equations near the equilibrium points tend toward the points with time, they are said to be locally stable. An equilibrium point is referred to as globally asymptotically stable if the behavior of the system at any point tends toward the equilibrium point as time tends toward infinity.

The stability of DFE and existence of other nontrivial equilibria can be determined from a ratio, known as basic reproduction ratio [20]. A very brief description of the essential conceptual results from mathematical modeling has been given in Table 1.

Parameters	Description
Disease generation time	Time from the moment one person becomes infected until that person infects another person
Equilibrium point	Can be categorized as a. disease-free equilibrium point when there is no infection in either the host or the vector or there is no pathogen and b. endemic equilibrium where the disease persists in the population. Both are steady state solutions.
Basic reproduction number	Number of secondary cases caused by one primary case introduced into a population that is wholly susceptible

Table 1. Glossary of important parameters associated with mathematical modeling of infectious diseases

8. Basic reproduction ratio

A key concept or parameter in epidemiology, the basic reproduction ratio, R_0 is being extensively studied during deterministic, non-spatial, unstructured modeling of in-host population dynamics of microparasitic infectious diseases, once they have been established. It is defined as the expected number of secondary individuals infected by an individual during his or her entire tenure of infectious period. Its derivation is applicable even when non-constant transmission probabilities between classes (i.e., non-exponential lifetime distributions) are assumed. If its value is greater than 1, the infection spreads across a non-zero fraction of susceptible population. If the spreading rate is too low and R_0 cannot cross beyond the threshold level, it is not feasible to affect a finite proportion of population and disease dies out in a finite time. In a contact network model, the disease cannot replenish itself and ultimately dies out after a finite number of waves, if $R_0 < 1$ with probability 1. Disease persists with positive probability, at least by infecting one person in each wave, if $R_0 > 1$. Keeping and maintaining the value of $R_0 < 1$ reflects the stability of the disease-free equilibrium and creates a condition for clearing of pathogen from the population and thus it is the goal of any public health initiative designed for containment or control of infection. Moreover, the estimation of R_0 plays a crucial role in understanding the outbreak and potential danger from emerging infectious disease. The concept of R_0 has also been developed for complex models like stochastic and finite systems, models with spatial structure and also macroparasite infections. Comparison of R_0 values, based either on their numerical values or area under the infectiousness curve, helps in estimation of relative intrinsic transmissibility of the pathogens [9], [10], [21], [22].

There are also alternative approaches of estimating R_0 from available incidence or epidemiological data which require simplifying assumptions for numerical estimation of some unknown parameters. It is assumed that the host population is homogeneous, mixes uniformly and is of constant size in a constant state. The number of contacts per infective is independent of the number of infectives. Infectivity and mortality do not depend on age, genetic make-up, geography. Moreover, it is assumed that all individuals are born susceptible and as soon as disease is acquired, they are no longer considered susceptible. Spreading pattern of the epidemics is controlled by the generation time-scale. All these assumptions may never be fully realized in a practical clinical setting. R_0 can be expressed as the ratio of the life expectancy and mean age of acquiring the infection. Thus, higher the R_0, lower is the mean age at infection. Another important relationship that can be derived is that the mean age at infection is the reciprocal of the force of infection. A key parameter, the coefficient of transmission for airborne diseases, can be determined from the value of the force of infection. Alternatively, R_0 can be estimated from the intrinsic growth rate of the infected class, which is highly dependent on collecting accurate data. Stochastic fluctuations can affect the value of growth rate. In case of vector-borne disease like dengue, R_0 was calculated from the survival function, assuming spatial compartments of varying vector density. For multiple classes of infectives, R_0 can be defined per infection cycle [6], [10], [21].

From sensitivity analysis, it has been found that different infection-and population-related factors may affect R_0 like, transmission rate, vector mortality, incubation period of the vector, the relative infectiousness after isolation [21].

For both measles and whooping cough in England and Wales from 1945 to 1965, R_0 has been found to be nearly 17. For the H1N1 epidemic in UK, R_0 has been estimated to be 1.4. Estimation of R_0 for SARS by different groups have mostly given the values in the range of 2-4, although a wide range of 1-7 has also been found in the literature. For smallpox, the R_0 was found to be in the range of $4 < R_0 < 10$. Though an upper bound has been found for pandemic influenza, no lower bound could be obtained. For AIDS, R_0 is always greater than 1, especially in African countries and it depends highly on the sexual behavior. For homosexual population in the United Kingdom, R_0 is close to 4 and approximately 11 for female prostitutes in Kenya [7], [13], [22].

8.1. Significance of basic reproduction ratio

The magnitude of R_0, along with the disease generation time, help in assessing the time scale of infection, implementing sustainable control measures at the most appropriate time and justifying implementation of costly approaches in management of infectious diseases. Low value of R_0 for any infection suggests that the epidemic can be controlled, either by adopting single or combined putative containment procedures [21], [22].

Condition for endemicity can be deduced from an idea of $R_{0.}$ Disease is said to exist in an endemic state when it persists in the population at a low and constant level of prevalence, for which there should be a continuous supply of susceptibles. This happens if deaths and births occur at equal constant rates keeping the population turnover rate at a fixed value. An outcome of this assumption is the negative exponential distribution of age. At endemic equilibrium, the relationship between the proportion of susceptible in the population and the basic reproduction ratio is inverse [6].

Though R_0 is the widely accepted and used indicator of control measure, it has been observed that different control approaches may produce same degree of reduction of R_0 but not same effect on the growth rate. Factors such as timing of secondary infections, negative impact of control measures on the population are not considered while implementing public health initiatives based on the basic reproduction ratio [21].

8.2. Alternatives to R_0

R_0 is a highly pathogen-centered parameter and recently, a host-centered parameter has been evolved, the basic depression ratio, D_0. An alternative parameter for heterogeneous population has been developed, type reproduction number, T which indicates the efficacy of the control measure against a particular subtype of host population, from which if infection is eradicated, the disease will not sustain at all [21].

In case of a population which is susceptible after acquiring immunity from a previous epidemic or due to vaccination, instead of R_0, R_{eff} or effective value of R_0 is used. R_{eff} is a time-dependent quantity that accounts for the population's reduced susceptibility. If R_{eff} is greater than one, the number of infected individuals grows and decreases if R_{eff} is less than one. Therefore, the critical proportion of susceptible is given by R_{eff} equal to one [11]. The parameter can be determined by fitting deterministic epidemiological model employing a generalized least squares estimation scheme [23].

In case of seasonally driven epidemics as with different childhood microparasitic infections, it is necessary to determine the number of susceptible left after a major epidemic (S_0). If S_0 goes above a critical threshold value, epidemic outbreak may recur in the next year or there will be a skip i.e., a year when epidemic fails to initiate [14].

9. Strategies for containment of an infectious disease

Barlett postulated that any infectious disease cannot be maintained if the population size is below the critical community size unless there is supply of susceptible or regular migration of the infected class from the adjoining places. This will ultimately lead to disease extinction. Disease is said to fade-out if the duration of disease extinction is more than the disease generation length [6]. Although, theoretically, it may be possible to estimate and predict the time for disease eradication from the population, practically it is not feasible. Therefore, in practice, attempts are made to prevent spreading of the infection.

Once the epidemiological data have been modeled into a reliable mathematical model, they can be used to identify population subgroups at high risk of disease and develop preventive interventions or measures according to time, place and person. These measures include education, immunization, quarantine regulations or social distancing to restrict interaction with others and treatment options. Mathematical modeling of intervention strategies can be done in two ways. In the first method, the goal is to assess the effect on the disease dynamics by changing the value of a constant parameter associated with the disease. This indicates the best parameter value for a given performance measure. In the second method, intervention measures are varied as a function of time and the objective is to determine the best parameter value for a given performance measure. Pontryagin's Maximum Principle (PMP) is applied for comparison of a wide range of time varying functions. The best strategy for mitigation of spreading of a contagious disease would be the one which evolves with time during different phases of infection and thus focuses on progressively changing classes of populations. Optimal control theory suggests the most effective mitigation strategy to minimize the risk of individuals being infected by applying and balancing vaccination and administering drug in a cost-effective manner. Based on this, vaccination has been found to be the most common strategy in reversing the epidemic growth of an infection within the population in the initial stages of an outbreak. But in absence of the strategy, due to some reason or other, medical practitioners either isolate symptomatic individuals or trace and quarantine contacts of symptomatic cases. These strategies require proper diagnosis of the symptoms of the disease in each and every individual. Efficacy of any implementation strategy is decided by the efficacy at which the infected person is isolated and the efficacy at which the persons with whom the infectious person came in contact can be quarantined. An infection can be sufficiently controlled if the values of basic reproduction ratio and the proportion of transmission occurring asymptotically can be reduced below a critical line. Since SARS is characterized by low R_0 and low infectiousness prior to clinical symptoms, effective isolation of symptomatic patients can sufficiently control an epidemic outbreak. For those diseases where the proportion of asymptomatic transmission is more than $1/R_0$, contact tracing should be added to the set of control measures used. This proportion can be determined from the longitudinal data on clinical symptoms and pathogen load within the patient. Mathematically, it has been deduced that influenza is more difficult to control than small pox. Moreover, quarantining and contact tracing would not provide any extra benefit in case of influenza because of very short incubation and infectious periods. AIDS has taken an alarming proportion because of high risk of pre-symptomatic transmission and under such circumstance, self-isolation and contact tracing would provide little respite [10], [22], [24], [25].

10. Vaccination

Implementation of proper and effective vaccination protocol is of primary concern to the epidemiologists and public health decision makers. Vaccination program is usually a government initiative applied on large spatial and temporal scales to reduce the level of complexity of disease. The ultimate goal of any vaccination program is to keep the value of basic reproduction ratio below unity by altering the various control parameters. Mathematical modeling of vaccination recognizes that linear transfer occurs between the susceptible and the removed compartments. For modeling purpose, important variables related to vaccination that should be included are vaccination rate, i.e. the rate at which the susceptible individuals are vaccinated and efficacy or the proportion of susceptible left unprotected even, after immunization [26].

Two schemes are being widely employed worldwide for prevention and eradication of vaccine-preventable infections-mass vaccination and pulse vaccination. Mass vaccination is usually carried out in infants before the mean age at infection. But, it may not always be practically the most effective approach for global disease eradication. Pulse vaccination, on the other hand, is a cheaper and a better alternative where periodic vaccination of a certain proportion of the population renders sufficient and enough protection against further spread of the disease as the percentage of susceptible is always maintained below the threshold level required for an epidemic to start. But, pulse vaccination suffers from the side effect of resonance. Impact of single- and multiple-dose vaccination on rubella eradication has been studied extensively in an age-structured model with constant transmission rate using Floquet analysis. It has been established that eradication likelihood is governed by the effective duration of immunity. Booster vaccination has also been studied, but, in less details. Permanent immunity is conferred by booster dose in contrast to partial immunity imparted by primary vaccines. A new threshold quantity, known as re-infection threshold in case of vaccination-induced partial immunity, indicates the condition when vaccination will not succeed thereby producing high levels of infection. Prevention or reduction in epidemicity is more readily achievable by booster vaccination, depending on the level of primary vaccination program, because it has the capacity to increase the vaccination coverage and herd immunity of the population as a whole. Outcome of a booster dose depends highly on precise timing of the additional vaccine doses as well as the proportion of individuals receiving the second-dose. During vaccination, decision of the individual or mass to undergo program greatly affects the efficacy of the program. Therefore, human behavior plays a significant role in ensuring success of the strategy [3], [6], [27].

An interesting thing to note while conducting mass scale immunization is that it is possible to protect the whole population from an outbreak even if there are some susceptibles in the population, at less than 100% immunization. This effect is called herd immunity. When $R_0 < 1$, the DFE is globally asymptotically stable resulting in disease eradication as observed in case of measles. Vaccination reduces the force of infection and increases the mean age at infection when the infection may be acquired. Vaccination desynchronizes local dynamics which will prevent migration of susceptible population from neighboring places and thus can facilitate extinction of the disease. However, vaccination of each and every individual in the susceptible class is practically not feasible and more so, in economically backward countries. Therefore, the critical fraction or proportion of population that needs to be vaccinated is to be determined. Moreover, desired degree of success may not be always obtained due to vaccination because of less than optimum coverage, irregularities in the supply of vaccines, use of low-efficiency vaccines or waning rate of vaccines. All these may lead to re-emergence of disease outbreak, sometimes with increased intensity, owing to the resurgence of the susceptible class finally resulting in serious side effects.

Vaccination coverage depends on the characteristics of the endemic equilibrium. At equilibrium, the replacement number, R is equal to the product of basic reproduction ratio and the proportion of susceptibles i.e. $R=R_0s^*$. The replacement number is defined as the average number of secondary infections produced by a typical infective during its entire course of infectiousness. Vaccination coverage of p reduces the proportion of susceptible to $1\text{-}p$. Higher the magnitude of R_0, higher is the vaccination coverage and is complicated by parameter such as vaccine efficacy. Therefore, for disease eradication to occur, $R=R_0s^*(1-p) < 1$ or $p > 1-1/R_0$. The critical vaccination coverage is expressed by the formula, $p_c=1-1/R_0$ and the value has been found to be 0.94 and 0.86 respectively for measles and rubella. An increase in the value results in a decrease of the spatial synchrony of disease dynamics. Smallpox has been successfully removed from the face of the earth because it possesses the least critical vaccination coverage. Vaccine efficacy of 0.97 represents that 3% of those vaccinated do not become immune.

Optimal vaccination coverage and frequency of pulse vaccination has been studied with the help of Pythagore theorem [6]. The important terminologies associated with vaccination has been presented in Table 2.

Parameters	Description
Herd immunity	Immunity and protection of the entire community achievable by vaccinating a proportion of the population and creating immune individuals
Basic reproduction number under vaccination	Number of secondary cases caused by one primary case introduced into a population in which a proportion has been vaccinated
Critical vaccination proportion	Proportion of population to be vaccinated to achieve eradication by maintaining Basic reproduction number under vaccination equal to one
Vaccine efficacy	Effectiveness of the vaccine to induce immunity
Eradication likelihood	Determined by effective period of immunity
Re-infection threshold	Occurs during transmission induced by partial immunity. It is a threshold quantity above which levels of infection will be high and vaccination fails

Table 2. Glossary of important parameters related to vaccination

http://dx.doi.org/10.5772/57387

11. Quarantine

Quarantine refers to intentional or forceful isolation of individuals suffering from diseases like leprosy, plague, cholera, typhus, yellow fever, smallpox, diphtheria, tuberculosis etc. The ultimate objective of the process is to reduce the average infectious period by isolating some infectives, so that they do not transmit the infection. To study the effect of quarantine, a new class Q of quarantined individuals has been included in standard SIS and SIR endemic models. They include those who have been removed and isolated either voluntarily or coercively from the Infectious class. The quarantine reproduction number, R_0 depends on the quarantine rate constant which governs the transfer rate out of the Infectious class into the Quarantine class [28].

12. Evolution of mathematical modeling

Epidemiological modeling has undergone numerous revisions and improvements to cope up with emerging new infections and discovery of new concepts and basis of existing infections. It is well-known that increase in model complexity by including more relevant biological details improves the accuracy. But it is practically not feasible to construct a fully accurate model. There will always be some factors related to host, pathogen, environment or population which cannot be estimated or predicted. Processes of random occurrence affect the degree of accuracy of model. Predictability of the model depends highly on a strong interplay between statistics and models for estimation of parameters from epidemiological data.

The key assumption of deterministic mathematical model is the existence of homogeneous and constant population, where it is assumed that, the death of a susceptible, infectious or recovered individual is immediately compensated by the birth of a new susceptible. In actual practice, heterogeneity is observed where the population can be divided into several homogeneous subpopulations or groups on the basis of mode of transmission, contact patterns, latent period, infectious period, genetic susceptibility or resistance as well as socio-economic, cultural, demographic and geographic factors. All these complexities can be suitably incorporated in a multi-group model and can prove effective in explaining the dynamics of sexually transmitted diseases such as gonorrhea or AIDS [29]. Population-level heterogeneities that, if included can improve the model's accuracy and predictive ability, include age, gender, behavior, genetic susceptibility [7]. Influenza infection is well-studied and well-modeled. But, there are still several aspects of the infection which have not been included in model construction like, the contribution of strain-specific cell tropism, pre-existing immunity, effect of host genetic factors on virulence and transmissibility of a particular strain. The model may be modified to determine the severity, duration and outcome of infection progression within an individual [30]. Moreover, drug resistance may develop. Therefore, a model with an immune response can be generated for better insight into the disease dynamics and the predictions from the model are different from those of a model formulated without an immune response. Two-phase solution can be used to study different viral infections. Study of models, specific for influenza or H1N1 require careful parameterization to match available data and it should reflect both statistical uncertainty and uncertainty in data itself [13].

A new rule, known as 20-80 rule has been proposed by researchers for certain infectious diseases which show unique features. According to the rule, 20% of the individuals are responsible for 80% of onward transmission and they are known as super-spreaders. This gives rise to variation in the number of secondary infections per infected individual which is denoted by Z. It is described by two parameters-mean R_0 among infections and dispersion parameter, K. A small K (<0.1) indicates that a small proportion of infected individuals actively transmit the pathogens whereas, a large K (>4) indicates that all infected individuals are equally responsible for onward transmission [19].

In multiple-host diseases, different hosts or reservoirs are involved. Dynamics of the disease itself may vary in the different hosts and the mode of transmission from one host to another is quite complex. All these factors should be borne in mind during study of these diseases [6].

In viral disease like Hepatitis B, there is a carrier state where the individual is not fully recovered and is able to transmit low level of infection throughout his life. Some diseases like chlamydial infection is characterized by infected individual who is asymptomatic but is able to transmit disease. Again, meningitis may remain benign for long within population but may exhibit sporadic symptomatic outbreaks [7]. Infectious diseases which are characterized by multi-factorial pathologies or where concurrent infections prevail in immune-compromised hosts usher in complexities in mathematical modeling [1]. A common feature of certain childhood infections is the periodical occurrence of high levels of infection of school-going children which necessitates the inclusion of a time-varying contact rate between susceptible and infected classes of individuals in the model, which is then known as seasonally-forced model and is recognized by a sinusoidal function. The concept of seasonality in the coefficient of transmission and temporal heterogeneity was introduced by Soper to account for the high amplitude outbreaks of measles in Glasgow. These types of diseases are characterized by strong annual, biennial and sometimes irregular oscillations. In India, polio has been found to occur annually. Measles is known to exhibit biennial occurrence for extended periods in London. It has been noticed that the same disease can have different temporal patterns during different epochs which may be attributed to changes in epidemiological factors, e.g. population birth rate, magnitude of disease transmission, and strength of seasonality [14]. Modeling of measles dynamics is best achieved by incorporation of an epidemic oscillator, which takes into account the birth rate variations and can analyze chaotic behavior of epidemic outbreaks. It has been observed that high birth rates drive measles dynamics to annual cycles and diminishing birth rates result in biennial patterns. Vaccination causes irregular cycles. Complex oscillations arise due to interactions between the externally imposed annual seasonality and intrinsic oscillatory dynamics of the infection itself [26]. The approach of "term-time forcing" should also be employed for temporally forced models of another childhood bacterial infection, pertussis or whooping cough. Though both measles and pertussis possess identical values for basic reproduction ratio, yet they exhibit different dynamics because the infectious period in whooping cough is longer than that of measles. School holidays during Christmas

http://dx.doi.org/10.5772/57387

does not affect severely the transmission of the disease [11], [27]. For better understanding of the model with periodic perturbations, bifurcation diagram proves beneficial [7].

Assumptions that have been discussed in a previous section hold true for developing countries where all individuals are exposed to similar death pressure, irrespective of age, due to the environmental conditions and lack of medical facilities. But the situation differs in developed countries where square shape age distribution is manifested. This can be attributed to availability of proper medical care. Modeling becomes somewhat complicated in analysis of macroparasitic infections owing to their inherent differences from the infections caused due to microparasites. In case of microparasitic infections, the internal dynamics of the pathogen within the host is not as crucial as the host's infection status. But, the complex life cycle of the macroparasite within the host necessitates inclusion of this parameter in modeling of macroparasitic infections. Moreover, disease transmission and pathogenicity are highly related to the load of the causative organisms within the host system [6], [7].

Furthermore, complex dynamics may be followed by the infections, where the causative agent can undergo mutation and can create a class of population, susceptible to the new strains. Previous infections in those cases confer only partial cross-immunity and thus, history of infection is important. Number of parameters in the model therefore, increases exponentially with the number of strains. In these circumstances, either reduced transmission approach or polarized immunity concept is applied [11]. Emergence of drug resistant strains is an issue of great concern which should be included in modeling disease dynamics. Sexually transmitted diseases unfold a different picture because of high risk of exposure of sexually active individuals, belonging to a particular age group.

Complexities may also arise in modeling of diseases in presence of an optimal control measure where there is a delay element between implementation of isolation and quarantining. Inclusion of delay increases the proportion of transmission occurring with an asymptomatic or pre-symptomatic infector and hence, necessitating adoption of stringent measure including contact tracing. Oversimplification may fail to estimate the efficacy of contact tracing in reducing the transmission. However, in this delay period, the patient may practice self-isolation depending on the nature and severity of the symptoms and the time scales involved [22].

In a modified SIR model with "skipping" dynamics for diseases like influenza, it has been shown that the immunity of hosts depends on previous exposure to the disease and immune memory. Due to mutational changes in influenza virus or antigenic evolution, hosts may be re-infected with the disease every few years, with years of 'skips' or gaps in between [31].

The simple SIR model has been extended to include the effects of saturation where the incidence rate is not bilinear in S and I but a general function $f(S,I)$. It is assumed that in presence of large number of infectives in the population, the number of contacts per time diminishes [3].

The simplistic SIR model has evolved into biphasic SIR model (B-SIR) to explain the key features of multi-ennial epidemic cycle. In this model, the SIR dynamics alternates between a relatively fast epidemic phase in which there is a significant increase in the number of infected as well as a rapid decline in the count of the susceptible and a slow build-up phase characterized by continuous replenishment of susceptible. This enables estimation of threshold(bifurcation) values at which there will be a switching from biennial to annual epidemic dynamics [14].

A likelihood-based methodology has been developed which assumes the generation interval to follow Weibull distribution and a specific infection network underlies the observed epidemic curve [23].

An agent-based model in the study of tuberculosis has revealed that recruitment of increased number of resting macrophages to the infection site in tuberculosis increases bacterial load. This suggests that the inflammatory response may be detrimental to the host [32].

Since, application of mathematical modeling approach shows that vaccination decreases the mean age at infection, it deduces that implementation of vaccination programs can actually increase the incidences of absolute number of serious cases, if the probability of disease complications increases with age. This is an interesting paradigm of mathematical modeling. In case of imperfect or ineffective vaccination, a backward transfer between the susceptible and recovered compartments must be considered because the vaccinated individuals may come back to the susceptible category or may become directly infected through nonlinear transmission. This behavior gives rise to bi-stability and backward bifurcation [26].

Exponentially growing population and incidences of mortality due to childhood infections in developing countries are not considered in modeling of infections where the host population is assumed to be of constant size. The component of heterogeneity also exists in cases of sexually transmitted diseases. This is further complicated by the fact that, unlike other infections, recovery from STD does not guarantee development of acquired immunity. The currently existing rationale of mathematical modeling may need to be modified while investigating mother-to-child diseases and diseases transmitted by multiple users of syringe as in AIDS [6].

A hierarchical dynamics has been observed in epidemic outbreaks of complex heterogeneous networks. Propagation of infection occurs via a cascade from higher to lower degree classes [10].

In most of the cases, epidemiological processes within the population and immunological processes involved within the individual host are considered separately, with no explicit interaction between the two. Infectious diseases, caused by RNA viruses are characterized by high mutation rate and short generation time of the viruses indicating that evolutionary processes occur rapidly and evolutionary outcomes depend on the fitness of viral mutants at different stages of viral lifecycles and interactions between viral variants. Moreover, ecological and epidemiological factors, such as host contact patterns, transmission routes, host movements also govern the success of viral transmission in a population. In this approach, three different time scales are considered-a fast time scale for within-host dynamics, an intermediate time scale for epidemiological process and a slow time scale for the environmental contamination [5]. Link between the evolutionary process at the pathogen level and the ecological processes at the host population level can be established by phylodynamics [11]. The phylodynamic approach can be successfully utilized in mathematical modeling of such viruses like dengue, human respiratory synctial virus, Hepatitis C, Toxoplasma etc. [19], [33], [34].

Several new modeling concepts are being explored for detailed description of diseases like AIDS, tuberculosis. These include differential infectivity (DI) and staged progression (SP) model [29]. For modeling of infectious diseases with long infectious period and where there are multiple alternative disease progression pathways and branching, or where there is considerable difference in virulence or when only a part of the infected population undergoes a treatment whereas the rest remains untreated, staged progression models seem to be the most suitable [35]. Individuals infected with HIV sequentially pass through a series of stages, being highly infectious in first few weeks after their own infection, then having low infectivity for many years, and finally becoming more infectious as their immune system breaks down and they progress to full-blown AIDS. Investigation of the influence of imperfect vaccine on HIV transmission by individuals in AIDS stage with the help of SP model revealed that the imperfect vaccine can eliminate HIV in a given community at vaccination reproduction number less than unity, but the disease will persist otherwise [36], [37]. Since, tuberculosis is characterized by presence of very long latent period and infectious period, time is not considered to be constant in modeling of the disease. The latent period and infectious period are divided into n-stages and stage progression model with bilinear incidence was formulated [39]. Characteristic features of DI and SP models have been given in a tabular form (Table 3).

DI model	SP model
Suitable for diseases where viral levels differ between individuals as in sexually transmitted diseases and also diseases where infectivity depends on parasite or viral loads in infected hosts or vectors e.g. malaria, dengue fever.	Suitable for modeling of diseases exhibiting variability of infectiousness with time as in AIDS or where time-scale of disease transmission is too long.
Infectives are divided into a number of a groups according to their infectivities. Total population size is assumed constant.	Total host population is partitioned into the following compartments: the susceptible compartment, the infectious compartment , whose members are in the *i*-th stage of the disease progression, and the terminal compartment. It is assumed that there is no recovery from the disease, and thus the only exit from the terminal compartment is death.
Infection-free equilibrium is globally stable and there exists a unique endemic equilibrium for these models	Disease-free equilibrium and unique endemic equilibrium have also been established with these models

Table 3. Characteristic features of DI and SP model

Healthcare-associated infections (HCAI) or nosocomial infections or hospital acquired infections are source of great concern in developed as well as developing countries. Such infections can be modeled using either deterministic or stochastic approach for evaluation of control policies. This requires sound model parameterization and sensitivity analyses [40].

Influenza control is a challenge since it is difficult to predict the predominant strain that will be circulating each season. Successful vaccination program can be designed from a model which includes the drift process (via the emergence of new strains), the co-circulation of existing strains and pre-existing immunity in the population. A good model is able to reproduce the herald wave phenomenon of strain persistence from one influenza season to the next in temperate regions [41].

Recently, multi-scale models are being developed which will help in predicting virulence, transmissibility, at the population level, susceptibility or resistance to drugs without conducting tough and time-consuming laboratory experiments. For development of these types of models, complete genome sequence of the pathogen should be made available, which will allow mapping from genotype to complex phenotypes.

Numerous modeling approaches contain data estimated from the literature and for such cases extensive sensitivity analysis may prove beneficial. In uni-variate sensitivity analysis, impact of variation of one parameter by a certain percent on the outcome of the model is measured while all other parameters are held constant. Such analysis can be graphically represented on a tornado plot. In multivariate analysis, impact of multiple parameters is studied through Monte Carlo simulations [38]. Other multilevel fitting schemes and Bayesian/Markov chain Monte Carlo frameworks may also be useful [30].

13. Conclusions

Infectious diseases pose a great threat to human civilization and world economy. Therefore, constant efforts are being made to prevent their occurrence, recurrence and spread. There are certain infections which do not manifest themselves as definite symptoms in the infected host for a long period of time but can be highly lethal at the end. Research is focused on development of economically viable new intervention strategies for any type of infectious disease with the aid of mathematical modeling. Symbiotic and synergistic relationship should exist between mathematicians and biologists for detailed analysis of the biological processes involved in host-pathogen interactions. Mathematical models involve assumption, abstraction, simplification and description of the most complex system of infectious disease, by the use of language of mathematics. Each element of host and pathogen can be monitored and varied simultaneously without actually performing any experiment to ascertain the role of the element in disease dynamics. Epidemiological modeling enables extrapolation of population behavior from individual behavior and long-term behavior from dynamics of early stage of infection following consideration of different epidemiological factors. Surveillance data, physicians' reports and data acquired from the hospitals are the sources for individual-to-individual chains of transmission. Despite the fact that mass human behavior becomes unpredictable at times, especially during a disaster, concerted rigorous approach adopted during model development can build up a strong framework for future planning. Extensive long-term data and refined mechanistic understanding of evolutionary and transmission dynamics has enriched the field of mathematical modeling and provided insights in shaping the global public health response to a pandemic. The foremost important contribution of mathematical epidemiology to healthcare professionals is the concept of basic reproduction ratio and epidemic threshold. From a medical or public health perspective, models are instrumental in policy-making, service planning, risk assessment and monitoring performance of infection control programs. Decision of whom, how and when to quarantine, vaccinate and initiate therapy can be planned and implemented successfully from the outcomes of a model of high quality. The source of complexity in models is the occurrence of huge variability in infection profiles, parameter values and time scales. However, complexity ensures model accuracy. Selection of type of model and its degree of complexity depends on the purpose of modeling and questions to be addressed. Failure to understand, forecast and control an epidemic outbreak in a particular locality can indicate that some of the key disease parameters and elements of biological complexity might have been overlooked while developing the model. One underlying reason for this may be traced to a key fundamental feature of mathematical model. Unless the model is tightly fitted to the experimental data, there remains a doubt on the reliability of the parameter estimates obtained from the model. At the end, it can be said that mathematical model helps in integrating several disease-related facts and factors into a cohesive structure, better visualization of a complex system, determining the plausibility of epidemiological explanations, prediction of unexpected interrelationships among empirical observations and prediction of impact of changes in the system.

Author details

Sutapa Biswas Majee* and Gopa Roy Biswas

*Address all correspondence to: sutapabiswas2001@yahoo.co.in

NSHM College Of Pharmaceutical Technology, NSHM Knowledge Campus, Kolkata-Group of of Institutions Kolkata, West Bengal, India

References

[1] A Sorathiya, A Bracciali and P Liò (2010). Formal reasoning on qualitative models of co-infection of HIV and Tuberculosis and HAART therapy. BMC Bioinformatics 11(doi:10.1186/1471-2105-11-S1-S67).

[2] N B Dimitrov and L A M Dimitrov (2010). Mathematical approaches to infectious disease prediction and control. In Infectious Disease Models Tutorials in Operations Research, INFORMS (ISBN: 978-0-9843378-0-4).

[3] S Funk, M Salathe and V A A Jansen (2010). Modeling the influence of human behavior on the spread of infectious diseases: a review J. R. Soc. Interface 7, 1247–1256.

[4] N Piazza and H Wang (2013). Bifurcation and sensitivity analysis of immunity duration in an epidemic model. Int. J. Numer. Analy. And Modeling Series B Computing and Information 4, 179-202.

[5] Z Feng, J Velasco-Hernandez and B. Tapia-Santos (2013). A mathematical model for coupling within-host and between-host dynamics in an environmentally-driven infectious disease. Math. Biosci. 241, 49-55.

[6] M Choisy, J F Guegan and P Rohani (2007). Mathematical modeling of infectious diseases dynamics in Encyclopedia of infectious diseases: modern methodologies. Edited by M Tibavrenc, John Wiley and Sons, 379-403.

[7] M J Keeling and P Rohani (2007). Modeling infectious diseases in humans and animals. Princeton University Press.

[8] H Squires and P Tappenden (2011). Mathematical modeling and its application to social care. Methods Review 7, 1-22. (ISBN 978-0-85328-452-9).

[9] D Easley and J Kleinberg (2010). Networks, Crowds, and Markets: Reasoning about a Highly Connected World. Cambridge University Press, (http ://www.cs.cornell.edu/home/kleinber/networks-book/).

[10] M Barthelmya, A Barrat, R Pastor-Satorrasc and A Vespignani (2005). Dynamical patterns of epidemic outbreaks in complex heterogeneous networks. J. Theor. Biol. 235, 275–288.

[11] B T Grenfell and F Lutscher (2004). Modeling the dynamics of infectious diseases In A series of PIMS lecture notes.

[12] M J Keeling and J V Ross (2008). On methods for studying stochastic disease dynamics. J. R. Soc. Interface 5, 171-181.

[13] M J Keeling and L Danon(2009). Mathematical modeling of infectious diseases. Br. Med. Bull. 92, 33–42.

[14] A Uziel and L Stone (2012). Determinants of periodicity in seasonally driven epidemics. J. Theor. Biol. 305, 88–95.

[15] N Masuda and P Holme (2013). Predicting and controlling infectious disease epidemics using temporal networks. F1000Prime Reports 5:6 (doi:10.12703/P5-6).

[16] R M Ribeiro and S Bonhoeffer (1999). A stochastic model for primary HIV infection: optimal timing of therapy. AIDS 13, 351-357.

[17] J E Pearson, P Krapivsky and A S Perelson (2011). Stochastic theory of early viral infection: continuous versus burst production of virions. PLoS Comput Biol. 7, e1001058(doi : 10.1371/journal.pcbi.1001058).

[18] N Dalal, D Greenhalgh and X Mao(2009). Mathematical modeling of internal HIV dynamics. Discrete and Continuous Dynamical Systems –Series B 12, 305-321.

[19] G Magiorkinis, V Sypsa E Magiorkinis A Katsoulidou, R Belshaw, C Fraser O G Pybus and A Hatzakis (2013). Integrating phylodynamics and epidemiology to estimate transmission diversity in viral epidemics. PLOS Comp. Biol. (doi : 10:1371/journal.pcbi.1002876).

[20] L C R F Lazhar (2012). Mathematical analysis of nonlinear epidemic models. J Math. Stat. 8, 258-263.

[21] J M Heffernan, R J Smith and L M Wahl (2005). Perspectives on the basic reproductive ratio. J R Soc Interface 2, 281–293.

[22] C Fraser, S Riley, R M Anderson and N M Ferguson (2004). Factors that make an infectious disease outbreak controllable. PNAS 101, 6146-6151.

[23] A Clinton-Arias, C Castillo-Chavez, L M A Bettencourt, A L Lloyd and H T Banks (2009). The estimation of the effective reproductive number from disease outbreak data. Math. Biosci. Eng. 6, 261-282.

[24] H Gaff and E Schaefer (2009). Optimal control applied to vaccination and treatment strategies for various epidemiological models. Math. Biosci Eng. 6, 469-492.

[25] E Hansen (2011). Applications of optimal control theory to infectious disease modeling. Ph. D. thesis, Queen's University, Kingston, Ontario, Canada.

[26] B Buonomo and D Lacitignola (2011). On the backward bifurcation of a vaccination model with nonlinear incidence. Nonlinear Analysis: Modeling and Control 16, 30–46.

[27] M E Alexander, S M Moghadas, P Rohani and A R Summers (2005). Modeling the effect of a booster vaccination on disease epidemiology. J. Math. Biol. (doi : 10.1007/s00285-005-0356-0).

[28] H Hethcote, M Zhien and L Shengbing (2002).Effects of quarantine in six endemic models for infectious diseases. Math. Biosci. 180, 141–160.

[29] A. Fall, A. Iggidr, G Sallet and J J Tewa (2007).Mathematical modeling of natural phenomena. Epidemiology 2, 55–73.

[30] C A A Beauchemin and A Handel (2011). A review of mathematical models of influenza A infections within a host or cell culture: lessons learned and challenges ahead. BMC Public Health 11, S7 (http://www.biomedcentral.com/1471-2458/11/S1/S7).

[31] R Olinky, A Huppert and L Stone (2008).Seasonal dynamics and thresholds governing recurrent epidemics. J. Math. Biol. 56, 827–839.

[32] D Kirschner, V DiRita, and J A Flynn (2005).Overcoming Math Anxiety: Malthus Meets Koch Mathematical modeling helps us to understand host-microbe interactions, including pathogenesis. ASM News 71, 357-362.

[33]] R Ke, J Aaskov, E C Holmes and J O Lloyd-Smith (2013). Phylodynamic analysis of the emergence and epidemiological impact of transmissible defective dengue viruses. PLOS Pathogens (doi : 10:1371/journal.ppat.1003193).

[34] H Chi, H F Liu, L C Weng, N Y Wang, N C Chiu, M J Lai, Y C Lin, Y Y Chiu, W S Hsieh and L M Huang (2013).Molecular epidemiology and phylodynamics of the human respiratory synctial virus fusion protein in Northern Taiwan. PLOS One (doi : 10. 1371/journal.pone.0064012).

[35]] A V Melnik and A Korobeinikov (2011).Global asymptotic properties of staged models with multiple progression pathways for infectious diseases. Math. Biosci. Eng. 8, 1019-1034.

[36] A B Gumel, C C McCluskey and P van der Driessche (2006).Mathematical study of a staged progression HIV model with imperfect vaccine. Bull. Math. Biol. 68, 2105-2128.

[37] J H Hyman, J Li, E A Stanley (1999). The differential infectivity model and staged progression models for the transmission of HIV. Math. Biosci. 155, 77-109.

[38] P M Luz, C J Struchiner and A P Galvani (2010) Modeling transmission dynamics and control of vector-borne neglected tropical diseases PLoS Negl Trop Dis 4, e761. (doi:10.1371/journal.pntd.0000761).

[39] Y Xue and X Wang (2012). Global stability of a SLIT TB model with staged progression. J. Appl. Math. Article ID 571469 (doi:10.1155/2012/571469).

[40] E van Kleef, J V Robotham, M Jit, S R Deeny and W J Edmunds (2013).Modeling the transmission of healthcare associated infections: a systematic review. BMC Inf. Dis. 13, 294. (http://www.biomedcentral.com/1471-2334/13/294).

[41] A Alfaro-Murilloa, S Towers and Z Feng (2013).A deterministic model for influenza infection with multiple strains and antigenic drift. J. Biol. Dynamics 7, 199–211.